TEACH Students to THINK Like a Nurse

TRANSFORMATIONAL Strategies that will PREPARE Students for PRACTICE

Keith Rischer, RN, MA, CEN, CCRN
Patricia Pence, EdD, MSN, RN

Praise for
TEACH Students to THINK Like a Nurse
TRANSFORMATIONAL Strategies that will PREPARE Students for PRACTICE

"Keith writes in the same fashion that he practices nursing: with excellence, passion, and a pure unadulterated fervor for the profession. Keith generously shares his nursing knowledge and lived experiences within the context of evidence-based knowledge and practices, while simultaneously urging the reader to self-examine his or her individual and collective commitment to the profession. This provocative book provides a deep dive into the clinical practices of nursing and helps each and every one of us to think and act more like a nurse!"

—Cynthia (Cindy) Clark, PhD, RN, ANEF, FAAN
Founder of Civility Matters© and author of *Creating and Sustaining Civility in Nursing Education*

"*TEACH Students to THINK Like a Nurse* provides nursing faculty with a much-needed 'how-to' formula for contextualizing classroom content so that it is situated in clinical practice. Thus, classroom and clinical content become better integrated and clinical reasoning is strengthened. In addition, the book challenges long held beliefs and assumptions about the value of NANDA as a diagnostic tool, the need to shift from a focus on critical thinking to clinical reasoning, and the impact of incivility on nursing education. The call for transformation in nursing education continues!"

—Carol Huston, MSN, MPA, DPA, FAAN
President, Sigma Theta Tau, the International Honor Society of Nursing, 2007–2009

"*TEACH Students to THINK Like a Nurse* approach to teaching students is reasonable, rational, and REAL! This book addresses the struggles many nursing educators face. I found his insightful chapter on nursing civility provides an avenue not only for student discussions, but also faculty. This is a book I will turn to again and again for insight and support."

—Lin Rauch, MSN, RN, BSEd.
Nursing Instructor, Western Technical College
La Crosse, Wisconsin

"*TEACH Students to THINK Like a Nurse* is written with sensitivity and passion for the art and science of nursing. Keith demonstrates how to enhance student critical thinking by interlinking the nursing process with the importance of identifying the relationships of clinical data to promote student clinical reasoning so vital to nursing. Invaluable tools are presented to enhance the nursing instructor's ability to promote student clinical reasoning in both the classroom and the clinical setting. A very helpful book!"

—Janice Eilerman, MSN, RN
Assistant Professor, Rhodes State College
Lima, Ohio

Praise for
Clinical Reasoning Resources on KeithRN.com

"I used the *Clinical Reasoning Questions to Develop Nurse Thinking* handout instead of our traditional care plan. Great success! The students loved it, I loved it, and they report feeling much better prepared for patient care."

—Rob Morris, RN, MSN
Nursing Faculty
College of the Sequoias
Visalia, California

"The handout *Clinical Reasoning Questions to Develop Nurse Thinking* really helped my fundamental students focus on what is most important and hit the floor running strong!"

—Dawn Page RN, MSN
Nursing Faculty
Copper Mountain College
Joshua Tree, California

"The handout *Clinical Reasoning Questions to Develop Nurse Thinking* helped my students initiate the reasoning process, and ensured better patient care starting with the first patient contact. It also reveals how each student is thinking at the beginning of the shift, and provides a vehicle for guiding their learning."

—Sherri Cozzens, MS, RN
Nursing Faculty
De Anza College
Cupertino, California

"I used the handout *Clinical Reasoning Questions to Develop Nurse Thinking* with my practical nursing students and they loved it! They felt better prepared to care for their patients."

—Priscilla Anderson, RN
Assistant Professor of Nursing
NHTI Concord's Community College
Concord, New Hampshire

"I recently used your Fundamental Reasoning clinical reasoning case studies and loved them! The students were able to see the importance and connection between patient history, clinical presentation and what to do with this information."

—Lynn L. McClellan, MSN, BSN, RN
Nursing Faculty
McHenry County College
Crystal Lake, Illinois

"Your clinical reasoning case studies are excellent and help develop critical thinking by having students determinewhat clinical data is relevant, how should the nurse respond and evaluate after nursing interventions to determine if a problem is present."

—Deb Aucoin-Ratcliff, DNP, RN
Nursing Faculty
American River College
Sacramento, California

"Your clinical reasoning case studies are challenging and an excellent resource for reinforcing knowledge and motivating my nursing students to pursue the "whys" of scenarios thus improving their ability to critically think."

–Nancy Mackey, RN, MS
Medical Academy/Practical Nursing Instructor
Inlet Grove Community High School
Riviera Beach, Florida

"I love the way your practice based approach to clinical reasoning ties everything together, while not losing sight of the person. Your clinical reasoning case studies not only challenge, but allow students to transfer knowledge to the bedside so students will be well prepared for practice."

—Meghan Picone, MSN, RN
PhD student at University of Massachusetts, Worcester
Mount Wachusett Community college
Gardner, Massachusetts

"I like how your clinical reasoning case studies break down the process of critical reasoning. Students just don't pick out abnormal information, they have to focus on what abnormal data is causing and contributing to which problem the patient is having, just like a nurse does in practice."

—Jodi A Nelson, MSN, RN
Nursing Faculty
Southeast Community College
Lincoln, Nebraska

"Your clinical reasoning case studies make students think like a nurse and challenge them to think critically by recalling essential knowledge."

—Ann S. Garton, MSN, RN, CNE
Nursing Faculty
St. Ambrose University
Davenport, Iowa

TEACH Students to THINK Like a Nurse
TRANSFORMATIONAL Strategies that will
PREPARE Students for PRACTICE

Authors: Keith Rischer, RN, MA, CEN, CCRN

Patricia Pence, EdD, MSN, RN

Copyright © 2017

ISBN: 978-0-9899369-8-9

Typeset in Times New Roman

Printed in USA

First Edition

Dedication

*Dedicated to every nurse educator who desires or has already
embraced a transformational vision for nursing education.
This book was written for you.*

Reviewers

Cynthia (Cindy) Clark, PhD, RN, ANEF, FAAN
Founder of Civility Matters© and author of *Creating and Sustaining Civility in Nursing Education*
(Reviewed chapter 25: Transforming Academia by Restoring Civility)

Becky Craig, RNC, MN, EdS, PhD
Nursing Instructor
Nursing Tutorial Lab, Perimeter College, Clarkston, Georgia

Janice Eilerman, MSN, RN
Assistant Professor
Rhodes State College, Lima, Ohio

Barb Hill, RN, MSN, CNE, CMSRN
Associate Professor
The Community College of Baltimore County, Baltimore, Maryland

Julie Hogue, RN, MSN
Department Chair
Illinois Valley Community College, Oglesby, Illinois

Carol Huston, MSN, MPA, DPA, FAAN
President, Sigma Theta Tau, the International Honor Society of Nursing, 2007–2009

Jill Lawson, MSN, APRN-FNP
Nursing Faculty
Barton Community College, Great Bend, Kansas

Patricia Pence, EdD, MSN, RN
Nursing Professor
Illinois Valley Community College, Oglesby, Illinois

Lin Rauch, MSN, RN, BSEd.
Nursing Instructor
Western Technical College, La Crosse, Wisconsin

Judith Rudokas, MS, MEd, RN
Nursing Faculty
Galen College of Nursing, Cincinnati, Ohio

About Keith Rischer

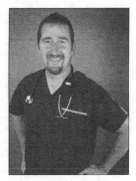

Caring in crisis attracted me to nursing over 30 years ago. I wanted to be a flight nurse/paramedic and chose to get my nursing degree right out of high school. I completed my EMT after my first year of nursing school and began to volunteer as an EMT in our community. I was so traumatized by getting lost on the back country roads with a critical patient in the ambulance, that I re-routed my career path and completed my two-year nursing degree in 1983 at a local community college. I entered a very tight job market as a registered nurse.

I started my nursing career as a psychiatric nurse at the local state hospital and went on to pursue my passion for emergency nursing. I then went into long-term care, pediatric home care, step-down NICU, cardiac telemetry, cardiac ICU, and finally, after 16 years, the emergency department (ED). I currently work in the critical care float pool of a large metro hospital and float between the ED, med/surg neuro ICU, cardiac medical ICU, cardiac surgical ICU, cardiac telemetry, and circulating/rapid response team. I am currently certified in my practice specialties of critical care and emergency department.

My applied strategies to teach clinical reasoning to nursing students have been published in the following nursing publications: 10th edition of *Kozier & Erb's Fundamentals of Nursing*, a chapter in the *Professional Issues in Nursing* 4th edition, "Can Clinical Reasoning Be Taught?" and an article on clinical reasoning for *Innovations in Nursing Education, Volume III*, published by the National League for Nursing and edited by Linda Caputi.

I am passionate about transforming nursing education by integrating clinical reasoning throughout the curriculum so students are prepared for real-world practice. I have created practical tools to help realize this transformation. My website, clinical reasoning resources, and blog are committed to be a part of the solution and to strengthen and support this needed change. I also have a passion to serve the poor through medical missions by using nursing and nursing education to share God's love and improve the quality of health care in the developing world.

About Patricia Pence

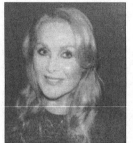 Dr. Patricia Pence, EdD, MSN, RN has been a nursing professor teaching first-year clinical and lecture courses at Illinois Valley Community College, in Oglesby, Illinois, since 2001.

Her educational background includes a certificate in Practical Nursing and an Associate Degree in Nursing from Illinois Valley Community College; a Bachelor's in Science in Nursing from Bradley University, Peoria, Illinois; a Master's in Nursing degree from Northern Illinois University; and a Doctoral degree in Education and Curriculum from University of Phoenix.

Her clinical practice in nursing spans over 28 years in constant care, medical-surgical nursing, home health, a skilled nursing unit, and director of nursing in long-term care facilities.

While teaching at Illinois Valley Community College, Dr. Pence has been recognized for her efforts to improve teaching and learning. She was awarded the Innovations in Teaching Award in 2004 and was the recipient of the Faculty Excellence in Teaching Award in 2016 at Illinois Valley Community College.

She received the Illinois Board of Higher Education Nurse Educator Fellowship Award in 2010.

She enjoys serving as a reviewer for *Nurse Educator* and the *Teaching and Learning in Nursing* journal. She has presented and published research on nursing student retention, emotional intelligence, motivation, plagiarism, using a skilled nursing facility for clinical practicum, and recently implemented a flipping active learning model in her nursing courses.

Contents

PART ONE
Transforming the Educator

_____

PART TWO
Transforming the Content

_____

PART THREE
Transforming the Classroom

_____

PART FOUR
Transforming Clinical Education

PART FIVE
Transforming Nursing Education

Appendices

Foreword

I attended a conference session on active learning five years ago that showed how nursing could be taught in ways other than the traditional lecture. I then spent several months changing my next lecture into an active learning course. I knew there would be hurdles to cross and kept an open mind to adapt each week based on what worked well and what did not. After only the second week, I realized my attempts at active learning were not going as I had hoped. Students resisted the needed change to engage in active learning.

I had heard of Keith and his innovative strategies to bring active learning that emphasized clinical reasoning. I called him to learn more about his clinical reasoning case studies and other resources available on his website. After implementing his clinical reasoning case studies in my classroom, I had the results I had hoped for! My students were willing participants, and engaged. My class was transformed from passive lecturing to meaningful active learning that involved solving clinical puzzles in a patient-based scenario. This was the genesis that would transform my nursing classroom into a clinical setting and I have not looked back since.

I then read *Educating Nurses: A Call for Radical Transformation.* Keith had stressed that the educational research presented in *Educating Nurses* provided the foundational framework for his clinical reasoning case studies. A new transformational vision is needed in nursing education. Continuing with the status quo was no longer acceptable. The exemplar teaching methods described in Educating Nurses was the stimulus I needed to develop other active learning strategies to complement Keith's clinical reasoning case studies.

My active learning strategies were later published in the 2016 *Teaching and Learning in Nursing* journal in an article titled, "'Flipping' a first-year medical-surgical associate degree registered nursing course: A 2-year pilot study." I also presented my work at the 2016 Organization of Associate Degree Nursing (OADN) convention. I met Keith at this convention and found him to be energetic and enthusiastic. His passion to empower nurse educators was palpable.

TEACH Students to THINK Like a Nurse is a practical guide and resource written for graduate students, novices, and seasoned nurse educators. It contains a new paradigm and vision to support the transformation of nursing education based on the best practice recommendations outlined in *Educating Nurses.*

TEACH Students to THINK Like a Nurse complements the student text, *Think Like a Nurse*, which Keith wrote to strengthen learning of students and new nurses. In *TEACH Students to THINK Like a Nurse,* you will find step-by-step explanations and guidance on HOW to implement a transformational vision for nursing education that includes an emphasis on clinical reasoning to bridge the current gap between theory and clinical practice. I highly recommend *TEACH Students to THINK Like a Nurse* if you are entering nursing education or seeking evidenced-based change in your teaching practice to engage and strengthen the learning of students.

—Dr. Patricia Pence, EdD, MSN, RN

Preface

My stomach was churning and I was so nervous I thought I was going to pass out! I was standing on the podium in 2012 before a packed room filled with over 200 educators at Elsevier Faculty Development Conference in Las Vegas, a national nurse educator conference. Even though I just completed my second year of teaching, I was invited to present how I had successfully transformed my classroom by incorporating the paradigm shifts in *Educating Nurses: A Call for Radical Transformation* by using clinical reasoning case studies I developed.

I made it through my 75-minute presentation and was humbled by the enthusiastic standing ovation I received afterwards. Little did I know it, but my life was about to change in ways I never expected. I received invitations to present my clinical reasoning strategies at colleges and conferences across the country. I quickly realized I could only be in one place at one time and needed to put in writing what I present so any educator could have access to the transformational strategies I developed to help students think more like a nurse.

Some would question if I am even qualified to write a book for nurse educators because of my academic inexperience. I believe I am uniquely qualified to write this book and that my lack of academic experience is an advantage. Let me explain. I am not beholden to the traditions of the past that hold many educators back by doing it the way it has always been done. This is what needs to change. Nursing education is broken and in need of radical transformation (Benner, Sutphen, Leonard, & Day, 2010). I view everything that is done in academia filtered through my lens of current clinical practice to facilitate needed change and transformation.

I have been a nurse for 35 years in a wide variety of acute care settings. I currently work at a large metropolitan hospital where I care for patients in critical care and the emergency department (ED). I am certified in these two specialty areas (CCRN & CEN). As a nurse educa-tor, I have a unique bifocal lens because I never left the bedside of direct patient care and continued to work in clinical practice every weekend. I infused this clinical salience into all that I taught including the clinical reasoning case studies and scenarios I developed. As a practicing nurse, I know what it takes to prepare students for real-world practice.

As educators, we must never lose sight of the fact that nursing is a practice-based profession. It is not academic tenure, terminal degree, years or even decades of academic experience that ensure your effectiveness as an educator. In order to effectively prepare students for real-world practice, current clinical realities need to be authentically integrated in nursing education, especially the classroom (Benner, et al., 2010). We must never lose sight that the endpoint of everything that is done in nursing education is to teach students to THINK like a nurse (Tanner, 2006).

TEACH Students to THINK Like a Nurse was written to champion a new paradigm and transformational vision for nursing education. By embracing new ways of thinking; transformation can be realized. No curriculum change is required! This book will help educators incorporate best practices from the nursing literature. If you are a new educator, it will help you transition successfully to the academic setting.

TEACH Students to THINK Like a Nurse is unique when compared to other books written for nurse educators:

- **Personal.** As a newer nurse educator who has remained current in practice, I share my journey and personal observations how the current academic-practice gap can be bridged to better prepare students for real-world clinical practice. Dr. Pence also shares her journey as an experienced educator who also successfully transformed her classroom.

- **Practical.** In addition to sharing WHY nursing education needs to change, this book reveals HOW it can be realized with numerous tools and strategies that have been successfully used by myself and educators across the country.

- **Contributions from nurse educators.** I solicited and received feedback from educators across the world who contributed practical, creative approaches they have successfully used to strengthen student learning in the class and clinical settings as well as pearls of wisdom to encourage new nurse educators.

Some may wonder if transformational change is attainable and if my experiences can be replicated. That is one reason I invited Dr. Patricia Pence to collaborate and contribute to this manuscript. As an educator with 16 years of experience, she was at one time stuck in the traditional ways nursing has been taught, but became "unstuck" by successfully implementing the best practice paradigm changes advocated in *Educating Nurses* and using the practical strategies advocated in this book.

Are you ready to embrace a transformational vision for nursing education and begin your own journey to step out and do things differently to strengthen student learning? Keep reading and let's take that first step of your journey together!

—Keith Rischer, RN, MA, CEN, CCRN

References

Benner, P., Sutphen, M., Leonard, V., & Day, L. (2010). *Educating nurses: A call for radical transformation.* San Francisco, CA: Jossey-Bass.

Tanner, C. A. (2006). Thinking like a nurse: A research-based model of clinical judgment in nursing. *Journal of Nursing Education, 45*(6), 204–211.

Introduction

Keith Rischer, RN, MA, CEN, CCRN

Nursing education needs to dramatically change. Nurse educators struggle to let go of the traditional model that may have worked in the past, but is no longer able to adequately prepare students for the complexities experienced in today's practice settings. I am not alone in these observations. Dr. Patricia Benner, a FAAN "living legend" who led the Carnegie Foundation's educational research detailed in *Educating Nurses* also came to the same conclusion. These are her observations (Benner et al., 2010):

- Nursing education is in need of radical transformation.
- The traditional ways of doing things are no longer working to prepare students for the demands of today's nursing practice.
- The current quality of nursing education needs to be improved to reflect current nursing practice.

In other words, business as usual is no longer an option. It is time to embrace a new vision and transformational paradigm of nursing education to better prepare students for professional practice by being able to think like a nurse.

Educating Nurses: A Call for Radical Transformation (2010) summarized the Carnegie Foundation's research findings of nursing education in the United States. This book was a wake-up call to challenge the status quo in nursing education. The Carnegie Foundation educational research findings contained in Educating Nurses identified that nursing education needs to be RADICALLY TRANSFORMED by implementing the following essential shifts of integration:

- Shift from covering decontextualized knowledge and content (textbook) to CONTEXTUALIZING classroom content so it is situated in clinical practice (at the bedside) so students can see why the content is relevant.
- Shift from sharp separation of classroom and clinical teaching to greater INTEGRATION of classroom theory and clinical content. They should not be kept in largely separate orbits in nursing education as it is typically taught.
- Shift from an emphasis on critical thinking to an emphasis on CLINICAL REASONING. Clinical reasoning is the ability of the nurse to think in action and reason as a situation changes over time by capturing and understanding the significance of clinical trajectories and grasping the essence of the current clinical situation (Benner, et al., 2010). Clinical reasoning is the essence of how a nurse thinks in real-world clinical practice.

Since *Educating Nurses* was published, progress has been made. Several states have implemented initiatives to transform nursing education. Other programs have implemented curriculum revisions and innovations in clinical education are taking place. But in order to see these changes last, it will depend on educators, nurses, and students to respond to the changes advocated in both education and practice settings (Benner, 2012).

But the quest to transform nursing education is far from over. Kavanagh and Szweda (2017) concluded that nursing education is losing ground in the battle for entry-level competency of graduate nurses into clinical practice. Of over 5,000 graduate nurses who were assessed, only 23 percent were able to demonstrate practice readiness by successfully evaluating a clinical scenario, identify the problem and use clinical reasoning to manage the problem correctly. Just because a graduate nurse passes the NCLEX, or a program has high NCLEX pass rates does not currently correlate to thinking like a nurse by graduates in the clinical setting.

I have worked with programs to implement needed change and have been encouraged by the passion and enthusiasm of educators that are committed to strengthen student learning. But some continue to resist change and ongoing work is still needed to close the practice–education gap once and for all.

Clinical Reasoning Curriculum

In order to better prepare students for practice and realize transformational change in your program, begin by changing the way you teach your current content (Benner, et al., 2010). Integrate clinical reasoning throughout the curriculum so students have opportunities to repeatedly practice clinical reasoning and think more like a nurse. The essence of this transformational paradigm shift is a "clinical reasoning based curriculum" that integrates this emphasis in all aspects of classroom and clinical content beginning with the first semester.

So where and how do you begin to integrate clinical reasoning in your program? This is an ongoing struggle. To see where you are in your journey, use the following reflection questions that capture the essence of what a clinical reasoning based curriculum practically looks like and assess your progress.

1. Emphasizes relevance, NOT content.

TMI (too much information!) is an ongoing problem in nursing education.

- Reflect: *Do you filter the content taught so it represents content relevant to bedside practice?*

2. Emphasizes DEEP learning of what is MOST important.

A&P. Pathophysiology must be DEEPLY under stood in order for students to make connections to the relationships of essential clinical data in practice.

- Reflect: *Do you emphasize and contextualize A&P in each presentation?*

F&E. What labs are most important and why? Applied understanding of F&E is more important than memorizing the "hypo" and "hyper" of the most common electrolytes!

- Reflect: *Do you contextualize F&E content to the most common scenarios that nurses may encounter?*

Pharmacology. To safely pass the most common medications, students must not memorize, but UNDERSTAND the mechanism of action.

- Reflect: *Do you integrate the most common medications in your presentations and briefly review the mechanism of action of these drugs?*

3. Content is contextualized to the bedside.

Nursing is a practice-based profession. Content or concepts that are taught must have a "hook" that contextualizes content to the bedside. Content-heavy lectures that highlight textbook content hinder student mastery of content that must be able to be applied, NOT memorized! If your program emphasizes concepts, then be sure to contextualize your concepts!

- Reflect: *In the classroom, do you contextualize content to the bedside using case studies or other active learning strategies?*

4. Emphasizes clinical reasoning as "nurse thinking."

Clinical reasoning is the ability of the nurse to think in action, reason as a situation changes, recognize relevant clinical data, and grasp the essence of the current clinical situation (Benner, et al., 2010).

- Reflect: *Do you teach clinical reasoning and other ways of nurse thinking besides nursing process and written care plans?*
- Reflect: *Do you use strategies during clinical practicum that bridge classroom learning with patient care?*

Why Change?

Why should nursing education change by implementing these paradigm shifts and emphasize clinical reasoning? What is the consequence if students are unable to think like a nurse by being able to clinically reason? They are NOT fundamentally prepared to provide safe and competent patient care (Romyn, et. al. (2009). To prepare students for the current challenges and complexities of patient care will require an "all hands on deck" approach to embrace a transformational paradigm shift in nursing education. This paradigm shift includes a renewed emphasis on preparing students for clinical practice and a transformational vision of nursing education and of nursing itself; how nurses see themselves, and their role in health care.

Because clinical reasoning mirrors the way a nurse thinks and sets priorities in clinical practice, it is imperative that every nurse educator reflect and ask the following question:

"What will be the ultimate consequence if a student in my program who graduates to be a nurse in practice fails to clinically reason and think like a nurse by identifying a change in a patient's status until it is too late?"

A patient will likely have an adverse outcome and may even die as a result. This is why nurse educators must not see clinical reasoning as just another trendy pedagogy, or active learning strategy. The inability of a new nurse to think like a nurse and clinically reason can potentially be a matter of life and death!

I See Dead Patients

"I see dead people" was a famous quote by Cole Sears from the hit horror movie *The Sixth Sense* in 1999. Fortunately, it was only a movie. Unfortunately, I have seen clinical situations as a rapid response nurse that foreshadowed a patient death as the result of the primary nurse's "failure to rescue" and clinically reason when there was a change of status that went unrecognized until it was too late.

Here is one of those scenarios. Jenny was a newer nurse who graduated a year ago. She had an elderly male patient named Ken. He had a perforated appendix, but it had been removed successfully two days prior and he was clinically stable. Around midnight, he became restless. His BP was slightly elevated at 158/90 and his HR was in the 100s. He had a history of mild dementia and was not able 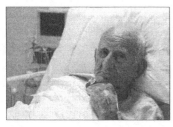 to readily communicate his needs, so Jenny gave him 1 tablet of oxycodone, assuming he was in pain. Two hours later, he continued to be restless and Jenny thought that she heard some faint wheezing. She noted that he was now more tachypneic with a respiratory rate of 28/minute. He did have a history of COPD and had an albuterol nebulizer PRN ordered, so that was given.

Two hours later, Jenny called me, as the rapid response nurse, to come and take a look at her patient. She was concerned but was unable to recognize the problem and wanted a second opinion. After Jenny explained the course of events that transpired to this point, I took one look at Ken and realized that he was in trouble. He was pale, diaphoretic, and his respirations had increased to 40/minute despite the nebulizer two hours ago. He was not responsive to loud verbal commands. The last BP was still on the monitor and read 158/90. I asked, *"When was the last BP checked?"* Jenny stated it was four hours prior. While obtaining another BP, I touched Ken's forehead. It was notably cold, as were his hands. The BP now read 68/30.

Recognizing that Ken was in septic shock, and that IV fluids and vasopressors would be needed to save his life,

I looked for an IV and found only one, a 24-gauge catheter in the left hand. This is the smallest size IV catheter and is typically used with infants and small children.

Ken needed a central line and there was little that could be done to initiate even the most basic life-saving treatments to rescue Ken on the floor. He was emergently transferred to ICU. Within 30 minutes Ken was intubated, a central line was placed, and three vasopressors—norepinephrine [Levophed], phenylephrine [Neosynephrine] and Vasopressin—were required to get his systolic blood pressure greater than 90 mmHg.

After this transfer was completed, I asked Jenny a simple clinical reasoning question: *"What was the most likely complication that Ken could experience based on his reason for being hospitalized?"* Jenny admitted that she hadn't thought about it because she was so focused on getting all of the tasks done with her four other patients.

Had Jenny asked herself this question while caring for Ken, but more importantly answered it, she would have been thinking like a nurse. She would have vigilantly looked and assessed for EARLY signs of the most likely complication Ken could experience because of his perforated appendix…SEPSIS. Although early signs of sepsis were present at midnight, it was not recognized until it was too late for Ken. He died the next day.

This story illustrates the tragic consequences of failure to rescue that is documented in the nursing literature (Clarke & Aiken, 2003). Unfortunately, this patient death is not an isolated incident. Preventable health care errors in hospitals are now the third leading cause of death in the United States (Makary & Daniel, 2016). This is WHY students must be practically prepared for real-world practice by UNDERSTANDING and APPLYING clinical reasoning to the bedside. To think, or not to think like a nurse, is literally a matter of life and death. Nursing education does not need to remain broken. All it takes is nurse educators who are willing to resist the "status quo" and do things differently to bring needed change that emphasizes clinical reasoning so students are taught how to think more like a nurse.

Transformation Is Possible

Transformation of nursing education is possible and within your reach. I liken this objective to the exodus of the Israelites from Egypt over four thousand years ago. A lack of faith and the reality of "giants" kept them from entering into the Promised Land, and, as a result, they wandered in the wilderness for 40 years. In the same way, your journey out of the current "wilderness" of nursing education is not going to be easy. You are going to face obstacles and giants that will challenge and test you. But numerous educators have successfully overcome the giants that include opposition from students and colleagues to do things differently.

Patricia Benner and the co-authors of *Educating Nurses* represent the leadership and direction that nursing education needs to follow in such a time as this. If nurse educators are willing to follow the educational best-practice recommendations of *Educating Nurses,* this is the path to transformation. Resist and go back to what is comfortable and the secure ways of the past will have disastrous consequences.

This book is uniquely structured to help any motivated educator successfully implement transformational change that will help students think like a nurse. Though tools and strategies are essential, transforming the educator and changing the way you currently THINK about nursing education is needed and is the focus of Part 1. Part 2 addresses the importance of transforming the content and what needs to be emphasized to strengthen student learning of what is most important. Part 3 addresses principles and strategies to transform classroom teaching, and Part 4 does the same with clinical instruction. We close with Part 5, transforming not only nursing education but the profession by emphasizing civility, addressing barriers that men in nursing education have encountered for over 150 years and recognizing the value and worth that nurses provide by caring and serving others. But before we go any further, whether you are a graduate student, new nurse educator transitioning to academia, or experienced nursing faculty, lets start with the key to successful change in nursing education—strengthening and transforming you, the nurse educator!

References

Benner, P. (2012). Educating nurses: A call for radical transformation—how far have we come? *Journal of Nursing Education, 51*(4), 183-184.

Benner, P., Sutphen, M., Leonard, V., & Day, L. (2010). *Educating nurses: A call for radical transformation.* San Francisco, CA: Jossey-Bass.

Clarke, S.P., & Aiken, L. H. (2003). Failure to rescue. *American Journal of Nursing, 103,* 42-47.

Kavanagh, J. & Szweda, C. (2017). A crisis in competency: The strategic and ethical imperative to assessing new graduate nurses' clinical reasoning. *Nursing Education Perspectives, 38*(2), 57-61.

Makary, M.A., & Daniel, M. (2016). Medical error- The third leading cause of death in the US. *BMJ, 353,* i2139. doi:10. 1136/bmj.i2139

Romyn, D. M., Linton, N., Giblin, C., Hendrickson, B., Limacher, L. H., Nordstrom, P., et al. (2009). Successful transition of the new graduate nurse. *International Journal of Nursing Education Scholarship, 6*(1), 1–17.

PART ONE

TRANSFORMING
THE EDUCATOR

My Journey

Keith Rischer, RN, MA, CEN, CCRN

"A journey of a thousand miles begins with a single step."

Lao-tzu, Chinese philosopher

I have been a nurse for 35 years in a wide variety of clinical settings including mental health, long-term care, pediatrics, and cardiac telemetry. I currently practice in the critical care float pool of a large metropolitan hospital where I bounce between critical care, emergency department (ED), and the rapid response team. Over ten years ago, I was torn between a career path as a nurse anesthetist, where I would make well over six figures, or become a nurse educator and make not as much. I decided to follow my heart and pursue my passion to teach and obtained my masters in nursing education in 2007. I continue to work part-time in the clinical setting and never left the bedside as a nurse educator. I evaluate everything that is done in academia through the lens of clinical practice as well as through the writings of leading nurse educators such as Patricia Benner and Christine Tanner. After my second year of classroom teaching, I began to feel disillusioned and discouraged. I did not know it at the time, but what I was experiencing was the well-documented academic-practice gap in nursing education. From my perspective, there was a clear disconnect between the realities of clinical practice and traditional nursing education. Content presented in the classroom and skills lab had little contextualization to practice. Textbook content was king. Classroom lectures were content heavy and students were clearly burdened and

highly stressed by the heavy load I was inadvertently placing on them.

Because I was a nurse in practice, I had not read nursing textbooks for over 20 years. I immediately noticed that the med/surg textbooks had gotten heavier, thicker, and were now in two separate volumes! From my vantage point, the amount of content that students were expected to master was unrealistic and was a barrier to student learning.

I did my best to FILTER and emphasize the MOST important content for my students based on what was most relevant to bedside patient care. Between content-heavy lectures and NANDA-driven care plans that required a correctly-worded three-part nursing diagnostic statement, I was discouraged. I felt this accepted norm hindered the ability of students to think like a nurse in clinical practice. As I observed other faculty members in our department, nobody openly challenged the status quo. As a new nurse educator, I was expected to go with the flow, even if I felt it was taking our students in the wrong direction!

First Steps

Everything changed when, over winter break in 2011, I read *Educating Nurses: A Call for Radical Transformation*. This book directly addressed the source of my discontent by giving me permission to decrease content saturation, bring clinical realities to class, and emphasize clinical reasoning. I quickly realized that I had to do something different! I spent the last half of my winter break reworking my traditional, content-heavy PowerPoint presentations so that they would incorporate and apply these paradigm changes in my classroom. I was determined to do what was needed to strengthen student learning. I developed a series of unique clinical reasoning case studies based on "Mr. Kelly" that put a series of cardiac topics I was teaching that spring semester into context.

I entered my classroom apprehensive and nervous. I was not sure how my first lecture would go over with my students on the topic of atherosclerosis and hypertension. I was going to do things very differently that day. I was NOT going to lecture the entire hour. I cut my PowerPoint presentation in half by emphasizing the most important content of my topic. Then I would have the remainder of class to present a unique clinical reasoning case study I had created on Mr. Kelly, a middle-aged/overweight man whose clinical presentations would capture each of the cardiac content topics I was teaching. Each case study was a practical implementation and integration of the essential shifts of integration from *Educating Nurses*. Students were going to APPLY contextualized content knowledge as well as PRACTICE clinical reasoning in the classroom.

I posted a blank student version of the case study I created a week earlier. Students knew that they were required to read the corresponding chapter of this content, work through the case study on Mr. Kelly either individually or in small groups, and then come prepared to discuss and work through the case study together in class. Students were skeptical. "Is this going to be on the test?" was a common concern.

As I completed my lecture and had almost 25 minutes left of class, I began reading the presenting scenario of Mr. Kelly:

Mr. Kelly is a 51-year-old male…who decided to have a physical when he recently became more easily fatigued, dizzy, and weak with mild activity. He currently has no health insurance. At the clinic, he had a routine physical exam and his BP was found to be 158/96 and 152/98 on two separate clinic visits. His labs were as follows…

The case study slowly unfolded with labs, vital signs, and assessment data that had specific findings that needed to be recognized as relevant and why they were clinically significant. In addition to contextualizing content, the essence of clinical reasoning and thinking in action was established. Nursing priorities, plan of care, and essential medication knowledge were identified. Students were clearly engaged in this case study and Mr. Kelly's story! Students in the back and throughout the classroom began to give their answers as they were called upon. Discussion, dialogue, and clarification took place as not every student response was correct. My role changed from "sage on the stage" to "guide on the side." The classroom no longer felt like a classroom, but more like the clinical setting. Students were discussing and applying clinical realities to practice.

Though there was some initial pushback by some students because of the extra work and desire to be "spoon fed" lecture content, I stayed the course, tying my remaining lectures to this new format. By the second lecture, students began to see the value of this applied learning because each case study emphasized content application. I did a simple survey at the end of the semester to see what students thought of this new approach. Student response was overwhelmingly positive. NOT ONE student said to go back to traditional content-heavy lectures but continue this emphasis on need-to-know concepts and clinical reasoning using case studies in the classroom!

One student comment summed it up for many:
"These clinical reasoning case studies were very helpful. I didn't feel like I was memorizing for the test. I felt like I was able to apply the information. It helped put knowledge into practice and made it clear why it was relevant."

Though I did not realize it at the time, what I had implemented in my classroom would be presented to a much larger audience of nurse educators in a matter of months.

National Spotlight

The same year, nationally-known nurse educator Linda Caputi was the keynote speaker at the annual Minnesota Health Educators spring conference. As a longtime advocate of applied clinical reasoning in nursing education, Linda's emphasis and passion for clinical reasoning from her presentation dovetailed with the essence of the findings of *Educating Nurses*. After she presented, I found her alone in the hallway and wanted to let her know how much I appreciated her presentation. I shared in passing that I had created and implemented a series of clinical reasoning case studies the last semester based on an emphasis of the paradigm shifts from *Educating Nurses* that my students found meaningful to their classroom learning.

She casually replied, "Could you send those to me? Here is my card." Unknown to me at the time, she was also on the planning committee of a large, annual national nurse educators conference (Elsevier's Faculty Development Institute in Las Vegas). She was interested in what I had developed, and after she reviewed my case studies, I was invited to speak and share my work in a well-received breakout session at this conference.

Next Steps

I quickly realized that many other nurse educators recognized the need to do something different to strengthen their students' learning. Knowing that there was an ongoing interest in clinical reasoning resources for nurse educators, I took the initiative to develop and build my website, KeithRN.com, in 2012. It contains numerous clinical reasoning case studies and related resources that emphasize and develop clinical reasoning and empower time-strapped educators to transform their content.

My practice-based approach to teaching clinical reasoning has been supported by prominent nurse educators including Patricia Benner, Carol Huston, and Shirlee Snyder, co-author of *Kozier & Erb's Fundamentals of Nursing. TEACH Students to THINK Like a Nurse* was birthed by my desire to put into writing the essence of what I present in my full-day workshops that I have since presented across the United States and Canada. This book will empower any nurse educator to pursue transformational change in the class and clinical settings through practical strategies that incorporate the paradigm shifts advocated by *Educating Nurses*.

Can my experience be your reality where you teach? Based on the feedback and testimonials that I have received from nurse educators and students, the answer is an emphatic YES! The reason is quite simple. It is NOT about me and mirroring my example. The practical strategies I have developed are established on a much stronger foundation, the lifelong work of pre-eminent nurse educator and scholar of this generation, Patricia Benner, one of the co-authors of *Educating Nurses*. Every nurse educator who has heard the call to do things differently must embrace the responsibility to become a transformational nurse educator and do what is needed to strengthen student learning. But I quickly realized that despite the best intentions to initiate needed change, I was about to encounter some unexpected obstacles in nursing education. I asked questions of students and faculty, and soon found out that there was trouble in paradise…

Trouble in Paradise

Keith Rischer, RN, MA, CEN, CCRN

"A major finding of our study is that a significant gap exists between today's nursing practice and the education for that practice…the quality of nursing education must be uniformly higher."
—*Educating Nurses: A Call for Radical Transformation,* p. 4

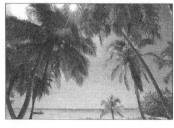

I entered nursing education with "rose-colored glasses." I worked hard and sacrificed much to complete graduate school so I could teach. Though I had visions (more like a mirage!) that this was going to be a "beach" experience with students who were eager to learn and hang on my every "pearl" of clinical wisdom, it did not take long for this idyllic vision of paradise in nursing education to come crashing down. It soon became apparent that there was trouble in paradise.

Though I experienced difficulties as a new nurse educator, I thought that they were unique to me. When I recently asked educators to share their greatest struggles through a random, open-ended survey, I received more than 200 responses. I was pleasantly surprised to see that many of the fears and struggles I had known as a nurse educator were NOT unique to me. My goal in sharing these findings with you is not to focus on what is wrong with nursing education, but to identify these struggles so they can be remedied. The remainder of the book will provide practical strategies to address these struggles so that nursing education can be strengthened and transformed.

Faculty Struggles

The majority of educators who responded to the survey identified four themes of struggles that are listed in order of prevalence:

1. Struggles with students
2. Struggles in the classroom
3. Struggles in the clinical setting
4. Struggles with faculty

Each struggle has the summary of educator responses and actual quotes that follow:

Struggles with Students

- Students who experience high stress/anxiety/burden
- Student entitlement
- Nursing school is not their highest priority.
- Unwilling to do the needed work/NOT buying the "flipped classroom"… wanting to be "spoon fed" as adult learners… "Just tell me what I need to know for the test."
- Getting students to read/come prepared for class
- Lack of respect/incivility from students

  "I should get a good grade because I paid for it!"

  "Students expect that the instructor will give them everything they need to know in order to pass an exam."

  "My biggest struggle is to get the students to do

the required work with a minimal amount of complaining."

"There is such a sense of entitlement that the student should do minimal work because they are already smart. Getting students to think like a nurse is a very difficult thing to do."

Struggles in the Classroom

- Need practical strategies to DECREASE content and increase APPLICATION
- How to decide what is most important content/simplify textbook learning
- How to implement active learning/flipped classroom effectively
- Strategies to develop priority setting, critical thinking, and clinical reasoning
- How to get students to think more like a nurse and connect theory to practice
- How to keep students engaged

  "Students are so reliant on PowerPoint. They believe group work is not as valuable."

  "I struggle to get students to buy into interactive classroom activities that bring the clinical into the classroom."

  "Transitioning to a flipped classroom. I embrace the concept but need help and creativity to make it happen."

Struggles in the Clinical Setting

- Too many students, too little time to spend with each student
- Guiding students to APPLY classroom content to practice. Some students not safe/failing in final clinical
- Simplify clinical paperwork so it is meaningful and not a struggle
- Students struggling to see the BIG PICTURE
- Transitioning students from being "task-oriented" to THINKING like a nurse
- How to develop critical thinking, clinical reasoning so they make correct clinical judgments
- Unable to make connections and recognize priorities

  "Getting the students past the focus on completing tasks and focusing on awareness of the total picture of the patient needs."

  "How to bridge the gap between what we teach and

what is being actually done in the clinical setting."

"Getting students to think critically and helping them put the pieces together."

Struggles with Faculty

- NOT enough time to keep up with ongoing demands
- CHANGE… Not feeling safe with other faculty to make needed change…Turmoil that change causes… Difficulty getting senior faculty on board
- Incivility to one another
- Lack of confidence in teaching ability… "Not knowing what I don't know"
- Working with faculty who are poorly motivated or inexperienced
- Lack of consistency between faculty members

  "Consistency among faculty to connect the threads of theory into clinical teaching and how caring is so important to provide for the holistic needs of clients."

  "Getting all faculty to understand and use clinical reasoning. Many are very small-minded and refuse to expand and explore the possibilities."

Student Struggles

I recently had an opportunity to ask nursing students from several different programs in Minnesota what their greatest struggle was as a nursing student. The following are their unedited comments. Consider their perspective and look for similar themes that may be present in your program to do what is needed to initiate and implement change.

These statements capture the essence of student concerns and struggles.

Struggles in the Classroom

"Lecture almost seemed like a waste of time because we had already read the book. I was not taught how to prioritize."

"Professors who lacked passion and did not teach the content but merely read off of PowerPoint slides."

"Classes NOT relevant to practice."

"Provide rationale for answers so I know the WHY."

"Too much memorizing facts and too little application and what/how to apply to clinical practice."

TMI (too much information!)

"How do you know what to study? It's impossible to memorize everything."

"Overload of information/overwhelming."

"We are taught so many subjects and then none in depth."

"We get so much information and thousands of pages to read. It is not possible to know it all."

"Information overload! Too many details without clear instruction on the critical data. Unrealistic reading expectations."

"We're rushed covering the huge content in a small amount of time."

Struggles in the Clinical Setting

"I did not have clinical instructors question or challenge me on doing what I'm doing."

"We spent way too much time with care plans and not enough learning about patient care and other important information."

"Too much time on care plans not on pathophysiology."

Though these findings are based on my personal observations, as I consult with educators across the country, these same themes are prevalent in programs today. Though progress is being made to improve the quality of nursing education, these reflections are a reminder of the work that yet needs to be done.

Though pursuing your passion as a nurse educator is exciting, it also will challenge and stretch you in ways you never thought possible. You will wonder at times if you really have what it takes to be a nurse educator. That is the topic of the next chapter.

Reflect

1. What faculty struggles do you currently experience?

2. What is the TOP faculty struggle that needs to be addressed to maintain your joy, purpose, and passion as an educator?

3. What can YOU do today to take action to help remedy this struggle?

4. What student struggles do you currently experience?

5. What is the TOP student struggle that needs to be addressed to maintain your joy, purpose, and passion as an educator?

6. What can YOU do today to take action to help remedy this student struggle?

Do You Have What It Takes to Be a Nurse Educator?

Keith Rischer, RN, MA, CEN, CCRN
Patricia Pence, EdD, MSN, RN

When I (Keith) wrote *THINK Like a Nurse: Practical Preparation for Professional Practice*, this book begins by asking students to reflect to determine if they had what it takes to be a nurse. Even though a student may have good intentions to be a nurse, a nurse in practice requires a certain set of traits and dispositions to be successful that students may or may not possess. A nurse educator is no different. In order to thrive in this role, you, too, must possess traits and abilities that are unique to academia. Cooley and De-Gagne (2016) identified four personal traits that lead to becoming a competent and successful nurse educator:

1. Dedication to the nursing profession
2. Obligation and responsibility to students
3. Diligence to teaching students well and responsibly
4. Understanding of the impact of their teaching

Additional expectations that students need in a nurse educator include:

- Demonstrate CARING and promote student personal growth
- Demonstrate RESPECT for students and prove yourself to be an educator who can be RESPECTED by students
- Be creative and use variety in how you teach
- Be APPROACHABLE as well as AVAILABLE to students
- Maintain healthy teacher-student boundaries
- Provide timely feedback to students (Schell, 2001)

What has prepared you best for teaching nursing students? Even though you may have years of clinical experience, this is not a guarantee that you will be an exceptional nurse educator. Knowing *what* to teach based on your experience does not mean that you will know *how* to teach students (Spencer, 2013). Novice nurse educators who have a strong clinical background may not necessarily have the expertise or educational preparation, and may have difficulty transitioning into a new teaching role. Being an excellent, experienced nurse will lay the foundation to prepare you to be an excellent educator. Your clinical experience and expertise with performing nursing skills, therapeutic communication, and care and compassion can help you gain confidence in teaching students these same skills during lab and clinical practice. Nursing education is a distinct discipline that requires clinical salience and educational preparation to effectively prepare students for nursing practice (Booth, Emerson, Hackney, & Souter, 2016). A lack of educational preparation can lead to stress, frustration, feelings of being overwhelmed, and difficulty during the transition from clinical practice to academia (Paul, 2015; Weidman, 2013).

So let's reflect and answer the following questions to see if you have what it takes to be a nurse educator!

Reflection Questions

1. What is your passion and motivating drive in life?

2. Why do you want to be a nurse educator?

3. Do you enjoy and find fulfillment in serving others?

4. What biases and attitudes may you possess?

5. Do you possess a strong work ethic?

6. Do you consider yourself a lifelong learner?

7. Do you have a natural aptitude for science?

8. How well do you perform under stress?

9. How well are you able to multitask?

10. Do you readily recognize your limitations and what you do/don't know?

11. How well do you handle responsibility?

12. How well do you communicate with others?

13. How much do you value relationships?

14. How well do you work together with others?

15. How well do you handle conflict with others?

Reflection Responses

1. What is your passion and motivating drive in life?

One practical way to determine your personal passion and motivating drives in life is to ask yourself, "What would I be willing to do even if I did not get paid because I enjoy doing it?"

One of the reasons nurses choose to become a nurse educator is because of their passion for teaching and developing others, even though it pays substantially less than clinical practice. Although your motivations may be to serve and teach students, it is worthwhile to prepare for the reality that teaching salaries may be less than what you anticipated. The lower salary for teaching compared to nurses in clinical practice has been a source of dissatisfaction reported by novice nurse educators and a critical barrier to filling vacancies (Oermann, Lynn, & Agger, 2015; Roughton, 2013). Will the reality of lower pay influence your decision to become a nurse educator?

When I was considering a change in career paths, I shadowed a nurse anesthetist for a day to see what this scope of practice would involve. At the end of the day, it left me bored and uninspired. Though nurse anesthetists are a valued and needed member of the health care team, it was not a good fit for me.

At this same time, I was reading *Wild at Heart* by John Eldredge when this quote literally jumped off the page:

> *"Don't ask yourself what the world needs. Ask yourself what makes you come alive, and do that. Because what the world needs are people who have come fully alive."*
>
> (Eldredge, 2001, p. 200).

I realized how much I enjoyed mentoring new nurses in the emergency department and watching the "lightbulb" turn on when what I shared was understood and incorporated into practice by other nurses. This quote gave me permission to pursue what I believe is my God-given passion and talent in nursing, the ability to teach. So, after completing my BSN, instead of pursuing the path of what I thought was NEEDED as a nurse anesthetist, I pursued my PASSION and entered a master's in nursing education program.

To transform nursing education, more than pedagogy needs to change. Transformation flows through the heart passions of the EDUCATOR. Everything that the educator communicates is influenced by what the teacher IS. Teaching is not merely the performance of an hour in class. It represents the outflow of the passions in the life of the educator. It takes years of clinical practice to formulate and deliver a powerful and authentic lecture, because it takes years in practice to make the nurse who is now the nurse educator. Authentic, transformational teaching is an outflow of a person's life.

Where are Nightingale's teachings? They are long gone and have died with the students that she taught over 150 years ago. But the woman who is Florence Nightingale is much greater than any of her best lectures. She lives forever as a passionate and transformational nurse educator even today. Your teaching is but a voice. Much of what you have spoken will be forgotten. But the person who communicates a passion for nursing and the value of serving others will live forever in the hearts of your students if you live this out in academia.

What about you? What makes you come alive as you consider becoming a nurse educator? If serving and teaching others is an internal passion of yours, then this is clearly an indicator that you are on the right path in your decision to become a nurse educator.

2. Why do you want to be a nurse educator?

When the road gets bumpy and you encounter unexpected obstacles in academia, you will question yourself and ask, "WHY did I ever choose this path?" When you know your WHY, you will be much more likely to persevere and transition successfully even when you encounter major turbulence. Your WHY reflects your primary motivation. So why do you want to be a nurse educator? You know what the expected and "right" answer is: "Because I want to teach students." But is this really true for you?

If the personal benefits are your primary motivation to enter/consider nursing education, carefully examine your choice to become a nurse educator. Nursing education is in need of radical transformation, and it may require extra time, energy, and giving of yourself to see it realized. Some faculty want to do only what is needed to maintain the status quo. This is no longer an option. Carefully reflect on your WHY, and pursue your passion wherever it may lead you.

3. Do you enjoy and find fulfillment in serving others?

The essence of nursing practice is serving others in a time of need. Serving others is not highly valued in our culture yet it is the essence of the mindset of not only the professional nurse, but also the nurse educator. The best nurse educators have a strong desire to serve their students. Nurse educators serve students, foster their students' personal and professional growth and development, while helping them learn how to serve others (Robinson, 2009).

The desire to serve needs to be present regardless of how the student may respond to you. Maintaining empathy remains important for academic practice. Can you still teach students even if it appears you are unappreciated? If you remain empathetic and do not take things personally, you will be an excellent nurse educator in practice.

As a nurse educator, you can bring the concept of serving to teaching and learning by applying these steps:

1. Provide a classroom and clinical environment where students feel comfortable, valued, and supported.
2. Tell students that their growth and success is the ultimate goal.
3. Acknowledge students who are having difficulty and be willing to work with these students in a way that will promote their success.
4. Create an environment where students are comfortable discussing their mistakes and errors. Work with the student to analyze the cause and create a plan to avoid future mistakes or errors.
5. Make time to listen and respond to students' concerns.
6. Be willing to change from traditional lecture to active, student-centered learning.
7. Reflect on teaching practice for improvement.
8. Collaborate and build consensus with students.
9. Implement strategies to promote healing for students who have experienced failure, incivility, or bullying.
10. Work toward building students' confidence, self-esteem, and success.

11. Create a sense of community where nurse educators and students learn together (Robinson, 2009).

4. What biases and attitudes may you possess?

Do you have assumptions about other people based on past experiences? For example, if you have had negative experiences with those of the opposite sex, or those of another religious or ethnic group, it's easy to generalize and transfer those assumptions to those from the same group whom you do not even know. Swanson in her research on caring (1991) identified one practical way that nurses can demonstrate caring to each patient is to "avoid assumptions" or preconceived judgments about them. Once an assumption or judgment of any kind is made, the nurse ceases to be authentically engaged and is unable to demonstrate caring to the patient.

As an educator, be aware of any assumptions you may have towards certain students (tattoos, piercings, personality, etc.) so that you can demonstrate authentic caring and advocacy for every student in your program.

5. Do you possess a strong work ethic?

Nursing is hard work. Being a nurse educator can be even harder at times. To be a successful nurse educator, you must embrace the hard work required and be willing to do what is needed without taking shortcuts to get by. Anticipate that there will be increased demands on your time at work and at home. Many novice nurse educators nationwide perceive that the academic workload is greater compared to nurses who do not teach in academics (Boellaard, Brandt, & Zorn, 2015; Candela, Gutierrez, & Keating, 2015; Roughton, 2013).

The increased amount of time to prepare a course, grade papers, and prepare tests is a barrier to transitioning into teaching (Cooley & DeGagne, 2016). The demands of teaching may cause difficulty with balancing family and other obligations (Bellack, 2016; Boellaard, Brandt, & Zorn, 2015; Roughton, 2013). Expect an intense workload and extra time to devote to your teaching role, especially if there is a shortage of faculty in your nursing department (Boellaard, Brandt, & Zorn, 2015; Roughton, 2013). Bellack (2016) recommends developing ways to maintain a balance between your academic and personal life.

A strong work ethic and the willingness to work hard were also emphasized as an important virtue of the professional nurse at the beginning of the modern era in the late 1800s. In her text *Nursing Ethics*, Hampton Robb (1900) wrote:

"A pupil (student nurse) should esteem it a piece of good fortune to be put on duty in the heavy wards, where one is always busy, where the work never seems to be done, and where there is so much in the way of nursing going on…Never be afraid to work and to work hard. Work pure and simple is not likely to do you harm…Never seek for the soft spots or the easy places in hospital work." (p. 69).

Though Hampton Robb's insight was addressed to nursing students, as a transformational nurse educator of her generation who collaborated to found the American Nurses Association, *America Journal of Nursing,* and what would later become the National League for Nursing, she embraced what it took to live this out. If you are saying to yourself, "Bring it on; I am willing to do the hard work that is needed to bring innovation in my generation," you can be assured you are on the right track to become an exceptional and transformational nurse educator!

6. Do you consider yourself a lifelong learner?

Do you love to learn for learning's sake? To be successful as a nurse educator, you must embrace being a lifelong learner to maximize the learning required to excel in this new role. If you are internally motivated and enjoy learning for learning's sake, you will thrive as a nurse educator. But it is not enough to be a lifelong learner. You need to be willing to put what you learn into PRACTICE.

For example, many nurse educators know about the need to radically transform nursing education after having read *Educating Nurses: A Call for Radical Transformation.* But some nurse educators resist and refuse to implement needed change despite having read the book.

Hold yourself to the same standards that you expect of your students. Programs expect students to embrace and even write papers on what is current evidence-based practice in nursing. In the same way, nurse educators must also embrace and then act on evidence-based teaching practice as well.

7. Do you have a natural aptitude for science?

Though nursing has its own body of knowledge or nursing science, the applied sciences of pharmacology, pathophysiology, and fluid and electrolytes are foundational to nursing. If you want to be an effective nurse educator you need to have an aptitude for the applied sciences of nursing, so that you can integrate it in your nursing courses and teach it effectively to your students.

Pathophysiology

Most of your nursing students have had pathophysiology as a required prerequisite for nursing. To teach nursing, you, too, need to know the mechanism of action for the most common medications, accurately interpret lab values, and understand the disease process of the patients you are responsible for in clinical. For example, understanding and then teaching the complexities of the inflammatory and immune response is foundational when caring for a patient who has sepsis. Heart failure is another common disease process that requires the nurse to know the physiologic differences between right-sided versus left-sided heart failure.

A common cardiac medication that is given for hypertension is atenolol, whose pharmacologic classification is a beta blocker. To understand what a beta blocker such as atenolol is blocking, students (and nurse educators!) must be able to know which nervous system (sympathetic or parasympathetic) beta receptors receive stimulation and the physiologic effects or expected outcomes when these same receptors are blocked. If a patient with acute or chronic renal failure receives opiate narcotics for pain control, how does this influence the dosage that the nurse would administer based upon the level of excretion by the body? Knowing that opiate narcotics are excreted primarily by the renal system, this knowledge is relevant and must be understood as well as adverse effects of over-sedation.

Pharmacology/Mechanism of Action

Since nurses administer medications every day, they need to possess a DEEP UNDERSTANDING of pharmacology. To ensure safe practice, nurse educators must teach students WHY patients are taking the medications and perform all necessary safety checks. This is more easily said than done. There is TMI in any nursing drug manual. Content categories include indications, mechanism of action, pharmacologic classification, time/action profile, contraindications, side effects, interactions, route

and dosages, nursing implications, and patient education. If a student has multiple medications to pass, what content areas of the drug manual should be taught as the most important?

Though all aspects of a drug manual are important and need to be known, I believe that the MECHANISM OF ACTION is the *priority* area to master. When the nurse understands how medication affects the body, the resultant nursing assessments will be self-evident and he/she will anticipate most common side effects. When the mechanism of action is deeply understood, the nurse does not need to consult the drug manual for this content, but will know it based on their applied knowledge. But to teach this essential content to students, it, too, must be understood by the educator.

Fluids and Electrolytes

A deep understanding of fluids and electrolytes (F&E) is fundamental to critical thinking in the clinical setting. This content is challenging because it requires application of chemistry, acid/base knowledge, and physiology. Just as anatomy and physiology are essential to understanding the mechanism of action, applied A&P must be integrated into F&E for practical application and contextualization to the bedside to occur.

Laboratory values provide a window to EARLY physiologic status changes that may not be initially evident in vital signs or assessment data collected by the nurse. Examples of this in clinical practice are TRENDS of an elevated serum lactate in any shock state, elevated neutrophils, bands, or WBCs that are seen in sepsis, or elevated serum creatinine in acute renal failure or severe dehydration.

For example, in acute kidney injury (AKI) or acute renal failure (ARF), would you be able to identify the relationship between AKI/ARF and elevation in creatinine, BUN, potassium, and decrease in CO_2 (serum bicarbonate)? Would you be able to anticipate the expected electrolyte derangements most often seen with dehydration caused by severe vomiting and diarrhea? WHY are they present? This is why educators must understand A&P and show students how to apply this content to clinical practice. When students are taught this level of understanding, they will be PROACTIVE and anticipate problems early because they will use knowledge and understand the WHY or rationale.

If this content is a struggle for you, honestly assess your current weaknesses and strengths as a nurse/nurse educator. Since you have embraced the importance of being a lifelong learner, apply yourself to master this content and make any identified weaknesses a strength!

8. How well do you perform under stress?

You already know that nursing practice can be stressful. Just as you managed multiple patients in the clinical setting, you will manage an entire classroom and/or multiple students in the clinical setting, meeting the unique needs of each student. If you have managed stress successfully in practice, you will likely do so in academia.

The clinical setting is where the rubber meets the road in academia. For me, it was the most challenging setting that had the highest levels of stress. Managing eight to ten students and the patients that my students were caring for, and prepping for each clinical pushed me to the brink! This was surprising to me because I was used to high levels of stress as an ED nurse. If you are new to nursing education, give yourself grace to be a novice nurse educator and acclimate to this completely different and often challenging environment. Remember, Benner's novice to expert theory (Benner, 1984) applies to you as a novice nurse educator. Though you may have been an expert nurse in clinical practice, you will take at least a couple steps backward and feel at times like a novice. Just give it time as you did in clinical practice to acquire the proficiency needed to develop as an educator!

9. How well are you able to multitask?

To handle the ongoing demands and stress of nursing practice, you need to multitask by managing and prioritizing competing tasks. This does not change once you are a nurse educator. This is most relevant in the clinical setting. Recognize the most important thing that needs to be done first and then go to the second, the third, and the fourth in succession. Though the ability to recognize what is most important in the clinical setting with multiple students is developed with clinical experience, reflect and determine how well you handle the stress of numerous pressing demands that seem to come all at once.

Expect numerous ongoing demands; PowerPoints to revise, test questions to write, student struggles, and active learning exercises that need to be completed. If you can successfully balance multiple platters in nursing as well as in academia, you will be well suited and thrive in nursing education!

10. Do you readily recognize your limitations and what you do/don't know?

If you are new to nursing education you must give yourself grace to be a novice educator. You do not know it all and will even make mistakes. Some educators struggle with being less than perfect and will resist any suggestion that they do not know what they really don't know. This is the opposite of humility, which recognizes one's weaknesses. This is also an example of role modeling humility to our students that we don't or will not know everything about nursing. This is okay. I tell my students as a nurse we need to know where to find the information. If you can accept yourself as less than perfect but willing to work hard to be excellent and the best nurse educator you can possibly be, you are well on your way to success.

11. How well do you handle responsibility?

As a practicing nurse, you literally hold the life of another human being in your hands. You must apply knowledge and identify a possible complication before it needlessly progresses. As a nurse educator, you are now responsible for teaching future nurses to do the same thing. Never lose sight of the fact that what takes place in the classroom and clinical settings ultimately impacts the patients students will soon care for after they graduate.

This responsibility is more pressing as an educator. Instead of just having your own practice that you are accountable and responsible for, you now are responsible for the students you teach in your program. This is an incredible responsibility. Be sobered by this reality, but use it to motivate you, not overwhelm you. Be accountable to your colleagues and embrace the responsibility that comes with teaching the next generation of students. Desire to be the best educator you can possibly be. This mindset and attitude needs to begin as you start your journey in academia and continue until you retire!

12. How well do you communicate with others?

Nursing is all about relationships. This includes nurse-to-patient, nurse-to-family, and nurse-to-nurse among others. Relationships are still central and just as important in academia. The relationships simply change. Educator-to-educator, educator-to-student, educator-to-department and institutional leadership. The ability to connect and relate effectively to others is also perceived as a caring behavior by your students. Conversely, if you are a loner, enjoy being by yourself, and are more comfortable behind a computer than talking with another person, this could be a challenge that will affect your ability to communicate effectively and relate authentically to your students.

The essence of incivility is a lack of respect for others. Make it a priority to adopt a more direct and respectful style of communication. This will be discussed in depth later in the book. Commit to never speaking negatively of another colleague in their absence. Grover (2005) identified eight skills that are essential for effective communication.

These skills include:
- Listening to the other person
- Asking open-ended questions to gain more in-depth information
- Asking closed questions to gain facts
- Clarifying in order to get more details
- Paraphrasing so that meaning can be interpreted
- Using facilitators to encourage continuing dialogue
- Assessing nonverbal communication cues
- Using silence to promote thinking

13. How much do you value relationships?

Your effectiveness as an educator ultimately hinges on the quality of the RELATIONSHIP that you have with your students. One practical way to intentionally engage with each student and relate to them on a person-to-person level is to take the time to uncover your students' unique stories. This level of disclosure can easily be integrated into the clinical setting. When you create a form to identify personal contact information in case of an emergency, add relevant personal details to learn more about your students. This can include details about the student's family, children, prior vocation, and any unique accomplishments.

When the student's story is known, something transformative begins to take place. The nurse educator begins to see the student on a personal level that builds and strengthens this person-to-person relationship and trust. But this level of disclosure needs to be reciprocated. As an educator, share your story, family, clinical experience, etc., as soon as possible at the beginning of the school year. When relationships in academia are built on mutual

respect, this can prevent incivility from being problematic in your academic culture.

14. How well do you work together with others?

We need one another! If you are a faculty member feeling the burn of a new semester, at some point you will stumble, fall, and need someone to pick you up so you can continue to persevere in nursing academia! *"Two are better than one, if either of them falls down, one can help the other up. But pity anyone who falls and has no one to help them up"* (Ecclesiastes 4:9-12). This timeless truth was written by Solomon, the wisest king in the history of ancient Israel. What was written more than 2,500 years ago remains relevant today!

The importance of working together was put in perspective when I presented my work on clinical reasoning at Elsevier's Faculty Development Institute in 2013. One word jumped off my closing statement that I feel is an exclamation point for those who desire to be a part of the needed transformation in nursing education.

"TOGETHER we can realize Benner's transforming vision of nursing education to not only promote the learning of our students, but more importantly better outcomes for the patients they care for."

Don't go it alone. Use the power of TOGETHER to TRANSFORM your department by doing the following:

1. **Encourage one another and pull them out of the pit PRN!** Life is hard, but academia is even harder. If you see your colleague struggling, or having a bad day, do not be passive or indifferent, but take initiative, and let them have your hand to grasp so you can help pull them out of their "pit"!
2. **Get your teaching team on the same page!** Begin by reading and discussing Educating Nurses TOGETHER. The implications of the educational research of the Carnegie Foundation must be addressed, discussed, and ultimately embraced!
3. **Business as usual is no longer an option!** Human nature tends to resist change. This is the time to get your team lead, or better yet, your department chair to be an advocate to transform your department TOGETHER based on the transformational paradigms from *Educating Nurses*. Leadership has the power to set a new HIGH bar.

15. How well do you handle conflict with others?

How you respond to this question will suggest whether you will be part of the problem or part of the solution to bullying and incivility endemic in nursing education. If you have conflict and disagree with another person, do you still value and respect their perspective and seek to find common ground? Are you able to step back and view this conflict from the other's perspective and any stress that may have influenced the conflict? Do you have strong conflict resolution skills?

If you experience conflict with another person, do you tend to interpret this conflict as an attack on yourself and think negatively of this person and share your critical concerns with others? Though this type of behavior may appear to be normal to some, it is unprofessional and must be called out for what it really is, bullying and disrespectful behavior that has the power to deeply wound and devastate another human being.

The most common overt bullying behaviors in nursing include isolating/marginalizing targeted faculty, personal slander, and withholding information that sets up another to fail (Clark, Olender, & Kenski, 2013). Be the needed change in nursing education by incorporating an attitude of valuing and respecting one another regardless of any differences. Remember that you will be working with educators, deans, directors, and others who have various passions, ideas, and personalities. Generational differences also influence each person's perspective on their work ethics and organizational commitment (Candela, Gutierrez, & Keating, 2015).

Nursing departments may consist of a mix of experienced and new faculty, baby boomers, generation Xers, and millennials who have different perspectives and values regarding academic work. I have observed experienced faculty question whether new faculty are ready to put the time and effort into learning and teaching a course. New faculty may feel overwhelmed with the time commitment required to prepare a course. Do not let these differing perspectives and values deter you from mentoring a new faculty member and working together as a team.

Here are some practical guidelines to live this out in all that you do:

- VALUE the perspective and expertise of ALL colleagues.
- RESPECT the unique attributes that members bring to a team.
- APPRECIATE the importance of all professional collaboration.
- VALUE TEAMWORK and the relationships within the team.
- VALUE different styles of communication used by patients, families, health care providers, and colleagues.
- CONTRIBUTE to resolution of conflict and disagreement. ("Pre-Licensure KSAS," 2014)

Reflect

1. What are your strengths as an educator?

2. What are areas for improvement?

3. What will you do to develop and make any identified weakness your strength so you can grow and strengthen your effectiveness as an educator?

References:

American Association of Colleges of Nursing [AACN] (2015). Nursing faculty shortage fact sheet. Retrieved at http://www.aacn.nche.edu/media-relations/FacultyShortage.FS.pdf.

Bellack, J. P. (2016). Advice for new (and seasoned) faculty: Reprise. *Journal of Nursing Education, 55*(9), 483-485.

Benner, P. (1984). *From novice to expert: Excellence and power in clinical nursing practice.* Upper Saddle River, NJ: Prentice Hall.

Boellaard, M. R., Brandt, C.L., & Zorn, C. R. (2015). Faculty to faculty: Advice for educators new to teaching in accelerated second baccalaureate degree nursing programs. *Journal of Nursing Education, 54(6)*, 343-346.

Booth, T. L., Emerson, C. J., Hackney, M. G., & Souter, S. (2016). Preparation of academic nurse educators. *Nurse Education in Practice, 19,* 54-57.

Candela, L., Gutierrez, A. P., & Keating, S. (2015). What predicts nurse faculty members' intent to stay in the academic organization? A structural equation model of a national survey of nursing faculty. *Nurse Education Today, 35*, 580-589.

Cooley, S. S., DeGagne, J. C. (2016). Transformative experience: Developing competence in novice nursing faculty. *Journal of Nursing Education, 55*(2), 96-100.

Derby-Davis, M.J. (2014). Predictors of nursing faculty's job satisfaction and intent to stay in academe. *Journal of Professional Nursing, 30*(1), 19-25.

Eldredge, J. (2001). *Wild at heart: Discovering the secret of a man's soul.* Nashville, Tennessee: Thomas Nelson.

Hampton Robb, E. (1900). *Nursing ethics.* Cleveland, OH: E.C. Koeckert.

Oermann, M.H., Lynn, M.R., & Agger, C.A. (2015). Faculty openings, shortage, and mentoring in associate degree nursing programs. *Teaching and Learning in Nursing, 10*(3), 107-111.

Paul, P.A. (2015). Transition from novice adjunct to experienced associate degree nurse educator: A comparative qualitative approach. *Teaching and Learning in Nursing, 10*(1), 3-11.

Peters, A. N. (2015). The concepts of incivility: A case study. *Teaching and Learning in Nursing, 10* (4), 156-160.

Pre-Licensure KSAS. (2014). QSEN.com. Retrieved from http://qsen.org/competencies/pre-licensure-ksas/#patient-centered_care

Robinson, F. P. (2009). Servant teaching: The power and promise for nursing education. *International Journal of Nursing Education Scholarship, 6*(1), 1-15.

Roughton, S. E. (2013). Nursing faculty characteristics and perceptions predicting intent to leave. *Nursing Education Perspectives, 34*(4), 217-225.

Schell, K: The process of innovative teaching in the generic baccalaureate nursing classroom: A cross-case analysis. Unpublished doctoral dissertation, Widener University, 2001.

Spencer, C. (2013). From bedside to classroom: From expert back to novice. *Teaching and Learning in Nursing, 8*(1), 13-16.

Swanson, K. M. (1991). Empirical development of a middle range theory of caring. *Nursing Research, 40*(3), 161–166.

Weidman, N. A. (2013). The lived experience of the transition of the clinical nurse expert to the novice nurse educator. *Teaching and Learning in Nursing, 8*(3), 102-109.

4

How to THRIVE, Not Merely Survive, as a Nurse Educator

Keith Rischer, RN, MA, CEN, CCRN
Patricia Pence, EdD, MSN, RN

What do you need to know to successfully transition to the academic setting? This chapter will share principles to help prepare not only those who are new to academia but those who are already educators. By successfully navigating the most common pitfalls, you will see that it really is possible to not just survive, but actually thrive personally and professionally as a nurse educator!

1. Make enough time
2. Take care of business...you!
3. Have realistic expectations
4. Pursue excellence
5. Use the power of passion
6. Be a lifelong learner
7. Find ways to recover from reality shock
8. Face and overcome your fears
9. Write down your goals
10. Always reflect
11. Understand learning theories

Make Enough Time

Time is a precious commodity as a nurse educator. The trap that many educators fall into when encountering the numerous and ongoing demands in academia is that what is most important in life (taking time to cultivate relationships) does NOT need to be done immediately. But the URGENT things or never-ending tasks on ones to-do list demand immediate attention and action. Without realizing it, we become slaves to the TYRANNY of the URGENT. By choosing to focus on the urgent, we can begin to neglect what is really MOST important in life.

In clinical practice, your work is left behind you when the shift is over. When I (Keith) began working as a nurse educator, I quickly realized that the work never leaves you! There are numerous urgent things that continually call and need to be done: Emails require a response, paperwork to grade, or presentations to develop. Though I was working full-time as a nurse educator during the week, I continued to work clinically every Friday and Saturday night. I was working 60-plus hours a week and, though I loved what I was doing in both education and clinical practice, I was a man in motion with the URGENT dictating my schedule. By the end of the school year, I was physically, emotionally, and spiritually drained. I was a slave to the tyranny of the urgent.

In the classic article "Tyranny of the Urgent" (1967), Charles Hummel insightfully stated that there is a constant tension in our life between the URGENT and the IMPORTANT. Filter each day by identifying what is "NICE to do" and what is "NEED to do." The urgent tasks that continually press are NICE to do, but the most important things in your life are the NEED to do and must become your priority. I have observed that the URGENT tasks will always be present in one form or another, but the things that are most IMPORTANT may not.

For me, the most important things in my life are RELATIONSHIPS. As a Christian, my relationship with God is my first priority. My wife, five children, and now two grandchildren follow closely. My work in clinical practice and with KeithRN is third.

Our five children have left our home and we now have an empty nest. In the past two years, one of my closest friends suddenly died of a massive myocardial infarction, and another has stage IV small cell lung cancer. The old Joni Mitchell song got it right, "You Don't Know What You Got 'Til It's Gone." What about you? What is most important to you? Do you consistently make time for it in your busy schedule? I would encourage you to make this a priority and schedule time for it, before it's too late.

Take Care of Business…You!

Motivation matters. Most educators teach because they love what they do. But unfortunately, this passion for teaching that makes you come alive can slowly fade and ultimately lead to burnout. The end result is that you become a "dead man or woman walking," putting in your time with no fire, only a trail of smoke. Nurses have one of the highest rates of burnout among all health care professionals. Don't become a casualty. Instead, determine to take care of yourself to go the distance in academia or you will be just another statistic.

Value of Self-Care

To maintain a healthy balance and prevent burnout in practice, educators must be proactive and embrace the necessity of self-care. Though academia will consume you with new challenges, do NOT let nursing education become your life! Pursue and fight for balance by establishing "margin" in your life. Margin is the space between your current demands and your limit to handle them (Swenson, 2004). Those blank spaces on the sides of each page of a book have a purpose, as do margins or blank spaces in your daily life. If you continually push yourself, you will soon find out that this cannot be sustained for the long haul of nursing education.

The perpetual "gerbil wheel" you experience as an educator with its incessant, ongoing demands requires you to be fully aware of the need to renew your body, mind, and spirit. If your "tank" of personal renewal is empty or dangerously low, this will directly affect your ability to be fully engaged and passionate as an educator. Many of the stresses in academia are NOT easily changed or within your direct control. You must learn to accept those things, but recognize that you have the power to directly control and change your RESPONSE to them.

Self-Care for Nurse Educators

I (Keith) tend to be an unbalanced, Type A, driven individual who sometimes does not know when to stop. I will virtually pour myself out and do whatever is needed to promote the learning of my students. Though this may benefit my students in the short term, it ultimately takes a toll on me in the long term. True wisdom is realized when we learn from the life lessons of others and do NOT repeat them ourselves. If you can identify with my struggle and disposition, I would like to share a few things I have learned along the way in the desire to strive for balance and margin in nursing education.

First, establish well-defined "margin" boundaries. As a new full-time nurse educator, I soon realized the reality and power of "job creep" and the ever-pressing demands of things that need to be done. This is one of the greatest distinctions between clinical practice and academia. In practice, you are paid by the hour and when your shift is done, so are you. But in academia this is hardly the case. There are always loose ends that need to be tied up, some more pressing than others.

A practical strategy to establish healthy boundaries and balance is to set STOP times in your evenings for all school-related work. Resist the temptation to keep going, just to finish off whatever is on your platter as the evening wears on. Communicate to staff and students that your weekends are sacred and you will NOT respond to emails until Monday unless it is urgent. Do what works for you but draw some lines in the sand, or the "tyranny of the urgent" will define your life in academia!

Burnout Warning: Nurses (and Educators!) at Risk

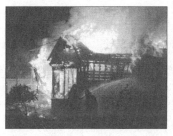

Burnout has been described as the progressive loss of the initial idealism, passion, energy, and purpose to enter the profession (Edelwich, 1980). It can also be defined as the loss of human caring, or stated another way, the separation of caregiving and caring (Benner & Wrubel, 1989). When a nurse initially enters the profession, he or she is motivated and engaged to begin this journey of a new career. If this same new nurse has unrealistic expectations or has not been prepared for real-world practice, the gap between individual expectations and the reality of clinical practice begin to widen, causing frustration and disappointment (Maslach, 2003). This can lead to job dissatisfaction, loss of confidence and enthusiasm. This is why it is so important to prepare students for real-world clinical practice and provide realistic expectations in various care settings after graduation. This could prevent unrealistic expectations that could eventually lead to burnout.

Slow Fade, Stage by Stage

When the consequences of burnout were summarized in the literature, the impact to nurses' emotional and mental health was dramatic. Nurses became hardened, oblivious, robot-like, depressed, frightened, and worn down (Swanson, 1999). It must be noted that nurse educators are at the same risk of developing burnout as a result of the inherent ongoing stress that is present in academia.

Burnout develops insidiously over time for nurses and nurse educators. This is another reason why reflection is essential to professional practice and needs to be encouraged. Burnout that is not identified until the later stages may take months or even years to fully resolve (Lyckholm, 2001). Burnout has five distinct stages that represent a predictable progression. Reflect on these stages yourself and teach your students the key characteristics of each stage to identify burnout EARLY and prevent needless progression.

Stage 1
- Mental and physical exhaustion
- Emotional emptiness
- Little or no desire to relate or engage with patients

Stage 2
- Indifference
- Cynical, uncaring
- Dehumanize patient and family

Stage 3
- Feelings of failure as a nurse
- Feelings of helplessness

Stage 4
- Feelings of failure as a person
- Self-hatred, isolation
- Increased absenteeism from work

Stage 5 (complete burnout)
- Performs responsibilities of nurse with no involvement, commitment, or enthusiasm
- Completely disengaged
- Contemplates leaving nursing (Spinetta et al., 2000)

My Story

Though I did not experience burnout in academia, I have experienced it as a nurse in the ED. When I first started in this clinical setting, it was a dream come true. The adrenalin rush that came with caring for critically ill patients and the wide range of clinical presentations provided a stimulating and invigorating environment for me. I became more proficient in clinical skills and critical thinking as I drew from my prior years of clinical experience in critical care. I was engaged and truly cared about what happened to each patient in my care. I enjoyed what I was doing so I began to pick up overtime on a regular basis because it was readily available. I became more physically and emotionally tired, but I did not realize it at the time. I was beginning to DRIFT.

Slowly but gradually over time, I began not to care. What I once enjoyed was now just a job and putting in my time. Patients became burdens. I had critical patients and some of them died as a result of their injuries or illness. I did not engage or truly care. When I began to reflect and saw how far I had fallen from my original motivation to care for others, I knew I had to do something dramatic to recapture my heart. I left the ED and renewed my passion for caring in an entirely different environment in acute care. In addition to a change of scenery, I also needed REST, which led to RESToration.

I have experienced in my journey the wisdom of Benner and Wrubel who wrote:

"It is a peculiarly modern mistake to think that caring is the cause of the burnout and that the cure is to protect oneself from caring to prevent the 'disease' called burnout. Rather, the loss of caring is the sickness, and the return of caring is the recovery." (1989, p. 473)

If you are a nurse educator and have also experienced

burnout in clinical practice or academia, do not hesitate to share the power of your story and what can be learned from it with your students. By being authentic and transparent, you are modeling the professional values you want your students to embody. What could you have done differently to prevent burnout? What have you done since to prevent it? By sharing your journey, your students will benefit and you will be an educator who will positively impact your students and make a lasting difference.

Have Realistic Expectations

When I (Keith) first became a nurse educator, I had numerous unrealistic expectations that almost set me up to fail. I thought all students would share my love for learning and nursing and that my well-polished PowerPoint lectures would keep them engaged for the entire lecture. I also thought that all students would value active learning that made them think and use knowledge in the classroom. If you have had any experience teaching, you know that these expectations were delusional thinking on my part.

As if student struggles weren't enough, I also experienced unexpected difficulties with colleagues. When I attended department meetings, it was obvious that some faculty did not respect or even like one another. Some faculty were targeted and their input and perspective was not valued or appreciated. Some faculty had a varying commitment toward teaching. When I suggested innovative strategies that could strengthen student learning, some were more interested in maintaining the status quo. Though each department is unique, never settle and accept an unhealthy status quo! Embrace your role to be a transformer that will move the ball forward to bring needed change in your department!

Students Do NOT Define You

I took my student evaluations seriously, but did my best not to take it personally. I have seen colleagues crushed and in tears from negative student feedback. I believe a better response is to reflect, look for THEMES of feedback that communicate a concern in your teaching, and see if the shoe fits. If not, let it go and take the shoe off. If there is more than one theme of similar concerns, take this at face value and see if there is an opportunity for growth.

Depending on the culture of your department, student evaluations and the fear of negative feedback pre-vent some faculty from bringing needed change. It is imperative that leadership recognize the need for change and support faculty who are courageous enough to do things differently! Leadership should be the final word of your evaluation as an educator, NOT students who as novice nurses have no idea what is required to prepare them for professional practice.

Pursue Excellence

Do you know what separates nurse educators who are passionate to bring needed change and make a difference from those who resist change and are content with the status quo? The desire to be excellent and excelling to be the best educator that you can possibly be. The final chapter of the nursing leadership textbook, *The New Leadership Challenge* by Grossman & Valiga, is a must-read for every nurse educator. It is titled "Leadership, Excellence, and Creating the Future of Nursing." Excellence is a choice and a habit. It does not just happen by chance or by accident. It is always the result of sincere effort and strong intention.

Excellence is inwardly motivated and is present because you cannot imagine doing anything less than your very best (Grossman & Valiga, 2013). Remember the old Gatorade commercials with Michael Jordan sweating Gatorade that correlated with the commercial message, "Is it in you." In the same way, the pursuit of excellence represents this inward motivation that is consistently demonstrated in those educators who will not settle for just getting by.

What Does Excellence Look Like?

Qualities associated with excellence are taking risks, being unconventional, and being on the cutting-edge of teaching and learning (Tagliareni, 2008). When daring to achieve excellence and bring about needed change, you must be willing to face less than satisfactory student evaluations, as well as become comfortable with insecurity and anxiety (Tagliareni, 2008; Valiga, 2010).

So how do nurse educators demonstrate excellence? Here are practical ways to bring excellence into your teaching practice:

- Develop innovative strategies based on evidenced-based literature that promote student engagement, instead of relying on tradition or your past experiences.
- Document the results of using effective strategies.

- Share your insights with other educators through a presentation or publication.
- Create a classroom where teachers and students learn together.
- Use strategies to develop effective learning.
- Focus on DEEP learning of the MOST important information, rather than covering content.
- Admit to students when you do not know the answer.
- Partner with students to determine learning objectives or assignments.
- Challenge yourself, your colleagues, and your students.
- Set high standards for student performance. (Ironside & Valiga, 2006; Valiga, 2010)

The National League for Nursing Task Force defined 30 characteristics or traits as Hallmarks of Excellence in Nursing Education (http://nln.org). The list above and the Hallmarks of Excellence are not all-inclusive, but can stimulate active dialogue among nurse educators to guide movement toward excellence in nursing programs. Reflect and ask yourself, "What does excellence mean to me? What risks am I willing to take toward achieving excellence?"

Role Model Excellence

Nehring (1990) identified that, from a student's perspective, being a good role model as a professional nurse is the most important characteristic that distinguishes the best from the worst-rated clinical faculty. Students value educators who demonstrate by their example that they enjoy nursing and teaching, are well prepared, demonstrate clinical excellence, are approachable, display self-confident, encourage mutual respect, and provide support and encouragement to students. Make it a priority to live out these values and be the nurse you want your students to aspire to become.

What does your example communicate? Do you demonstrate the values and ethics of the nursing profession that include caring, compassion, and respect consistently in all that you do? If there is a lack of integrity demonstrated by faculty due to an inconsistency between what is taught and what is modeled, students will readily recognize it. They are more likely to model what they see lived out. Tanner (1990) recognized the power of the "hidden curriculum." It is not what is in the syllabus that students really learn, but the values and example that are role-modeled to students that influence the formative development of students.

What Is the Culture in Your Department?

When nurses work on units where excellent nursing is the norm, nurses strive to continually reach the level of excellence they see in their nurse colleagues. But the converse is also true. When nurses practice on a unit where the standard of care is poor or merely average, the other nurses are satisfied with merely maintaining the status quo and doing just enough to get by (Grossman & Valiga, 2013). What is the culture in your nursing department? How would you honestly describe it? Are educators on the same page pursuing excellence and applying educational research to practice and encouraging others through their example to be the best for their students? Do educators strive for transformation through continuous growth, improvement, and understanding? Do faculty trust the recommendations made by committee members that are sound and well thought out? (Ironside & Valiga, 2006). Or are faculty in "silos," doing just what is needed to get by, regardless of how it may impact student learning?

Vince Lombardi, the former coach of the Green Bay Packers, said, "The quality of a person's life is in direct proportion to his or her commitment to excellence, regardless of the chosen field of endeavor." Pursuing excellence affects not just the quality of the nurse educator you will become, but all areas of your life! Make it a priority to pass the mirror test. Honestly look at yourself in the mirror each day knowing that you have done your very best in all that you do as a nurse educator.

Use the Power of Passion

What is it that separates those who are successful in everything they do and those who are not? Is it intelligence, education, or social status? No. The most important characteristic of your success as a nurse educator will be your passion. Passion is "the essence of excellence" (Valiga, 2003, p. 276). You must have a burning desire to be the best and overcome any obstacles that may be in front of you. If you have this burning passion, even if you are average or ordinary in your abilities, you can and will achieve and accomplish great things! This is why nurturing and cultivating passion is so important (Maxwell, 1999).

Passion is the first step to accomplishing your goals.

Those who live extraordinary lives have great desire. Passion makes the impossible possible. If you have a burning fire in your heart, this will lift everything in your life (Maxwell, 1999). This is why passionate educators excel. Passion is also contagious. If you possess this fiery passion, you will impact and influence your students and colleagues and lead by lived example.

What Is Your Temperature?

Do you desire to be the best nurse educator you can be? Or are you overwhelmed and just want to survive each day? To be passionate, the following are practical strategies to see this realized in your life (Maxwell, 1999):

- **Take your temperature**. How passionate are you about nursing education? Does it show? Ask those around you, including your students and trusted colleagues, about your level of desire and if it is hot, cold, or waning.
- **Return to your first love.** Too many educators allow the tyranny of the urgent and stress of nursing school to get them off track and steal their joy and passion. Look back to when you were just starting out as a nurse educator. Try to recapture this enthusiasm. Then evaluate your current passion in light of those former desires.
- **Associate with people of passion.** Birds of a feather really do flock together. If you've lost your passion and desire, you need to get around some "fire-lighters"! Because passion is contagious, make it a priority to have friends and colleagues who will infect you with passion instead of stealing your joy with their negativity.

There are numerous barriers that prevent change in nursing education. Transformational change is hard and requires additional time and energy. It is the passionate nurse educator who possesses not only the energy, but also the commitment and DESIRE to see it realized. It is NOT that transformation is too hard; the greatest barrier is that nurse educators do not want or DESIRE it badly enough.

Be a Lifelong Learner

Your journey of learning does not end once you are a nurse educator. It has only begun. You must have a thirst and desire to learn and grow as an educator throughout your career in order to provide the best current and evi-

dence-based teaching your students deserve. Health care, nursing, and nursing education are continually changing based on new research. Change is a given.

To keep abreast of change requires continual learning. Treatments and nursing procedures change with evidence-based practice findings. Embrace this reality. But when you enjoy the journey, you will have the aptitude that will lead to your ongoing success and professional development as a nurse educator. Make it a priority to subscribe to relevant nursing journals that will keep you abreast of current research findings and feed your knowledge as a lifelong learner.

Incorporating Evidence-Based Practices into Your Practice

As a nurse educator, you likely have your students complete an evidence-based practice assignment. Nurse educators not only have a responsibility to keep abreast of clinical best practices, but just as important, if not more so, is educational evidence-based practice. This is why the recommendations of the Carnegie Foundation to improve nursing education contained in *Educating Nurses: A Call for Radical Transformation* must not be seen as optional to embrace; it is educational evidence-based practice that must be implemented.

To keep abreast of changes and opportunities to incorporate evidence-based practice, read appropriate and relevant nursing journals. As a nurse educator, my favorite journal is *The Journal of Nursing Education*. For practice, *The American Journal of Nursing (AJN)* is an excellent resource that is relevant for all clinical practice settings. *Nurse Educator, Journal of Nursing Education,* and *Teaching and Learning in Nursing* are excellent journals to maintain educational best practice. One of the blessings of being an educator is access to every journal relevant to nursing and nursing education through your institutional library database.

Find Ways to Recover from Reality Shock

Reality shock is when you first enter nursing education and feel unprepared and overwhelmed. What does reality shock look like? Feelings of fear, anxiety, and lack of feeling prepared. If you can identify with these feelings, know that you are not alone! Because of a lack of educational experience, the full force of reality shock will intensify the normal stress and anxiety that any person experiences when starting a new position. You don't need to know everything as a new educator! Now is the time to develop realistic expectations. It will take at least one to two years to learn and grow in your new role.

How to Cope

It is one thing to experience the painful feelings that accompany reality shock; it is another to cope and to overcome them. The following are some practical strategies that you can incorporate to help you cope and overcome reality shock as a new nurse educator.

- Develop meaningful relationships with your mentor and new co-workers.
- Share your struggles and feelings with a trusted nurse colleague or mentor. This is another reason to establish meaningful relationships with others in your department.
- Know how to access practical resources that will develop you as a nurse educator. (Patricia Benner and her body of work became my mentor as well as the book *Educating Nurses: A Call for Radical Transformation.*)
- It is normal to experience some dissatisfaction with your new role and work environment. Have realistic expectations and be kind to yourself!
- Pattern your practice after educators who are excellent role models.
- Use reflection to identify what is going well and what can be improved. Celebrate and acknowledge what you are doing well and do not focus on the negative!
- Keep a journal so you can reflect on your practice and acknowledge your feelings. This will help you to see the progress you are making on your journey!
- Identify and manage conflicts as they arise. Be direct with communication. Do not allow inevitable conflict with co-workers to steal your joy and exacerbate reality shock (Ferris, 2012).

Face and Overcome Your Fears

Fear is one of the primary emotions present when you embark on a new journey as an educator as well as a red flag that reality shock is present. Some of the fears that I (Keith) experienced entering academia included:

- Fear of the unknown

- Fear of doing things differently
- Fear of student and faculty acceptance

When I conducted a survey of my readers, asking, "What is the most significant barrier to realize transformation in nursing education?" the most common response was the unwillingness of faculty to change. You need to dig beneath the surface to understand WHY faculty struggle with and even resist change. I believe the primary reason is fear. To thrive and bring needed transformation to academia, reflect and determine what specific fear(s) that may be holding you back. Once this fear is identified, it can be confronted and will lose its power to keep you from being successful as an educator.

Let me share an example from my life that demonstrates how facing your fears can actually be liberating and life changing. My daughter Nikki was traveling with me in Southern California and she found a Groupon for half off skydiving and was excited to do something she had always wanted to do at a discount. I had absolutely no desire to follow in her steps, but was glad to see her go for it. But as she enthusiastically pursued her passion to jump off a plane, I began to confront my fears. What was I afraid of? Jumping out of a plane at 14,000 feet could be a lot of fun and something I could cross off my "bucket list." But it could also kill me!

Realizing that this was a once-in-a-lifetime father-daughter experience, I decided to go for it at the last minute. As a result, we shared an awesome experience together. I will never forget the deep fear I felt being connected to my jumper who had a belt connecting me to him. I hoped the parachute was packed correctly and would open as planned. But the most gut-wrenching aspect of this jump was facing my fear of possible death. Looking down 14,000 feet through the open jump door of the plane and rolling out the door on the count of three made me seriously want to reconsider, but it was too late. Once I jumped out of the plane, I was free-falling for a full minute at 120 mph and was exhilarated by this incredible experience! The chute opened, and I could now enjoy the ride and the view as I drifted gently to earth.

Here are five principles derived from my "near-death" experience that can help you face and overcome your fears in academia:

1. **Identify your specific fear.** Though I have no fear of heights, that fear was palpable as I prepared to

jump out of an open door at 14,000 feet. If you or other colleagues you work with are struggling to implement needed change, there is a reason! Dialogue with your colleagues and explore what is holding you or them back. Once the fear or barrier to change has been identified, it is time to take the next step.

2. **Overcome the fear.** I had to decide if my fear was going to hold me back from what could be the ultimate experience of my life. Fears are meant to be overcome if they are barriers to change. Are your fears rational or irrational? You need to work with experienced colleagues for guidance. Once the fear is identified, you must decide how to respond and develop a plan to do things differently.

3. **Find supportive colleagues who are willing to jump with you.** If my daughter had not encouraged and supported me to "go for it," I would have never left the ground. You need the support of colleagues who will encourage and support you as your friend and mentor. Identify those supportive colleagues and you are on your way to making a difference! Had I not been strapped to an expert jumper, there is no way I could have taken a life-threatening plunge. The experts in academia who have been instrumental when I first took the transformational "plunge" are Patricia Benner and Christine Tanner. Their insight, wisdom, and evidence-based practice will provide expert support and guidance for you, too.

4. **Take the plunge!** Though I had come as far as being inside the plane at 14,000 feet, I still had to decide whether I had the courage (or folly!) to jump out. Facing your fears and talking about transformation is NOT the same as doing it. You must commit to take the plunge. Commit to implementing needed change and do not look back!

5. **The time is now!** Though I could have rationalized my fear and said I will jump out of a plane another time, I knew it was then or never. Because so much is riding on the need to transform nursing education, including student learning and the lives of patients that students will care for, recapture that sense of urgency and make it a priority to do what is needed today.

As you face your fears and step out to bring needed change, commit to see it through. I can promise a few bumps and some student resistance along the way. But if you face your fears and persevere with transformational change, you will be THAT educator students will contact after graduation and say, "THANK YOU! Though you made me think and work hard to apply my learning to be the best nurse possible, you were the educator who prepared me well for professional practice!"

Write Down Your Goals

There is a part of me that does not like to write down personal goals. I rationalize that if I don't write them down, I do not have to feel like a failure when I fail to meet them. But those who write down their goals and review them regularly are much more likely to meet them. Patient goals/outcomes using nursing process are taught to be:

• Specific
• Measurable
• Realistic
• Time limited

Use this same process for writing out goals for transforming your content. Don"t write, "I will use more active learning in my classroom," State, "I will use a case study or group learning activity that situates clinical realities for 15-30 minutes for every hour of every classroom lecture." When you write your goal in this manner, you will know whether it was met or not. Every lecture may not be realistic for some. Then rewrite the goal so it not only stretches your abilities, but is able to be consistently attained!

To accomplish your goals as an educator, you must have a target. Have a clear sense of direction of where you want to go at the beginning of the school year and you are well on your way to bring about needed change and accomplish what is most important.

Always Reflect

To improve your craft as a nurse educator, honestly and authentically reflect to determine what went well and what did not with your teaching. Just as REFLECTION is central to clinical practice, it remains relevant to you as an educator. I was crushed by some of the student evaluations I received as a new nurse educator. I had to remind myself that students are NOT the final determinant of the effectiveness of my teaching, but their input needs to be considered.

Though students can rate their satisfaction with

your teaching methods and organization, they are unable to judge the accuracy, depth, and educational best practices. Keep student comments in perspective. Student comments reflect their views at one point in time in the program. Students realize only later WHY a course or assignment was taught the way it was that proved critical to their learning (Oermann, 2017). Evaluating how students respond to your teaching is essential in continuing to improve in all that you do in the class or clinical settings.

To be proactive with student evaluations and improve the effectiveness of your teaching, ask your students the following three questions midpoint in the semester (Oermann, 2017):

1. Are you satisfied with your learning in this course?
2. What is going well in this course?
3. What recommendations do you have to improve the course?

Though Tanner's model of clinical judgment (2006) is patient-practice based, it can be applied and adapted to the practice of nurse educators. Step four of Tanner's model includes the importance of reflection-IN-action. This is the ability to accurately interpret the patient's response to an intervention in the moment as the events are unfolding. In nursing education, the nurse educator needs to assess the student's response to the effectiveness of what and how content was taught.

Three Reflection Questions

After every classroom lecture or when implementing a new active learning strategy, use these three questions to help you transfer what went well and leave behind what did not, next time you teach.

1. **What can I learn from this?** Be honest and determine if student learning actually improved with any new approaches or techniques used in your classroom. Though a new approach may look good when presented in an educator conference setting, this does not mean that it will be a hit in your class or clinical.
2. **What would I do differently (if applicable) using this pedagogy?** Be willing to be flexible and change if needed. If you did something new and obtained the desired response, then stick with it and persevere. Fine tune as needed.
3. **How can I use what I have learned from this situation to improve student learning in the future?** Use what has been learned to see if it could be improved to strengthen and engage student learning for next semester. Adjustments are to be expected!

Every nurse educator as well as nurses in practice should adopt the motto of the Home Depot, "Never stop improving!" Reflect and determine what went well and contributed to student learning and what did not this past semester. Using these three reflection questions influenced by Christine Tanner's model of clinical judgment can help you refine and improve your practice as an educator to strengthen student learning.

Understand Learning Theories

Nursing theory was not my favorite class as a graduate nursing student, but I was surprised by how much I understood the bigger picture of nursing practice when theory was applied to nursing. In the same way, when different theories are understood regarding how students learn, it will strengthen your ability to teach and make it stick when these theories are applied in your teaching.

Following is a quick summary of relevant learning theories to integrate into your practice (Billings & Halstead, 2016):

Cognitive Learning Theory

Emphasizes the mental structures of learning that include perception, thinking, understanding, and knowledge acquisition. Learning is defined as processing information and is experiential. Nurse educators can apply this to practice by making learning ACTIVE instead of passive and developing students' ability to THINK more like a nurse. Content presentation is not enough; students must discover meaning by USING knowledge.

Situated Learning and Situated Cognition

This is the standard of nursing education that must be realized to bring needed transformation (Benner et al., 2010) by integrating clinical and classroom experiences. Situated learning takes place in the context of the clinical setting. The primary objective is bringing clinical to class so students can develop skills relevant to practice and are better prepared when they are in the actual clinical setting. Case studies, role play, and simulation are examples that emphasize APPLICATION to clinical practice.

Adult Learning Theory

Adults learn best when information is perceived as important and relevant and they are asked to use their prior life experiences to apply knowledge and solve problems. Adult learners are also self-directed. Because adults fear failure, work to create an atmosphere of trust and respect to facilitate student empowerment by guiding students in a collaborative relationship. Learning activities should include independent study and inquiry as well as reflective journaling.

Novice to Expert

Benner (1982) states that nursing expertise develops over time and passes through five stages. In order to progress and develop, there is no substitute for clinical experience to strengthen and develop expertise. Educators must identify the level of the students they are working with to develop realistic expectations based on prior clinical experience. This theory will be discussed in depth later in the book.

Caring Theory

The concepts of Watson's (1989) caring theory emphasize the practice of loving-kindness, authentic presence, and cultivation of one's own spiritual practice. These concepts can become the framework for a caring curriculum in academia that can include addressing ways to eliminate adversarial relationships with students and faculty, and maintain open, honest, caring, and supportive relationships. Integrating questions that highlight the importance of caring in the context of patient care are addressed in detail later in this book.

Neuroscience Theory

Current research findings have revealed that the brain continues to adapt and change even as an adult as new neuronal connections are made. It's called neuroplasticity (Kalia, 2008). REPETITION of key content can speed processing time through neural networks.

Brain-based Learning

Focuses on optimal conditions for the brain to learn. The way the brain learns is influenced by multiple factors including the time of day, nutrition, and stress (Jensen, 2008). Once these factors are taken into account, learning can be maximized by enhancing the conditions when the brain learns best. Brain-based learning is fostered through activities that require knowledge construction (I have a case study tool that can develop this and is addressed later in the book) and making connections to prior knowledge. Case studies and simulation are effective tools to develop.

Steps to Transition Successfully as a New Educator

If you are new or have recently transitioned to nursing education, the following practical strategies will help you transition from clinical practice to academia:

1. **Get a mentor.** Make this a priority if you are new to academia. Identify faculty who are excellent, experienced, and model the essence of the nurse educator you aspire to be. Your mentor can be official or unofficial, depending on where you work and the orientation process. A good mentor will imprint the intangibles of nursing education that will positively influence your professional development in this new setting. If you are an experienced educator, embrace the responsibility to take a new educator under your wing. Make yourself available and schedule regular times to meet to discuss struggles and challenges before they become a crisis. Welcome, guide, nurture, support, and positively impact the transition of novice nurse educators (Bellack, 2016; Weidman, 2013). Paul (2015) proposed that these topics for orientating novice nurse educators are NEED to know. Be sure that these topics are included in your department orientation for new educators.
   - Strategies to handle student behaviors and unprofessionalism
   - Orientation to simulation and laboratory equipment
   - Learning theories and teaching techniques
   - Expectations for the course and student performance
   - Guidelines and logistics for clinical
   - Changes in the NCLEX
   - Available student resources
   - Evaluation processes

2. **Network with other faculty and find a solid support system.** A healthy department is comprised of positive and meaningful relationships with col-

leagues. Make it a priority to engage with your colleagues and take advantage of opportunities to go out after work or any outside activities planned by other staff. Identify faculty who are supportive so you have someone who not only understands academia, but can share your thoughts, feelings, and struggles as a nurse transitioning from practice to academia.

If you are not already on LinkedIn, make it a priority to set up a profile and begin to establish an online network of nurse educators. Start with colleagues you already know and those you personally meet at educator conferences. The power of online networking begins when you search for educators who have presented at conferences or authored journal articles or books. Once they accept your invitation you are in the "circle" and can message them with any question or comment you have and receive a response. There are also nurse educator groups that you can be a member of and participate in forums that will also be a source of support.

3. **Speak up and contribute.** New nurse educators who are current in clinical practice are the greatest asset to any nursing program. Their input and perspectives strengthen the content and curriculum of the program and must be valued and considered. Educators who are recent or current in practice can be the bridge and catalyst to bring a practice-based emphasis to the program and realize transformational change.

4. **Take care of yourself.** Take time for adequate rest and do not feel guilty if you need to call in sick. By practicing self-care you will be less likely to burn out and will persistently carry the passion to prepare the next generation for professional practice.

5. **Give yourself grace to be a new nurse educator.** Just as it was essential to give yourself grace to be a new nurse after graduation, this also applies once you enter academia for the first time. Remember that it takes at least two years to be competent and comfortable in practice (Benner, 1982). As you transition to a completely different role, this principle now applies to you! There is no substitute for experience in academia. Expect to struggle as you learn how to write test questions, develop lectures, and bring relevant active learning to your content. This will

change, and your proficiency and comfort level will increase over time as you acquire needed experience!

6. **Assume the best of your colleagues.** You will be stressed and pulled in ways you never thought possible as an educator. As a result, you may find it all too easy to assume the worst of those around you. Be slow to make judgments about your colleagues. Get a thick skin. You will work with colleagues and primary care providers who will irritate you and may rub you the wrong way. Don't take every interaction personally and give grace to others for being stressed, tired, and not always kind and gracious with every interaction they have with you. Remember that you, too, will need this same grace extended to you at times as well!

7. **Get certified as an educator**. Once you have been an educator for two years or more, make it a priority to pursue your certification as a nurse educator (CNE). Just as in clinical practice, certification validates your knowledge and expertise as an educator. Obtaining your CNE recognizes the unique knowledge, skills, and abilities needed to be successful as an educator.

Reflect

1. How do you prioritize your schedule to ensure that the most important things get done each day?

2. What are the most urgent things in your schedule that keep you from the most important?

3. How do you pamper or take care of yourself in a practical way that communicates that you are a person of value and worth?

4. How have you encouraged or brought needed change to your department by your example of excellence?

5. What have you learned in your journey to keep your passion burning in nursing/academia?

6. What journals do you subscribe to, what websites do you regularly review to maintain your passion for lifelong learning?

7. What expectations have you had to change since you entered academia?

8. What obstacles or struggles do you anticipate or have experienced in teaching?

9. What was your primary emotion as a new educator? Have you overcome it?

10. How have you overcome your fear of change? Was it worth it and what did you learn in the process?

11. What goals will you pursue to bring needed change to your program?

12. What went well this past semester in your class or clinical setting? What not so well? What will you do differently to strengthen student learning?

13. Who is your mentor in academia? What have you learned from this relationship?

References

Benner, P. & Wrubel, J. (1989). *Primacy of caring: Stress and coping in health and illness.* Menlo Park, CA: Addison-Wesley Publishing Company.

Benner, P., Sutphen, M., Leonard, V., & Day, L. (2010). *Educating nurses: A call for radical transformation.* San Francisco, California: Jossey-Bass.

Billings, D.M., & Halstead, J.A. (2016). *Teaching in Nursing: A guide for faculty* (5th ed.). St. Louis: MO, Elsevier.

Ferris, T. (2012). Reality shock. Retrieved from http://newgraduatenurses.weebly.com/reality-shock.html

Grossman, S.C., & Valiga, T.M. (2013). *The new leadership challenge: Creating the future of nursing.* (4th ed.) Philadelphia, Pennsylvania: F. A. Davis Company.

Hummel, C. (1967). Tyranny of the urgent. Retrieved from http://www.my279days.com/wp-content/uploads/2010/08/Tyranny-of-the-Urgent.pdf

Jensen, E. (2008). *Brain-based learning: The new paradigm of teaching* (2nd ed.). Thousand Oaks, CA: Corwin Press.

Ironside, P. M., & Valiga, T. M. (2006). Creating a vision for the future of nursing education: Moving toward excellence through innovation. *Nursing Education Perspectives, 27*(3), 120-121.

Kalia, M. (2008). Brain development: Anatomy, connectivity, adaptive plasticity, and toxicity. *Metabolism, 57,* S2-S5.

Lyckholm L. Stress, burnout, and grief. In: *ASCO Curriculum: Optimizing Care—The Importance of Symptom Management.* Alexandria, VA: Kendall/Hunt Publishing Co.

Maslach C. (2003). *Burnout: The cost of caring.* Cambridge, Massachusetts: Malor Books.

Maxwell, J.C. (1999). *The 21 indispensable qualities of a leader: Becoming the person others will follow.* Nashville, TN: Thomas Nelson.

Oermann, M. (2017). Student evaluations of teaching: There is more to course evaluations than student ratings. *Nurse Educator 42*(5), 55-56.

Spinetta, J. J., Jankovic, M., Ben Arush, M. W., et al. (2000). Guidelines for the recognition, prevention, and remediation of burnout in health care professionals participating in the care of children with cancer:

report of the SIOP Working Committee on Psychosocial Issues in Pediatric Oncology. *Medical and Pediatric Oncology, 35*(2), 122–125.

Swanson, K. M. (1999). What is known about caring in
nursing: A literary meta-analysis. In A.S. Hinshaw,
S.L. Feetham, & J.L.F. Shaver, eds. *Handbook of
clinical nursing research.* Thousand Oaks, California:
Sage Publications.

Swenson, R. (2004). *Margin: Restoring emotional, physical, financial, and time reserves to overloaded lives.*
Colorado Springs, CO: NavPress.

Tagliareni, M.E. (2008). Change as a dialogue, opportunity, and courage to embrace the new. *Nursing Education Perspectives, 29*(2), 42.

Tanner, C. A. (2006). Thinking like a nurse: A research-
based model of clinical judgment in nursing. *Journal
of Nursing Education, 45*(6), 204–211.

Valiga, T. M. (2003). The pursuit of excellence in nursing
education. *Nursing Education Perspectives, 24*(5),
275-277.

Valiga, T. M. (2010). Excellence—Does the word mean
anything anymore? *Journal of Nursing Education,
49*(8), 427-428.

Watson, J. (1989). Transformative thinking and caring
curriculum. In E. O. Bevis & J. Watson (Eds), *Toward
a caring curriculum: A new pedagogy for nursing*
(51-60. New York: National League for Nursing.

5

Words of Wisdom from Experienced Educators

I asked educators to share what they wish they had been told as they began their journey and transition from clinical practice to nursing education. Their insights have been tested, tried, and refined through their academic experience. Whether you are just getting started or have years of experience, take time to carefully consider these reflections that will encourage, guide, and inspire you as a nurse educator!

"Be patient with yourself as you adjust to a very new role as a nurse educator. It will be challenging and very fulfilling; however, it is not a walk in the park. Allow yourself at least two years to fully acclimate."
—Kate Johnson, PhD, RN, CNE
Assistant Professor of Nursing
Westfield State University
Westfield, Massachusetts

"Be yourself; students can spot an imposter a mile away."
—Judith Belanger, RN, MSN, CNE
Associate Professor of Nursing
University of New England
Portland, Maine

"Organization and a good mentor are key to success. As an educator you need to be organized in the material *you are presenting to the students, in the classroom, and on exams. Having a good mentor who knows the 'ropes' and is willing to share their knowledge will benefit not only the new educator, but is essential for the success of the program."*
—Mary Terwilliger, PhD, RN
Nursing Instructor
Clarion University of Pennsylvia
Clarion, Pennsylvia

"Get a mentor and read all you can about teaching techniques."
—Gina Briscoe, DNP, RN, CNE
Nursing Instructor
Calhoun Community College
Huntsville, Alabama

"Find a mentor! It is so important that you have a seasoned faculty member to help guide you into the role of nurse educator and give constructive feedback."
—Kristy Snyder, MSN, RN
Nursing Instructor
Neosho County Community College
Ottawa, Kansas

"When you begin to doubt yourself, remember that you are bringing your years of experience and wisdom to this

new role that students do not possess. You cannot know everything but do your best to understand what you are responsible for teaching."

—Susan E Lewis, DNP, MSN, RN
Nursing Instructor
Delaware Technical Community College
Dover, Delaware

"You can't teach students everything, so make it a priority to teach them to be safe and think critically."

—Shelly Jack, BSN, RN
Nursing Instructor
University of Arkansas Community College
Morrilton, Arkansas

"Use reflection regularly. Appreciate the fact that as a novice educator you are learning and have room to grow. Listen to student feedback with an open mind and consider their ideas and incorporate them into your teaching. Be willing to step out of your comfort zone to bring needed change to the classroom and clinical setting."

—Ann Scott, MSN, RN
Nurse Educator
Surry Community College
Dobson, North Carolina

"You can't know everything and your students will respect you for telling them when you do not know the answer. I tell my students no one can know everything about everything and that if someone claims to you should probably not trust anything they say!"

—Julie A. Collins, MSN, RN
Nurse Educator
Surry Community College Dobson
North Carolina

"Relax. You don't have to "cover" everything and students won't retain everything you try to "cover."

—Mary Anne Murtha, MSN, RN
Instructor of Nursing
Penn State College of Nursing
Philadelphia, Pennsylvania

"Give yourself a chance to grow as a new nurse educator. As educators in a new role, you now have new soil

underneath you, but your roots will become well established in the world of academia. In just a matter of time, you will flourish and see the beauty of your efforts as you educate the next generation of nurses."

—Bret Hess, MSN, RN
Lecturer
Nevada State College
Henderson, Nevada

"Forget everything you thought you knew about teaching, read Patricia Benner's Educating Nurses: A Call for Radical Transformation and contextualize the material you teach to the bedside. Don't give out too much information, just what is most important and be passionate about your subject matter."

—Gwen Reed, MS, BS, RN, Paramedic, CEN
Nurse Educator
Gillette College
Gillette, Wyoming

"Focus on the essentials and help students learn to clinically reason. Demonstrate your passion for nursing."

—Elaine D. Goehner, PhD, RN, CPHQ
Professor and Chair, Entry Level Masters Program
Azusa Pacific University
Azusa, California

"You must be flexible. Each semester a situation will come up that you have never dealt with before. How you choose to let it affect you will define your success."

—Shannon Mckinzie, MSN, RN
Nursing Instructor
Mercy College of Nursing and Health Sciences
Des Moines, Iowa

"Develop a trust relationship by taking the time to get to know your students. Each will be unique in their individual learning needs as well as their response to challenges, their emotions, feelings, and the need for you to listen and support them."

—Claudette Abounader, MS, ANP
Assistant Professor of Nursing
Utica College
Utica, New York

"If you don't know the answer to a question, look it up or find the answer together."

—Laura Mallett, MSN, RN
Nursing Faculty
Neosho County Community College
Chanute, Kansas

"Remember that you can't teach students everything you know. We are there to provide the groundwork and help them learn to think like a nurse. The rest will come with experience."

—Natalie Bogue, BSN, RN
Practical Nursing Instructor
Arkansas Northeastern College
Blytheville, Arkansas

"No matter how fearful you are, be strong and appear to be confident. The first impression that students have of you will stick. You want to capture their attention, gain their trust in your ability as an instructor, while building a climate of encouragement, respect, and a free exchange of ideas."

—Kathleen Veprek, RN, MSN
Nursing Instructor
Northern Arizona University
Flagstaff, Arizona

"Be patient with yourself and don't be afraid to seek guidance from experienced faculty."

—Renay McCarley, DNP, RN, CNE
Associate Professor
Mercy College of Nursing and Health Sciences
of Southwest Baptist University
Bolivar, Missouri

"You don't have to know everything. I work through the chart with a student and say, 'This is a treasure hunt.' Then we work to connect the dots together. Coming alongside a student rather than directly 'grilling' them makes it a much better learning experience."

—Kate Whalen, RN, MSN
Clinical Instructor
Walla Walla University School of Nursing
College Place, Washington

"When I first started in nursing education, I always felt that when things did not go well or students failed that it was my fault. If a student says 'you' flunked me! That is really not the case because the student is responsible for their own behaviors. The student didn't do what was necessary to be successful."

—Jonda Hennosy, RN, MSN
Nursing Instructor
Hocking College
Nelsonville, Ohio

"Don't try to 'change the world'— or your course —all at once. Use materials from experienced instructors who have previously taught the course, and you'll figure out what works and what doesn't. Once you find your groove, you can start making changes that work for you, your teaching style, and your students' learning styles. When you start to see your students thriving, you'll be energized to continually strive to improve and change your teaching practices, and you'll begin to develop an arsenal of different ways to facilitate learning."

—Sherri Cozzens, MS, RN
Nursing Faculty
De Anza College
Cupertino, California

"Hang in there! It takes about 2-3 years to get grounded. The first year is the hardest, second year gets much better, and by the third year, you are comfortable and realize that you can really make a difference in student lives."

—Jeanie Ward, RN, NSN, CNE
Professor of Nursing
Austin Community College
Austin, Texas

"You are the expert. Use your clinical experiences as you teaching tools."

—Raul Salas, MSN, RN
Course Coordinator Level I
Delgado Community College
Charity School of Nursing
New Orleans, Louisiana

"You need to have hope in something outside yourself and your department."

—Emily Day, MPH, RN
Nursing Lab Coordinator
Crown College
St. Bonifacious, Minnesota

"Do not overwhelm or bore the students with too much information. Try to accommodate different learning styles in each lecture and get them moving with active learning."

—Linda Olsen, MSN, RN
Nursing Instructor
Mid-State Technical College
Wisconsin Rapids, Wisconsin

"Don't stop being a change agent and stay strong when you experience opposition because academia as a whole is a slow arduous process. Your accomplishments can be measured one student at a time, and before you know it you will have touched many."

—Rebecca L Potter, MSN/ED, RN
Nursing Consultant

"Relax and remember that you are the expert. Try to keep one day and one step ahead of your students. Ask questions of your peers because they are your best resources. Then find a mentor who shares your philosophy of teaching."

—Kathryn Ryno, RN, MSN
Adjunct Allied Health Faculty
Bay College
Escanaba, Michigan

"Always share your love of nursing with your students. If you have passion for what you are doing, the students will see that and will come to respect you more as an educator."

—Cassandra Werle-Rice, MSN, RN
Assistant Professor
Park University
Parkville, Missouri

"It is not going to be easy, but it is going to be worth it!"

—Cynthia (Cindy) E. Young, MSN/RN
Adjunct Faculty
Elgin Community College
Elgin, Illinois

"Find a colleague with similar interests who will challenge, mentor, support, and listen to you. The first couple of years it is important to have the support of individuals with a similar background, interests, or philosophy. This provides you with someone to bounce ideas off, encourage new concepts in the classroom, and provide someone who understands your struggles and career issues. Teaching in a silo is not healthy."

—Miranda Peterson, DNP, RN, CNE
Nursing Instructor
Western Kentucky University
Bowling Green, Kentucky

"1. Don't think you have to be perfect or do it all yourself. 2. Ask for help and don't be afraid to look dumb. 3. Don't think you have to know it all. It is SMART to tell a student, 'I don't know that. Please look it up and tell us all what you found out.' 4. Don't tolerate being bullied. Call it as you see it and ask the perpetrator to stop."

—Judy Evans, MSN, RN, CNE
Professor of Nursing
Colorado Mountain College
Glenwood Springs, Colorado

"Take it one day at a time! Educating students is so worth the time and effort it takes, you will receive great inspiration and knowledge that you impart to your students!"

—Stacy Rust, MSN, BSN
Nursing Instructor
Great Basin College
Elko, Nevada

"Have patience with yourself and seek out a seasoned mentor to work with you for the first year or two. Teach your students how to think like a nurse using their mind, mouth, heart and hands. Always remember, the student comes to you thinking like a student and will leave you thinking like a nurse. You are privileged to be witness to such personal and professional growth."

—Allison Shields, MS, RN
Instructor of Nursing
Fitchburg State University
Fitchburg, Massachusetts

"Find resources that will help enhance students' ability to clinically reason. Although you should be prepared, you do not need to know everything before you teach a class. Everything they learn does not need to come out

of your mouth. Lecturing for hours on end is not effective and 'death by PowerPoint' can and does happen. Concrete-thinking nurse educators will produce concrete-thinking new graduate nurses. Resources like case studies and scenarios will help the students connect the dots early on. Help them to see the bigger picture and facilitate their learning. If we maintain this mindset, the students who graduate will be safe, competent and ready to care for complex patients."

—Tara Devila, MSN-Ed, RN, PHN
Adjunct Faculty
Azusa Pacific University
Azusa, California

"Be confident. Remember that you are an experienced nurse and you know more than the students."

—Lynn Landseadel, MS, RN-C, CNE
Nursing Instructor
Rasmussen College
New Port Richey, Florida

"The rewards of being an educator are many. Always be open to new ideas, keep up with the latest information, and do not be afraid to try new teaching strategies."

—Argie Clifford, MSN, MHA, RN
Nursing Instructor
Moorpark College
Moorpark, California

"Be humble! You are probably an expert clinician, but new to the academic world. You will teach nursing based on your program's curriculum and add fascinating anecdotes from your practice, not the other way around! Learn your program's curriculum, ask questions, rely on your mentors, and enjoy your new role!"

—Suzanne Clarke, MPH, RN, CNE
Associate Professor
St. Catherine University
Minneapolis, Minnesota

"Connect with the students on a personal level. Be approachable."

—Joëlle Wolf, MSN, RN, CMSRN, CNE
Associate Professor
Southern Adventist University
Collegedale, Tennessee

"Never fear saying, 'I don't know, let's investigate that together.' Students respond well to 'human' instructors. Always remember that students are not friends. After graduation they can be friends."

—Danielle H. Kishkill, RN
Nursing Instructor
Eastwick College
Ramsey, New Jersey

"When teaching in the clinical setting, you need to change your focus from caring for the patient to helping students learn and assessing their learning As an educator, your 'patient' is now the student and while you still want to ensure the patient receives the appropriate nursing care, YOUR responsibility is the student."

—Heidi Monroe, MSN, RN-BC, CAPA
Assistant Professor of Nursing
Bellin College
Green Bay, Wisconsin

"Give yourself time to become a quality educator; just like it may take a few years to feel comfortable and confident as a nurse, it is the same for the educator role. Listen to the more experienced educators, as they will help you transition faster, which means having a mentor is extremely helpful. Lastly, when you're struggling with a decision or dilemma related to students, let the rules and policies guide you."

—Judith Thompson, RN, CMSRN, MN
Nursing Instructor
Richmond Community College
Hamlet, North Carolina

"Realize it takes time to be fully comfortable in the academic role, so don't give up! The first semester you are just getting your feet wet and may feel completely overwhelmed. As Patricia Benner would say, you are moving from being an expert in your previous role to being a novice in your new role. By the second semester you will be tweaking the things that didn't work, refining your approaches and strategies, and getting a little more comfortable. Finally by your third semester you should be feeling pretty good about your teaching. Also, don't be the 'sage on the stage.' Be the 'guide on the side.' Use lots of interactive strategies, case studies, clickers, group work, etc. It's a lot of work to transition from straight lecture to using more interactive approaches, but once you do it, you will have a livelier, more interesting class!"

—Pam Walker, MSN, RN, CNE
Associate Professor of Nursing
Goodwin College
East Hartford, Connecticut

"Lead by example. Show and share with the students the type of nurse you are and why nursing is so important to you."

—Dana Deere, RN, MSN
Nursing Instructor
California State University
Fullerton. California

"Get your students to be active in their learning (they are responsible for their learning, not you) and don't try to teach them EVERYTHING; stick to the truly 'NEED to know.'"

—Laura Kubin, PhD, RN, CPN, CHES
Associate Professor
Texas Woman's University
Denton, Texas

"There seems to be a pervasive thought among those in academia that if you are a 'good' clinical nurse, you will be a good educator; that the transition will be seamless and you will just intuitively 'know' how to teach. Realize that as with initially becoming a nurse, there is much to learn in becoming an effective educator. Be gentle and patient with yourself during this learning process."

—Maryanne Bletscher, MS, RN, AOCN
Nursing Instructor
Good Samaritan School of Nursing
Portland, Oregon

"You must possess compassion and have a commitment to be creative in teaching. Embrace the responsibility and be approachable to your students."

—Raijah A Rahim
Dean, Faculty of Nursing & Allied Health Sciences
Open University
Malaysia

"When prepping for your lecture, read the text the night before, or morning before the lecture. It seems like a 'no-brainer' but those challenging questions the students ask are usually related to a lack of understanding from what they 'think' they read and what they have seen in practice. Even after 10 years, I still read the sections I am discussing in class and it saves me every time!"

—Lisa Harding, RN, DNP, CEN
Professor of Nursing
Bakersfield College
Bakersfield, California

"Students seem to know when you are new to the role and they will test you. Don't take it personal. Know that your first year will be tough and be sure to stay connected to the experienced faculty and check with your colleagues. It is always better to say, 'I have to check about that,' rather than be rushed to a response that might not be consistent with school policies."

—Judith M. Pelletier, MSN, RN, CNE
Director, Division of Nurse Education
Upper Cape Cod Regional Technical School
Bourne, Massachusetts

"Remember to search for the strength of each student. Find out what makes them curious. It is curiosity that will make them great Nurses clinically."

—Laura Walton, RN, BScN
Masters Student Clinical Nurse Educator
Health Sciences Center
Winnipeg, Manitoba, Canada

"Get involved in the process and the committee work in your department. The best way to learn is to do the work. As a new faculty member I joined the curriculum committee and learned the practical application of everything I learned in my master's degree. It was the best thing I did as an educator."

—Jodi A Nelson, MSN, RN
Nursing Instructor
Southeast Community College
Lincoln, Nebraska

"Focus on the must know, the basics, the A&P, Patho and Pharm. Help the students apply the information, talk them through what might be happening in the patient's *body when they have disease A, B, and C and are on 25 meds."*

—June Parham, RN, BScN
Clinical Placement Instructor
Faculty of Health & Community Studies, NorQuest College
Edmonton, Alberta, Canada

"Be true to your professionalism and the caring of the profession of nursing."

—Melissa Guidry, MSN, RN
Faculty Associate Degree Nursing Program
Laredo Community College
Laredo, Texas

"Be a lifelong learner and be more prepared than your students are."

—Leigh Moore, MSN, RN, CNOR, CNE
Associate Professor of Nursing
Southside Virginia Community College
Alberta, Virginia

"Students cannot learn unless the instructor controls the classroom; only one person talks at a time, usually the instructor. Treat students as ADULTS. The adult learner wants to be challenged with interesting information and exercises! Don't treat fundamental students like children. Start decision-making and appropriately demanding assignments from Day #1. Never forget to involve other team faculty and the dean for ANY 'problem' students. For some reason, many adult students start acting like elementary school students when in nursing school. Expect adult behavior at all times, and remind them that they are adult students."

—Thomas Oertel, DNP, RN, NP
Professor, Nursing Education (retired)
Grossmont College
El Cajon, California

"Be very familiar with the required clinical objectives and try to correlate these experiences with theory."

—Sheila Kennedy-Stewart, MSN, RN, CMSRN
Adjunct Instructor Southwestern Oklahoma University
& Oklahoma City Community College

"Be a lifelong learner and be more prepared than your students are."

—Leigh Moore, MSN, RN, CNOR, CNE

Associate Professor of Nursing
Southside Virginia Community College
Alberta, Virginia

"Be the teacher you are meant to be. Stay student-centered and don't worry too much about what others think."

—Anntippia Short, MSN, RN, CNE
Professor of Nursing
Santa Monica College
Santa Monica, California

"Demonstrate compassion for your students like you have for your patients. Recognize and alleviate their anxiety and they will perform better."

—Deborah Kemper, MSN, RN
Clinical Instructor, Staff Education Coordinator
Siena Heights University, Hospice of Lenawee
Adrian, Michigan

"Remember that teaching is NOT a democracy. You are in charge of your classroom and the clinical experience."

—Cathy Leppold, MSN, RN
Nursing Instructor
Arkansas State University
Jonesboro, Arkansas

"Hold the students accountable for professionalism, and be supportive to their learning needs."

—Mabel Morton, RN, MSN
Adjunct Clinical and Online Instructor
Southeast Community College
Lincoln, Nebraska

"Remember that every student learns differently so diversify your teaching strategies."

—Nancy Mackey, RN, MS
Medical Academy/Practical Nursing Instructor
Inlet Grove Community High School
Riviera Beach, Florida

"Do not take everything students say personally."

—Chris M. Wood, OP, RN, PhD, GNP
Assistant Professor
Grand Rapids Community College
Grand Rapids, Michigan

"Use the objectives to guide learning and what you teach. Develop a plan for students to attain the objectives, then let them know how each requirement helps them to get where they need to go. If you do this, they will have buy-in, if you don't, they may perceive assignments as 'busy work.'"

—Deb Aucoin-Ratcliff, DNP, RN
American River College & Samuel Merritt University (adjunct)
Sacramento, California

"Know your lecture inside and out! Research the subject matter and develop a true passion for it! The students can and will pick up on your passion and become more involved in the learning process."

—Daniel Eaton, MSN, RN
Instructor of Nursing
Penn State University
University Park, Pennsylvania

"Don't be afraid to show students that you care about them and their success. It's possible to remain objective about their skill set and still genuinely care about them as individuals. I have found that it's easier to provide constructive criticism when they know you truly care about them and want them to succeed."

—Janine Johnson, MSN, RN
Associate Professor
Mott Community College
Flint, Michigan

"Rely on your most trusted and experienced colleagues to hear you out and process painful/stressful situations. Ac-ademia can be frustrating and exciting. It'll be a delight to see your students turn into colleagues later on. Dive right in ... I found it to be the biggest splash of my life!"

—Marina Espiritu Lutz, MSN, RN
Nursing Instructor
Neumann University
Aston Township, Pennsylvania

"Keep it simple for students! If you are not upsetting the students, then you are not doing your job! (Meaning to keep them on their toes.) Don't make friends with the stu-dents and don't friend them on social media sites until they have graduated."

—Patricia C. Williams, MSN, RN
Practical Nursing Program Coordinator
Hagerstown Community College
Hagerstown, Maryland

"I am always positive when I counsel students who are failing. I have found that 100% of the time students are successful when I tell them, 'You can do it!' and 'Make you and your family proud!' Students say they have become successful because they wanted to make me proud."

—Dawn M. Zimmerman, DNP, MSN, RNC, CNE
Nursing Instructor
Trinitas School of Nursing and Rutgers University
New Brunswick, New Jersey

"Your hands-on hospital experience is priceless, students love hearing your stories. It helps them realize they can do this job, too!"

—Sarah Poole RN, BScN, MSc Forensic Nursing
Nursing Instructor
Saskpolytech and the University of Regina
Saskatchewan, Canada

Reflect

1. What words of wisdom encouraged you?

2. What words of wisdom do you need to never forget?

PART TWO

TRANSFORMING THE CONTENT

In any practice-based profession including nursing, there are three apprenticeships. The three professional apprenticeships that embody nursing practice include:

1. Ethical comportment and formation. Developing the dispositions and actions the profession values and represents, including caring, compassion and professional behavior.
2. Knowledge, science, and theory of the profession, including pathophysiology, pharmacology, and F&E
3. Clinical reasoning and knowledge required for practice (Benner, et al., 2010)

As I reflected on these three apprenticeships using my lens as a nurse in practice and nurse educator, I began to see how these three apprenticeships parallel the primary structural components of a home that include the foundation, walls, and roof. To visualize the professional development that is needed as every student progresses through nursing education and learns the responsibilities of the professional nurse, I will use the metaphor of building a house. This is not just any house or a static structure, but a unique, vibrant, "living" house. To build this "living" house, it requires the active and intentional engagement of the nurse educator as well as the student. Both must fulfill their responsibility to see this structure take shape to be the best it can possibly be.

In order to prepare the way for transformation, you must face head-on the mountain of content in your program and develop a clear sense of salience or what is most important in each apprenticeship and the content that is taught. In this section, I highlight what is essential regarding the "art" of nursing; pathophysiology, pharmacology, and fluids and electrolytes, and what must be known to think more like a nurse with an emphasis on clinical reasoning.

Laying the Foundation: The "Art" of Nursing

6

Keith Rischer, RN, MA, CEN, CCRN

"The spirit in which she does her work makes all the difference. Invested as she should with the dignity of her profession and the cloak of love for suffering humanity, she can ennoble anything her hand may be called upon to do, and for work done in this spirit there will ever come to her a recompense far outweighing that of silver and gold."

—Isabel Hampton Robb, 1900 Founder of the American Nurses Association, *American Journal of Nursing*, and National League for Nursing

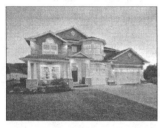

Each student metaphorically represents a "living house" that is an ongoing work in progress as the three apprenticeships of the professional nurse are developed in nursing school. To be strong and last over time, this "house" must have a firm and stable foundation. The ethical apprenticeship or the art of nursing is this foundation for every student. Caring behaviors, nurse engagement, and professionalism in practice must be present or your student's nursing practice will be on an unsteady foundation before it even begins. Once the foundation is strongly established, it is time to build.

The apprenticeship of knowledge, theory, and the science of the profession comprise the walls of the living house of professional practice. This includes a DEEP understanding of the applied sciences of nursing that are contextualized to the bedside: pharmacology, fluid and electrolytes, and anatomy and physiology. Finally, the roof of the house is the ability of the student to think like a nurse. This brings four elements — nursing process, critical thinking, pattern recognition, and clinical reasoning—to the bedside.

If the student's "living house" is established on a shaky foundation because they lack the professional and ethical comportments that include caring, compassion, or professionalism in practice, it will soon come crashing down like a house built on sand. But if this "living" house is built on a rock-solid foundation of caring, compassion, nurse engagement, and professional behaviors, his/her practice will be strong and students will build the remainder of the house (applied sciences/clinical reasoning) that will make them an exceptional health care professional.

To lay the foundation of the "living" house in each student, three separate building blocks are required:

- Building Block #1: Caring and Compassion
- Building Block #2: Holistic and Spiritual Care
- Building Block #3: Professionalism in Practice

Building Block #1: Caring and Compassion

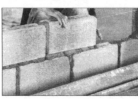

Caring practices are central to nursing. What it is to nurse cannot be separated from what it is to care for and about others. To see nursing curriculum revolutionized, caring must become a core value. (Tanner, 1990). How educators integrate caring and compassion in the curriculum is crucial. Though the importance of caring to nursing practice can be taught in the curriculum, what cannot be taught is a heart motivation to serve others as a caregiver. If students lack empathetic caring, their practice will reflect this and be devoid of life. But if students are truly caring and engaged in the story of each patient they care for, they will be nurses who make a difference in all that they do!

Caring behaviors are not only for students to demonstrate. Nurse educators must authentically care for students as well. Student learning is strengthened when it takes place in the context of a meaningful relationship that is predicated on caring. Students have an innate need and desire for the educator to care for them and to be personally invested in their success (Story & Butts, 2010). Watson (2003) noted that caring begets more caring. When educators clearly communicate caring, students reciprocate and a circle of caring is created. Make it a priority to listen to students' concerns, be authentic, fair, and convey availability. By communicating caring, your lived example can be a powerful model of the core values of the nursing profession to the next generation of caregivers.

Why is caring central to the role and identity of the professional nurse? There is a historical basis for this emphasis, though it is not addressed in most fundamental textbooks. Though most fundamental nursing texts start the history of nursing with Florence Nightingale and the modern era, this is inaccurate. Nursing history began over 2,000 years ago. In order to put the centrality of caring and compassion in context, the entire range of the history of nursing needs to be known, including where it began and the worldview that gave value, dignity, and worth to caring for the sick. These values that motivated others to care are timeless and remain relevant and need to be emphasized today so students are able to recognize the relevance of caring to the profession.

Caring and the History of Nursing

Though caring for the sick occurred in numerous cultural settings, including India, Rome, and Greece in the BC era, from the first century AD to the late Middle Ages, caring for the sick was primarily a ministry of the Christian church performed by lay deacons and deaconesses and later through convents and monastic orders (Berman, Snyder, & Frandsen, 2016). Showing compassion and caring for the sick was founded on the teachings and example of Jesus, who demonstrated high

regard for human life through His model of service, sacrifice, and teaching that *"So in everything, do to others what you would have them do to you, for this sums up the Law and the Prophets."* (Matthew 7:12). His example of healing and giving personal attention to the sick and "untouchable" has strongly influenced nursing and the value given to caring for the sick (Pavey, 1952). Caring and compassion did not derive from a vacuum, but has a definite source and origin.

The first organized group of nurses was established in response to His teachings and example (Dolan, Fitzpatrick, & Krohn Herrmann, 1983). Phoebe, a deaconess in the first century church whom the apostle Paul refers to by name in his letter to the Roman church (Romans 16:1), was a nurse who took care of both men and women (DeWit, 2009). While pagan religions seldom offered help to the sick and dying, the early Christians were willing to nurse those in need of care regardless of their religion (Blainey, 2011). The Christian emphasis on compassion and caring for others gave rise to the development of nursing and hospitals after the end of the persecution of the early church in the third century AD (Knight, 2012).

Early Middle Ages

In the Byzantine (eastern Roman) Empire beginning in AD 325, construction of a hospital began in every cathedral town. Some hospitals maintained libraries and training programs, and doctors compiled their medical and pharmacological studies in manuscripts. Byzantine hospital staff included a chief physician, nurses (deaconesses), and orderlies. Thus, in-patient medical care and what would be considered a hospital today, was an outgrowth of Christian mercy and Byzantine innovation (McClellan & Dorn, 2006). To care for the sick was often self-sacrificing in this era, because exposure to diseases could be incurable and result in death for caregivers (Wilkinson & Treas, 2011).

Middle Ages

During the Middle Ages, nursing and caring for the sick was centered in monasteries. By the twelfth century, Constantinople had two well-organized hospitals, staffed by doctors who were both male and female. Facilities included systematic treatment procedures and specialized wards for various diseases.

1600s to 1800s

The Renaissance through the eighteenth century was literally the Dark Age in the history of nursing. Catholic religious orders were disbanded and suppressed in Protestant Europe. As a result, hospitals and the care provided deteriorated. By the nineteenth century, with the exception of a few nursing orders of nuns, nursing was disorganized and corrupt. Author Charles Dickens portrayed the worst of nursing in this era in the character of Sairey Gamp, a self-serving alcoholic nurse in his novel *Martin Chuzzlewit.* Dickens also addressed the substandard care that was provided by alcoholics, prostitutes, and women who were uncaring and immoral (Shelly & Miller, 2006).

In the mid-1800s, a German Lutheran pastor, Theodor Fleidner, responded to the pressing needs of the poor and sick in his community, and his church began to care for them. Over time, this ministry grew into the Kaiserwerth Institute and became a large organization that included a hospital and training programs. When Florence Nightingale felt God calling her to service, she began her studies at the Kaiserwerth Institute and then at Catholic hospitals in Paris (Shelly & Miller, 2006).

Caring and Compassion

Caring has traditionally been viewed as the essence of nursing practice and the most important characteristic of a nurse (Leininger, 1988) and a distinct, dominant, central, and unifying focus for nursing practice (Leininger, 1991). Caring as a recognized core value in nursing was also emphasized at the beginning of the modern era by influential nurse educator Isabel Hampton Robb, who later went on to found the American Nurses Association, the *American Journal of Nursing*, and what would later become the National League for Nursing. In 1900, she wrote the following in her textbook for students *Nursing Ethics*:

"The spirit in which she does her work makes all the difference. Invested as she should with the dignity of her profession and the cloak of love for suffering humanity, she can ennoble anything her hand may be called upon to do, and for work done in this spirit there will ever come to her a recompense far outweighing that of silver and gold." (Hampton Robb, 1900, p. 36)

While Hampton Robb stated in the language of her day that nurses should provide care by embracing *"the dignity of her profession and the cloak of love for suffer-*

ing humanity," it is important to recognize that this must NOT be treated as an abstract philosophical platitude. This ethic must not only be embraced, but lived out in practice (Benner, 2013).

Defining Caring and Compassion

Caring and compassion are essential components of the foundation that must be established in each student's practice. So how do you define caring in the context of nursing and make it concrete for nursing students? In *The Primacy of Caring,* Patricia Benner and Judith Wrubel captured the essence of caring beautifully.

CARING DEFINED
The ability to recognize the value and worth of those you care for and that the patient and their experience MATTER to you (Benner & Wrubel, 1989).

Compassion literally means to "suffer with" another. This is a feeling of deep empathy and sorrow for someone who is stricken by misfortune, accompanied by a strong desire to alleviate the suffering. The nurse must actively demonstrate this ethic in the clinical setting for every patient cared for. Though the emphasis in nursing education is knowledge acquisition and skill development, this in and of itself is not enough; every student must CARE and have COMPASSION for the patients they care for.

Patricia Benner also affirms that caring is central to nursing practice. *"Nursing can never be reduced to mere technique...the nature of the caring relationship is central to most nursing interventions"* (Benner & Wrubel, 1989, p. 4). *"The nurse is both a knowledge worker and one who cares...knowledge is dangerous if it is divorced from caring"* (p. 400). Caring is an essential component of expert practice that has the power to not only impact the patient but enriches the nurse in the process (Benner & Wrubel, 1988).

Benefits of Caring

The patients of a caring, engaged nurse have better outcomes (Swanson, 1999). Why? Caring gives the nurse a heightened sense of awareness and guides the evaluation of nursing interventions by recognizing subtle changes in the patient's condition. In this context of caring, the nurse is paying close attention to the patient's body language, facial expressions, and tone of voice and is interpreting the significance of what is being communicated (Benner & Wrubel, 1989). When the head and heart are integrated and fully engaged in practice, the nurse clearly communicates verbally and nonverbally that each person matters. She or he recognizes EARLY changes that may signify a change in status.

In one study, the degree of critical thinking and the emotions of caring and emotional engagement by students had a positive clinical relationship. The higher the degree of caring measured in students showed an improved disposition to critical thinking. This study recommended emphasizing caring behaviors in the curriculum to improve the adoption of critical thinking in nursing students (Pai, Eng, & Ko, 2013).

Some patients lose hope and a sense of connection to others because of their illness and do not feel that they matter. When the nurse demonstrates that the patient matters by caring, this has the power to reintegrate the patient with his or her world. Caring behaviors also create healing environments that positively influence and improve patient outcomes. The benefits patients receive when they experience caring by the nurse include enhanced healing, decreased length of stay, increased well-being, and physical comfort. Caring influences nurse engagement, which makes the nurse notice the effectiveness of interventions and detect subtle signs of patient improvement or deterioration (Benner & Wrubel, 1988).

Practicing in a caring manner also benefits the nurse and enhances the nurse's well-being, both personally and professionally. The nurse feels more connected both to his or her patients and colleagues and is more satisfied with bedside care (Swanson, 1999). Patients can readily detect a nurse's nonverbal communication that contradicts caring behaviors. Students need to remember that the influence and significance of eye contact, body language, and tone of voice are nonverbal actions that can communicate caring and contribute to a patient's well-being (Benner & Wrubel, 1989). Some patients lose hope and a sense of connection to others because of their illness and feel that they do not matter.

When the nurse demonstrates that the patient matters to him/her, this has the power to reintegrate the patient with his/her world. Being approachable and available is central to effective nursing care and essential ingredients

to patient recovery (Orlick & Benner, 1988). When the head and heart are integrated and fully engaged in practice, the nurse clearly communicates in both verbal and nonverbal communication that each person matters and is more likely to recognize EARLY changes that may signify a change in status and mitigate "failure to rescue."

QSEN and Caring
Patient-centered care is the first competency of the Quality and Safety Education for Nurses (QSEN) that situates the value of caring and compassion. QSEN defines caring and compassion by its recognition that patient-centered care happens when the nurse *"recognizes the patient or designee as the source of control and full partner in providing compassionate and coordinated care based on respect for patient's preferences, values, and needs"* ("Pre-Licensure KSAS," n.d).

The underlying attitudes that are required by the nurse to provide patient-centered care according to QSEN include seeing health care situations through the patient's eyes, respect, encouraging individual expression of what the patient needs, and valuing active partnership with the patient and family in all aspects of care ("Pre-Licensure KSAS," 2014). This captures the essence of empathetic caring that can guide educators to use this framework to integrate caring in your program.

Caring and Critical Thinking
Empathetic caring has been shown to improve the critical thinking of nursing students. In one study, a structural equation model was used to test the relationship between caring behavior and critical thinking skills. This study identified that nursing students with a higher frequency of caring behaviors that were measured had a statistically higher score (p<.001) on levels of critical thinking related to nursing practice (Pai, Eng, & Ko, 2013).

This study recommended that nursing education should emphasize caring in the curriculum to improve disposition toward critical thinking of nursing students and strengthen clinical reasoning. Critical thinking can be predicted and correlated by the degree of caring behaviors demonstrated by students. One reason cited is that emotions and level of engagement influence how clinical data is interpreted (Pai, Eng, & Ko, 2013). Interpretation is also the first step (Tanner, 2006) required by the nurse to make a correct clinical judgment.

Empathy

A nurse who demonstrates empathy will provide patient care that improves patient outcomes and develop meaningful nurse-patient relationships (Williams & Stickley, 2010). Empathy can be defined as placing yourself into the experience of the patient (Kelly, Lepo, & Frinzi, 2011). Empathy desires to relieve the suffering of another and meet the other as a fellow human being. Empathy involves not only understanding how a patient may be feeling, but involves a level of self-awareness by the nurse to communicate this understanding to the patient. Therefore, empathy is a critical component of the therapeutic nurse-patient relationship (Webster, 2010).

Helping people during periods of vulnerability and distress is the essence of what it means to be "good" as a nurse in practice (Benner, Hooper-Kyriakidis, & Stannard, 2011). Are we teaching our students to have eyes to see that every patient they care for is their "neighbor" for whom they are called to have mercy and compassion? This timeless truth is found in the parable of the Good Samaritan taught by Jesus and has been an influential example for nurses to emulate (Walsh, 1929).

A religious leader of the Jews asked Jesus, *"Who is my neighbor?"* Jesus shared a brief story of a man who was severely beaten, left for dead, and was lying on the side of a road. Two religious leaders saw the man, but ignored his plight. They even walked on the opposite side of the road. But the Samaritan, when he saw the man, was moved with compassion. He responded by acting to alleviate his suffering and took him to a place to be cared for. Jesus then asked this religious leader a question that is relevant to all who provide care for those in need today. *"Which of these three do you think was a neighbor to the man who fell into the hands of robbers?"* The religious leader replied, *"The one who had mercy on him."* Jesus then replied, *"Go, and do likewise"* (Luke 10:29–37).

Influential nurse educator and scholar Patricia Benner validates this truth as relevant to nursing today:

> *"As nurses, we have been given the ministry and tradition of compassionately caring for strangers, of loving our neighbors as ourselves. We do not have to have great will power to do this, or even great determination and motivation. We do need knowledge and skilled know-how, but we need to be open to see every patient as an opportunity to demonstrate this compassion to those we do not yet know."* (Benner, 2012)

Hampton Robb (1900) also recognized the value of this ethic when she wrote that the nurse will receive a "recompense far outweighing that of silver and gold" through compassionate care for others. To teach students to practically demonstrate empathy to their patient, the nurse must make it a priority to UNDERSTAND the plight and experience of those being cared for (Scott, 2009). In the clinical setting, students need to place themselves in the patient's shoes and attempt to identify and understand what the patient is experiencing from this perspective. In one three-year research study, Sweeney (2012) identified that 96 percent of patients had fears and anxieties about being in the health care setting.

Nurse Engagement

Skillful nurse engagement complements caring and compassion and is also basic to nursing practice and care. The nurse must remain clinically curious and responsive to the patient's story and situation. When distracted and not engaged, the nurse will be unable to invest the energy needed to recognize relevant and urgent clinical signs that may require intervention. When nurses are not engaged with the patient and their clinical problem, patient outcomes will suffer (Benner, Hooper-Kyriakidis, & Stannard, 2011).

The importance of nurse engagement was also identified in Sweeney's (2012) research on empathy. Patients made it clear that they wanted a nurse who was completely engaged in the clinical setting and focused on the patient and their needs. To be engaged in practice also implies that the patient is your priority, focus, and motivation for all that is done as a nurse.

Know Each Patient's Story

Each patient is unique and has a story that the student must know. It is not enough to know the primary medical problem and the pathophysiology of this problem. The nurse comes to know his or her patients through the stories they share about their health care experiences and who they are as a person (Benner, Tanner, & Chesla, 1996). These stories are important because they are unique and represent the journey that gives context to the current clinical scenario. This is an important component of the art of nursing that involves making meaningful connections through listening to and learning from the patient's story (Pesut & Herman, 1999).

When the patient's story is known and understood by the nurse, the next step is to frame the patient's story. Framing creates meaning out of the patient's story and helps distinguish the central or core problem from those that are peripheral. Framing the current clinical situation is like having a lens through which the nurse views the patient's story and is best done through the use of reflection (Pesut & Herman, 1999). It also helps distinguish the patient as an individual, rather than an illness or diagnosis.

Make it a priority to encourage your students to engage with and know the story of each patient in their care. This will help them frame each patient appropriately and correctly enhance their ability to be thorough in thinking and make correct clinical judgments. This is an excellent example of how the art of nursing must be incorporated into every aspect of the nurse's practice and why it is relevant to everything that the nurse does.

How to Obtain the Story

Because students are inexperienced, they tend to focus on the TASKS of patient care and do not tune in to the PATIENT they are caring for (Benner, 1982). In order to frame the patient's current clinical scenario correctly, students must make an effort to engage person-to-person and allow this patient and his/her story to matter to them as a nurse. Patients don't care how much students know until they know how much they care. The patient's story can only be known and framed when caring and trust have been established and the patient feels safe sharing with the nurse.

In order to do this, teach students to avoid all assumptions or judgments and relate to them person-to-person. To obtain the story while the student is providing care, sit at the patient's bedside, put down the stethoscope, make eye contact and let the patient lead and share his/her story so you can frame the current situation.

Use the following questions as discussion starters:

- Tell me about your family (spouse, children, grandchildren, etc.)
- Tell me about your work and what you do (or did) for a living.
- Were there any contributing factors that may have influenced your need for care?
  - Financial
  - Personal stress
  - Chemical dependency (ETOH, etc.)

After collecting this information and framing the patient's story, each student can incorporate a framework of clinical reasoning that will guide the step-by-step thinking required to rightly interpret the clinical data that is collected.

Building Block #2: Holistic and Spiritual Care

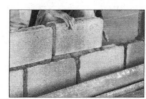

Holism teaches that each individual is more than the sum of his or her parts. Each person is multidimensional and has unique characteristics that cannot be separated from the whole. This philosophy and worldview has been foundational to nursing going back over 2,000 years, and reinforced as central to nursing practice by Nightingale and current nursing theorists and leaders today. Thus, professional nurses are taught to embrace holistic care in practice by caring for all aspects of each patient's being.

When compassionate care is provided, the nurse impacts the patient's physical and emotional needs. Holistic care also involves supporting spirituality as defined by the patient. For some students, spiritual care may conjure up images and expectations of religious practices or prayer and going way out of their comfort zone. Though spiritual care may include prayer, it is much more.

The essence of spiritual care is caring and serving the whole person: the physical, emotional, social, and spiritual aspects of their being (Murphy & Walker, 2013). Nursing students need to see spiritual care as a thread to naturally weave into the tapestry of care that they provide for each patient (Wilt & Smucker, 2001). Spiritual care is a key component of holistic care, but is not taught in the curriculum of most programs (Murphy & Walker, 2013). Reflect and determine if your program is doing all it can to integrate spiritual care in the curriculum especially at the fundamental level.

Spiritual Care

Nurses need to provide care that encompass the mind, body, and spirit. Providing spiritual care is a patient-centered care strategy advocated by QSEN and The Joint Commission practice guidelines. Yet, spiritual care is uncomfortable for most students who hesitate to "go there" when providing patient care. In one study, 92 percent of nurses felt inadequately prepared to meet their patients' spiritual needs (McSherry & Jameson, 2011). In order to empower future nurses to provide spiritual care, nursing programs need to incorporate this essential content in the curriculum (Labine, 2015).

A practical, holistic approach to providing spiritual care in nursing recaptures the perspective that all that is done for the patient by the nurse can represent spiritual care. For example, taking a set of vital signs becomes an opportunity for presence and spiritual assessment. The student can further intentionalize spiritual care by thinking with every interaction, "What are this patient's needs, fears, anxieties, or questions?" Every interaction is filled with meaning as the student engages the "entire" patient (Murphy & Walker, 2013).

Because HOPE and MEANING are key components of spirituality, spiritual care can be defined as helping a patient to find/make MEANING out of his/her experience and find HOPE. Practical interventions that students can use include listening, encouraging the expression of feelings, compassionate presence, open-ended questions, instilling hope, and prayer (Murphy & Walker, 2013). Though spiritual care is clearly within the nurse's scope of practice, most students as well as nurses in practice are uncomfortable with this responsibility.

Contributing factors to this discomfort for some may include the dominant physical/medical model in health care, secular-humanistic worldview of educational and health care institutions as well as a lack of emphasis on spiritual care in nursing education. In one survey, 87 percent of nursing programs do not have specific content on how to practically incorporate spiritual care in practice (Murphy & Walker, 2013). Remind students that they can positively affect and meet the patient's physical and emotional needs by providing compassionate care.

Those most comfortable with spiritual care find their own faith and spiritual traditions personally meaningful and relevant. When it comes to spirituality, you cannot give to others if you do not have something within to give. Just because a student may not be a participant of any faith tradition or may even be an atheist or agnostic, he or she must recognize that if spirituality or a faith tradition is important to the patient, it must also be central and important to the nurse!

FICA Spirituality Assessment Tool

The FICA Spirituality Assessment tool is an evidence-based spirituality assessment guide that provides students with a structured approach to begin a conversation about spirituality and providing spiritual care. FICA addresses questions in the following areas:

F-Faith or beliefs:
- What are your spiritual beliefs?
- Do you consider yourself spiritual?
- What things do you believe in that give meaning to life?

I-Importance and influence:
- Is faith important to you?
- How has your illness or hospitalization affected your personal belief practices?

C-Community:
- Are you connected to a faith center in the community?
- Does it provide support/comfort for you during times of stress?
- Is there a person/group who assists you in your spirituality?

A-Address:
- What can I do for you?
- What support can health care provide to support your spiritual beliefs/practices?

By using this tool, a student can determine the patient's spiritual strengths and determine how those strengths can be used by the patient to promote healing. Students can design nursing interventions related to the provision of spiritual care (Williams, Voss, Vahle, & Capp, 2016). In order to increase the effectiveness of this tool, students may need to be taught therapeutic communication related to spirituality. Students would benefit by developing communication skills on how to respond to stories of spiritual pain, listening, nurturing resilience, reframing, and encouraging religious practices (Taylor, 2007).

Nursing Process and Spiritual Care

Though students are taught to use the nursing process to provide a framework to care for physical needs, each step of the nursing process can also help guide students to provide spiritual care.

Assessment

Because matters of the spirit are more nuanced and not as tangible as physical needs, the nurse must look at the present clinical situation and nonverbal communication or statements of losing hope that may indicate a spiritual concern or crisis. If there is a potential spiritual concern, the following questions that center on hope can be used when a spiritual assessment needs to be done by the nurse:

- What is your source of strength or support?
- Do you believe in a power greater than yourself?
- What gives you hope?
- Where have you found strength in the past? (Wilt & Smucker, 2001)

Diagnosis/Priority

Determine the nursing priority by understanding and interpreting what has been collected. The NANDA nursing diagnostic statement that addresses a need for spiritual intervention is spiritual distress. The essence of spiritual distress is that the spirit of your patient is clearly troubled and deteriorating. Spiritual distress is present when your patient begins to openly question the purpose and meaning of life or the existence of God (Smucker, 1996). In this scenario, the nursing goal would be to help the patient find meaning, hope, and rediscover his/her purpose in life. Nursing interventions to address spiritual distress include providing compassionate care, active listening to concerns, and making referrals to chaplaincy.

Implementing

The primary role of the nurse includes facilitating and connecting the patient and/or family with spiritual support such as chaplaincy or the patient's pastor/rabbi/priest/imam. In one study, the interventions that patients found most meaningful when they needed spiritual care was when the nurse helped to enable transcendence of the present situation so they could see the bigger picture, provide hope, and establish an authentic connection with the caregiver (Conco, 1995). When patients feel cared for, their spirit is also touched. This is another reason why caring and compassion are so important to nursing practice.

Evaluating

If a patient experiences spiritual distress, the nurse can help the patient find meaning, hope, and rediscover his/her purpose in life. Though successful resolution of spiritual distress will likely involve pastoral or chaplaincy support, the nurse is on the front lines. When a patient is in crisis and you are "it," the nurse must be prepared!

Patient Presentations

Not every patient will have a clinical presentation that will require the nurse to provide spiritual care. This is the exception, not the norm. But there are specific clinical situations that often have a high correlation to a potential crisis of the spirit that the nurse must recognize and intervene as needed.

These clinical scenarios include:

- Patients who have been recently diagnosed with a life-altering or terminal illness such as cancer
- Patients who are transitioning to hospice care
- Patients who are facing decisions regarding withdrawal of aggressive interventions such as dialysis
- Patients who are facing major surgery
- Patients who have lost hope
- Patients who are depressed
- Patients who are anxious

Power of Presence

It is the LITTLE things that the nurse does that are, in reality, the BIG things that make a lasting difference. Students need to be reminded of this regularly. One example of this axiom is the power of nurse presence. Most students are unaware that their physical presence, while providing care, can meet the emotional and even spiritual needs of each patient in their care.

But what does it mean to be "present"? To be present means that the nurse is AVAILABLE and ACCESSIBLE and this is clearly communicated to the patient. Presence can also be defined as "being with" and "being there" for the specific purpose of meeting their needs in a time of need. Other ways to define or explain presence include caring, nurturance, empathy, physical closeness, and physical touch (Rex-Smith, 2007).

Being present also implies a spiritual presence, to be attuned with the situation in such a way that it becomes spiritually transcendent when you quiet your mind to hear, see, and feel not only your current thoughts and feelings, but those of your patient (Dossey, 1995). When truly present, the nurse experiences what the patient is feeling (Faas, 2004). This is also the essence of empathy applied to practice.

To practically integrate the power of presence while providing patient care, encourage students to recognize the value of the unique person they are about to meet. As students introduce themselves, they should establish eye contact and let go of any assumptions or all the tasks that need to be completed that day. Let the patient tell you his/her story. Allow the patient to lead you on their journey. The nurse is a companion with the patient on their current journey (Wilt & Smucker, 2001).

Presence is a nursing intervention that can be used in situations where there is nothing more that can be done but BE THERE by being supportive, physically close, offering a touch, or sitting in silence (Rex-Smith, 2007). Sitting quietly in times of need can communicate so much more than any words, even if it is for just a moment. In contrast, a "non-present" nurse would be aloof, outside the situation, or preoccupied with other thoughts though physically present (Benner & Wrubel, 1989).

This is the tension students will experience as novice nurses who are focused on the "tasks" to be done. They may not be able to recognize the importance to be "present" in a way that communicates caring. Presence is also a nursing intervention recognized by the Nursing Interventions Classifications (NIC). Specific NIC presence interventions include:

- Demonstrate accepting attitude.
- Verbally communicate empathy or understanding of the patient's experience.
- Establish patient trust.
- Listen to the patient's concern.
- Touch the patient to express concern as appropriate.
- Remain physically present without expecting interactional responses. (Cavendish et al., 2003)

Power of Touch

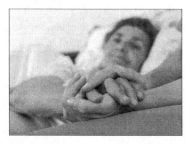

Caring and acceptance can be communicated through physical touch, especially by those in our culture who are considered "untouchable." An example of the power of physical touch to bring healing and acceptance is powerfully demonstrated in the life and ministry of Jesus. He was approached by a leper who desired healing. In the context of this man's experience, he was "untouchable" and had never experienced the warmth and acceptance of human touch since he was diagnosed with leprosy and became a leper. Instead, he had to proclaim and raise his voice to say, "Unclean! Unclean!" as people quickly moved out of his way to avoid his presence as he left the leper colony. This was his lived reality every day of his life. Recognizing not only his need to be healed, but also his deep unmet emotional need of acceptance that only human touch could communicate, the very FIRST thing that Jesus did before He brought needed healing, was to reach out and TOUCH the man who was "untouchable" and "unclean" (Matthew 8:1–4).

What can nurses learn from this example? Who is "untouchable" and "unclean" today in health care settings? What about those with HIV/AIDS, the homeless, or the increasing prevalence of patients with contact precautions that require the nurse to wear a gown and gloves every time they enter the room? What do you think the patient over time feels experiencing this? Teach students to recognize the power of touch and be sensitive to the needs of those in contact precautions as well as anyone else whose illness has a similar stigma and is considered "untouchable" or "unclean" by cultural norms today.

Building Block #3: Professionalism in Practice

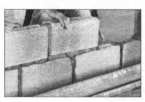

From my vantage point, there is a lack of professionalism in the nursing profession today. We are health care professionals, but our behavior often betrays this truth with the prevalence of incivility, bullying, and disrespectful behavior that is well-documented as a problem in our profession. Because incivility and entitlement have become normalized in popular culture, many students may be unaware that they are being unprofessional. Though it is not easy, these behaviors must be identified and respectfully addressed by faculty if they become apparent.

Faculty need to emphasize professional behavior and the values of the ANA Code of Ethics EARLY in the curriculum. When educators do this, it reinforces professional standards, clarifies expectations of professional behavior, and facilitates early intervention when students deviate from professional values and behaviors. Each student will bring their own set of values to your program. Therefore, it is essential that nurse educators nurture and instill professional values so their personal value system becomes identified as a member of the nursing profession. Only then will the patient, student, and the profession be well served (Fowler, 2015).

The foundational professional behaviors that we want to see lived out in our students before they leave our programs can be boiled down to CARING, COMPASSION, and RESPECT. These core values are also a part of our code of ethics. Provision 1 states:

"The nurse practices with compassion and respect for the inherent dignity, worth, and unique attributes of every person." (American Nurses Association, 2015)

Are your students aware of the ANA code of ethics and the values it calls each nurse to embody? These same principles that we are called to demonstrate toward our patients must also be shown to one another.

Character Matters

Florence Nightingale recognized the importance of personal character and virtue to those who would aspire to become a nurse. Nightingale identified the following character traits as central to nursing (Woodham-Smith, 1951). Though written more than 150 years ago, they remain relevant today. Have your students reflect on these questions about each essential character trait and see if these values are present:

- **Truthfulness/honesty.** Do you consistently tell the truth regardless of the consequences or only when it's convenient? Are you willing to cheat on an exam to get a passing grade?
- **Obedience.** Do you find it easy to follow the directions of those in authority over you?
- **Punctuality.** Are you on time for class and clinical learning? How about your current job or appointments?
- **Sympathy.** Are you able to identify easily with the pain and suffering of others or are you distant and aloof?
- **Humility.** Do you readily recognize your limitations as a student learner? Are you comfortable asking questions to validate your knowledge base?

Building on Nightingale's legacy, the American Nurses Association has identified the following values and character traits as essential to the professional nurse (American Nurses Association, 2015):

- **Integrity.** What are you like when nobody is watching? Are you the same or different?
- **Accountability.** Are you willing to allow others to hold you accountable for areas that may be a weakness for you?
- **Credibility.** Are you known to those close to you as being honest and trustworthy?
- **Advocacy.** Are you willing to take a stand for what you believe is right even if others may not agree with you?
- **Compassion.** Do you identify with the sufferings of others in such a way that you "suffer together" with them? This is the essence of what it means to be compassionate.
- **Respect.** Do you see others as having infinite value and worth regardless of their socioeconomic status or ethnicity? Do you have a high regard for the value and sanctity of every human being?

Excellence Matters

Excellence means that you have a strong desire to excel and be the best that you can possibly be. This ethic is true for both students and educators! Excellence is inwardly motivated and is present because you cannot imagine doing anything less than your very best. If students are content to be average and just good enough to get by, remind them that they are selling themselves short and will not live up to the potential they could be as a person and nurse (Grossman & Valiga, 2013). Encourage your students to push themselves to do what is needed and sacrifice to be the best nurse they can possibly be.

Excellence is also a CHOICE and a habit. It is always the result of sincere effort and strong intention. Help students to incorporate the pursuit of excellence into everything they do (Grossman & Valiga, 2013). For the health care professional, excellence needs to be a way of life. Excellence begets excellence, for ourselves and for those we work with.

Historical Examples to Emulate

Do not underestimate the power of a role model to contextualize the "art" of nursing and what you want your students to embody. This role model of excellence needs to begin with you! But build on this and use the following historical role models to inspire students to recognize the value of serving the needs of others as a professional nurse. I chose three individuals from three different historical time periods who capture the essence of the foundational values of our profession who compassionately and sacrificially served and cared for others that can provide an opportunity for students to imprint and learn from their example.

St. Camillus de Lellis

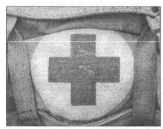

St. Camillus de Lellis (1550–1614) was a male caregiver from the Middle Ages. St. Camillus entered a Franciscan monastery after he recognized that he was not living a life worthy of God and desired to turn his life around. While needing hospital care for a chronic infection, he was concerned about the lack of compassion by caregivers he saw in practice and vowed to be different. As he cared for others, he recognized that good nursing depended on loving humanity, and he believed nursing would be better if it was not influenced by being paid for services provided (O'Lynn, 2012).

He made it his primary goal to gather men who would care for others, who were motivated by love for humanity and would let the wages take care of themselves. As he looked about the streets of Rome, he realized that it was the sick outside the hospital who needed care. He set up the first hospice service in Rome and began to focus his ministry on caring for the dying and providing comfort. His order was known as the Brothers of the Happy Death, since they brought compassion and comfort to those who were dying.

Some of the caregivers of his order became ill and died of the plague. The remaining men in his order continued to sacrificially serve and care for others. This order was formally titled the Congregation of the Servants of the Sick (the Camellians) and still exists today, providing health care in 35 countries. His example of caring, service, and sacrifice embodies the spirit of the nursing profession and remains relevant today. This order had a unique symbol that identified their order of male care-

givers; the RED CROSS that remains the universal symbol of health care today (O'Lynn, 2012)!

Florence Nightingale

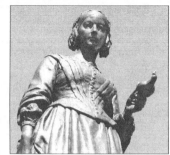

At the age of 17, Florence Nightingale (1820–1910) felt that God had spoken to her and called her to service. Nightingale was influenced by a belief in God that motivated her to transform health care and the nursing profession (McDonald, 1999). Her desire to serve and obey God through her life is evident in this passage from her diary at the age of thirty, *"Today I am 30, the age Christ began His mission…now Lord, let me only think of Thy will, what Thou willest me to do, O Lord, Thy will, Thy will"* (Widerquist, 1992, p. 51).

As a young woman who sensed God leading her to devote herself to works of charity in hospitals, she recognized the need for health care training. However, her parents were wealthy and respectable, and caring for the sick in England was not practiced by respectable women. Nurses in this era routinely came to work drunk, and sexually immoral conduct was present even on the patient care wards.

Therefore, she left England and went to Germany and obtained her health care training at the moral and respectable Lutheran deaconesses. She willingly chose to sacrificially serve during the Crimean War, caring for the wounded, making rounds as the "lady with the lamp," and educating nurses. Nightingale demonstrated God's care for humanity when she wrote:

"I have not a moment. The whole Army is coming into the hospitals. The task will be gigantic. Alas how will it all end? We are in the hands of God. Pray for us. We have at the moment five thousand sick and wounded. My only comfort is, God sees it, God knows it, God loves us." (Dossey, 1999, p. 121)

She implemented numerous reforms to lower the 73 percent mortality rate from diseases alone and wrote a one-thousand-page report of statistics she compiled during this time. Nightingale established her schools of nursing after the war based on her "evidence-based practice" (Lewis Coakley, 1990). Despite poor health later in life, Nightingale continued to devote herself to nursing research, using her gifts and passion as a statistician. As the first nurse educator and researcher of the modern era, her legacy includes the value and importance of applied research to practice and how it can lead to better patient outcomes (Berman & Snyder, 2011). Nightingale's life clearly demonstrates that faith, service, and nursing can and do complement one another in practice.

Agnes Gonxa Bojaxhu

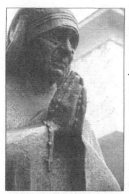 Though not a trained professional nurse, one caregiver who is worth emulating is Agnes Gonxa Bojaxhu (1910–1997). Never heard of her? I am sure you have if I use her more commonly known name of Mother Teresa!

Like Florence Nightingale, Agnes responded to the call of God on her life to serve others. At the age of 18, she joined an Irish community of nuns with missions located in India. While teaching at the high school in Calcutta, she received further clarity of the call to serve Christ in the poorest of the poor and received permission to start a school for the children of the slums. She then started her own order, The Missionaries of Charity (active in 133 countries), whose primary task was to love and care for persons nobody valued, the sick and dying homeless poor ("Mother Teresa—Biographical," 1979). Her primary mission was not about the work; it was all done for Jesus. She served sacrificially in this capacity until her death at the age of 87.

Out of her heart of love for God and love for others, the following quotes capture the essence of the example of her life. Regardless of your faith tradition, these principles have relevance and embody the essence of compassionate caregiving:

- *"Do ordinary things with extraordinary love."*
- *"It is not how much we do, but how much love we put into that action."*
- *"Let us touch the dying...and let us not be ashamed or slow to do the humble work."* ("Her own words," n.d.)

Vocation vs. Occupation

Each of these caregivers from the past has a common thread of vocation as the primary motivation to care for others. Vocation can be defined as doing all that is possible and whatever is necessary for the good of the patient. Others, including Nightingale, have spiritualized vocation by referring to it as a divine "calling." In the first nursing textbook of the modern era, Notes on Nursing, Nightingale (1859) writes, *"Every nurse...must have a respect for her own calling, because God's precious gift of life is often placed literally in her hands"* (p. 71).

Tanner (2004) affirms that nursing is a calling that requires each nursing student to recognize the importance of renewing their body, mind, and spirit. Nursing as a vocation remains relevant today and can guide students to care deeply for their patients. This vision of nursing makes values, faith, and the patient the primary motivation to care for others. Financial compensation is a secondary motivator to be a caregiver (O'Lynn, 2012).

Nursing is a now a well-paid profession. There is nothing wrong with being financially compensated for accepting the responsibilities to be a professional nurse. But what every student nurse who enters the profession needs to carefully examine is her or his PRIMARY motivation to enter nursing. When nursing becomes all about me and what I get out of it (salary, benefits, pension, etc.), nursing begins to drift from the foundational virtues and ethics the profession has historically represented.

Reflect

Building Block #1: Caring and Compassion

1. How do you emphasize the importance of caring in your content and/or curriculum?

2. What caregiving role models do you use or could you use as examples that you want your students to aspire to and be like?

Building Block #2: Holistic and Spiritual Care

How are your students being prepared to provide spiritual care?

3. What could you do differently to strengthen this aspect of holistic care?

Building Block #3: Professionalism in Practice

4. How do you emphasize self-care and principles to decrease student stress and burnout?

5. Using the symptoms present with each of the five stages of burnout, what stage (if applicable) do you observe in your students? In yourself?

6. How do you promote professional behaviors with your students?

7. What are the URGENT things in your schedule that keep you from what is really MOST important?

8. What changes do you need to make to your schedule to make time for what is MOST important?

References

American Nurses Association. (2015). *Code of ethics for nurses with interpretive statements*. Silver Spring, MD: Author. Retrieved from http://www.nursing world.org/codeofethics

Benner, P. (2012). International Nurses Christian Fellowship speech.

Benner, P. (2013). Teacher curiosity, passion, engagement and self-cultivation—Essential for transformative education. Retrieved from http://www.educat ing nurses.com/articles/teacher-curiosity-passion-en gagement-and-self-cultivation-essential-for-transfor mative-education/

Benner, P., & Wrubel, J. (1988). Caring comes first. *American Journal of Nursing, 88*(8), 1073–1075.

Benner, P., & Wrubel, J. (1989). *Primacy of caring: Stress and coping in health and illness*. Menlo Park, CA: Addison-Wesley Publishing Company.

Benner, P., Sutphen, M., Leonard, V., & Day, L. (2010). *Educating nurses: A call for radical transformation*. San Francisco, CA: Jossey-Bass.

Benner, P., Hooper-Kyriakidis, P., & Stannard, D. (2011). *Clinical wisdom and interventions in acute and critical care: A thinking-in-action approach*. (2nd ed.). New York, NY: Springer.

Berman, A., & Snyder, S. (2012). *Fundamentals of nursing*. (9th ed.). Upper Saddle River, NJ: Prentice Hall.

Berman, A., & Snyder, S. (2016). *Fundamentals of nursing*. (10th ed.). Upper Saddle River, NJ: Prentice Hall.

Blainey, G. (2011). *A short history of christianity*. Penguin Viking.

DeWit, S. (2009). *Fundamental concepts and skills for nursing*. St. Louis, MO: Saunders Elsevier.

Dolan, J., Fitzpatrick, L., & Krohn Herrmann, E. (1983). *Nursing in society: A historical perspective*. 15th ed. Philadelphia: W.B. Saunders, p.43.

Dossey, B. et al. (1995). *Holistic nursing: A handbook for practice*. Rockville, MD: Aspen.

Fowler, M.D.M. (2015). *Guide to the code of ethics for nurses with interpretive statements* (2nd ed.) Silver Spring, MD: American Nurses Association.

Hampton Robb, E. (1900). *Nursing ethics*. Cleveland, OH: E.C. Koeckert.

Her own words. Motherteresa.org. Retrieved from http://www.motherteresa.org/layout.html

Kelly, K.J., Lepo, A.W., & Frinzi, C. (2011). Empathy

and nursing education from mirror neurons to the experience of empathy: 21st century nursing education. *International Journal of Human Caring, 15*(4). 22-28.

Knight, K. (2012). Catholic Encyclopedia: Hospital, retrieved from http://www.newadvent.org/cathen/07480a.htm

LaBine, N.L. (2015). Teaching the spiritual dimension of nursing care: A survey of associate degree nursing programs in the southeast united states. [dissertation]. Johnson City, TN: East Tennessee State University.

Leininger, M. (1988). Leininger's theory of nursing: Cultural care diversity and university. *Nursing Science Quarterly, 1*, 152–160.

Leininger, M. (1991). *Culture care diversity and universality: A theory of nursing.* New York, NY: National League for Nursing.

McSherry, W., & Jameson, S. (2011). An online survey of nurses' perceptions of spirituality and spiritual care. *Journal of Clinical Nursing, 20*(11-12), 1757-1767.

Mother Teresa—Biographical. Retrieved from http://www.nobelprize.org/nobel_prizes/peace/laureates/1979/teresa-bio.html

Nightingale, F. (1859). *Notes on nursing: What it is and what it is not.* London: Harrison.

O'Lynn, C. (2012). *A man's guide to a nursing career.* New York, NY: Springer Publishing Company

Orlick, S., & Benner, P. (1988). The primacy of caring. *American Journal of Nursing, 88*(3). 318–319.

Pai, H,. Eng, C., & Ko, H. (2013). Effect of caring behavior on disposition toward critical thinking of nursing students. *Journal of Professional Nursing, 29*(6), 423-429.

Pavey, A. E. (1952). *The story of the growth of nursing.* London: Faber and Faber Ltd.

Pre-Licensure KSAS. (2014). QSEN.com. Retrieved from http://qsen.org/competencies/pre-licensure-ksas/#patient-centered_care

Scott, B.A. (2009). *Thinking as a nurse.* Bloomington, IN: iUniverse.

Shelly, J.A., & Miller, A.B. (2006). *Called to care: A Christian worldview for nursing.* Downers Grove, IL: InterVarsity Press.

Story, L., & Butts, J.B. (2010). Compelling teaching with the four Cs: Caring, comedy, creativity and challeng-

ing. *Journal of Nursing Education, 49*(5), 291-294.

Swanson, K. M. (1999). *What is known about caring in nursing: A literary meta-analysis.* In A.S. Hinshaw, S.L. Feetham, & J.L.F. Shaver, eds. *Handbook of clinical nursing research.* Thousand Oaks, CA: Sage Publications.

Sweeney, C. (2012). *160 ways to empathize.*

Tanner, C. A. (1990). Clinical education, circa *2010. Journal of Nursing Education, 41*(2), 51–52.

Tanner, C. A. (2004). The meaning of curriculum: Content to be covered or stories to be heard? *Journal of Nursing Education, 43*(1), 3–4.

Tanner, C. A. (2006). Thinking like a nurse: A research-based model of clinical judgment in nursing. *Journal of Nursing Education, 45*(6), 204–211.

Taylor, E.J. (2007). *What do I say? Talking with patients about spirituality.* Philadelphia, PA: Templeton Foundation.

Walsh, J. J. (1929). *The history of nursing.* New York, NY: Kennedy & Sons.

Watson, J. (2003). Love and caring: Ethics of face and hand—An invitation to return to the heart and soul of nursing and our deep humanity. *Nursing Administration Quarterly, 27,* 197-202.

Webster, D. (2010). Promoting empathy through a creative reflective teaching strategy: A mixed-method study. *Journal of Nursing Education, 49*(2), 87-94.

Widerquist, J.G. (1992). The spirituality of florence nightingale. *Nursing Research, (41)*1, 51.

Wilkinson, J. M. & Treas, L. S. (2011). *Fundamentals of nursing.* (2nd ed.). Philadelphia, PA: F.A. Davis Company.

Williams, J. & Stickley, T. (2010). Empathy and nurse education. *Nurse Education Today, 30*(8), 752-755.

7

Strategies and Tools to Teach the Foundation

Keith Rischer, RN, MA, CEN, CCRN

"As nurses, we have been given the ministry and tradition of compassionately caring for strangers, of loving our neighbors as ourselves...we need to be open to see every patient as an opportunity to demonstrate this compassion to those we do not yet know."

—Patricia Benner, RN, PhD, FAAN, FRCN

Building Block #1: Caring and Compassion

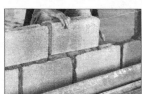 In order to revolutionize clinical education, students need experiences and activities that will help them to care like nurses (Tanner, 2002). In this chapter I will share activities I have developed and used with my students that provide practical guidance to help develop and build the foundation of the "art" of nursing in your students so that they will be empowered and equipped to care like nurses.

Two Caring Questions

Novice nursing students are focused on what needs to be done for their patient and are task oriented (Benner, 1984). When I taught fundamental clinical, some students seemed to forget at times that there is a person in the bed! This observation was validated by a recent study that showed that first-year students were more likely to be focused on tasks and equipment, and the patient was almost invisible. Performing procedures and skills successfully was more important (Ostrogorsky, T.L. et al., 2015).

One nurse educator observed that caring behaviors appear to be in decline with nurses in practice and wondered why. She felt that the way that nursing is currently taught may be part of the problem. Nursing curriculum emphasizes the medical model, moving nursing practice toward diagnosis-centered care. Communication skills and holistic care become minimized (Serber, 2014). Caring and holistic care need to be emphasized in the curriculum.

To integrate caring behaviors and make them intentional in your clinical setting, I created two open-ended questions that require students to reflect upon and then answer those questions that address empathy, caring, compassion, and nurse engagement in the context of the patient in their care. Use these questions each clinical as students provide care, or use them as a post-conference reflection that students can take turns answering.

1. **What is the patient likely experiencing/feeling right now in this situation?**

   This question emphasizes empathy, which is the ability to imagine and put oneself in another's place with the intention to understand what another is feeling or experiencing. Empathy is a synonym of compassion and represents another perspective to situate compassion to nursing practice.

2. **What can I do to engage myself with this patient's experience and show that they matter to me as a person?**

   This question begins with an emphasis of nurse engagement and what can be practically done to demonstrate this. The last half of this question is derived from Patricia Benner, who defines the essence of caring as a nurse when "you recognize the value and worth of those you care for and that the patient and their experience matter to you" (Benner & Wrubel, 1989).

My students expected me to ask these questions each clinical day. Even if I was not able to ask them personally, they were always prepared to answer them. This simple strategy kept caring on their radar regardless of how task oriented they may be as a novice nurse. Consider incorporating these two questions into your clinical setting. The way that your students respond to each patient using these questions will vary. As you encourage each student to intentionally engage with each patient and their personal story, clinical situation, family dynamics, and culture/ethnic traditions, each will be well on her/his way to cultivating caring and providing the best possible care for their patients! I also have adapted these two questions in my clinical reasoning case studies so that this emphasis can be reflected on and practiced in the classroom. This will be discussed later in this book.

Can Caring Be Taught?

This is the million-dollar question! Are caring behaviors in nursing students innate, or can caring be taught? One of the characteristics of a novice nurse is not only an emphasis on tasks, but difficulty in establishing priorities and recognizing what is relevant because of clinical inexperience (Benner, 1984). Nursing is both a science and an art. Many nursing programs allude to the importance of caring in their handbook or mission statement, yet do not incorporate teaching caring in the curriculum. Since caring is the central core and essence of nursing's culture, knowledge, and art, it becomes the moral responsibility of nurse educators to study theories of caring, read the literature on caring, then practice, and teach caring to students (Bevis, 1989). If caring behaviors are not clearly taught, defined, and evaluated as part of the educational process, do we have the assurance that students will be centered in caring while in school and then in practice?

Caring is a behavior that can be taught and learned (Cronin & Harrison, 1988), but not all nurse educators share a consistent belief that caring behaviors can actually be taught (Nelms, Jones, & Gray, 1993). Simonson (1996) discovered that in order for caring to be effectively taught, it needed to be "caught" by being modeled to other faculty and then to students. Tanner (1990) recognized that caring is learned by students when they experience caring practices between faculty and students. She also identified that the hidden curriculum may be most important in terms of what students learn. This is manifested in part by the manner in which faculty interact with students and the socialization of how to think and feel as nurses.

Tanner (1990) warned that the language of health care institutions is dehumanizing and detached. Therefore, it is imperative that students are helped to retain their caring practices in these settings and have them continuously nurtured and cultivated. How can nurse educators accomplish this objective? When I first began teaching clinical as an adjunct, I developed a caring tool based on Kristen Swanson's "Empirical Development of a Middle Range Theory of Caring" that prepared students to have a "plan of caring" in addition to their written care plan.

Swanson's Middle Range Theory of Caring

I was introduced to Kristen Swanson's caring theory during my graduate studies in nursing education. Swanson based her theory on the foundational caring theory work of Jean Watson and Patricia Benner. Swanson validated their observations by building her caring processes through qualitative research in a perinatal context. Mothers who had a critically ill infant in the neonatal intensive care unit (NICU) or had experienced the death of their baby through miscarriage or stillbirth were asked what the nurse did to show that they cared. Swanson identified five qualitative themes that mothers perceived as caring behaviors from nurses (Swanson, 1991). These themes of caring transfer to any patient-care setting despite the perinatal context from which they were derived.

In addition to each theme, Swanson also identified three to five caring interventions for each theme that described what the nurse did to demonstrate caring. These caring interventions can be taught to students to give them practical tools to integrate and cultivate caring behaviors in the clinical setting. To illustrate this strategy, I will use the following caring interventions Swanson identified: "conveying availability" and "avoid assumptions."

Conveying Availability

"Conveying availability" is one of the caring interven-

Swanson's Caring Processes and Their Definitions:

1. **Maintaining Belief (Esteem)**
   - Sustaining faith in the other's capacity to get through an event/transition and face a future with meaning
2. **Knowing (Empathetic Understanding)**
   - Striving to understand an event as it has meaning in the life of the other
3. **Being With (Emotionally Present)**
   - Being emotionally present to the other
4. **Doing For (Enact For)**
   - Doing for the other as he/she would do for oneself
5. **Enabling (Empowering)**
   - Facilitating the other's passage through life transitions and face a future with meaning (Swanson, 1991)

tions from the "Being With" theme. When the nurse "conveys availability" to a patient, this communicates caring (Swanson, 1991). So instead of saying to your patient, "Here is the call light," the student can also convey availability by stating, "Here is the call light; do not hesitate to call me. I am available if you need me." Both statements involve making the call light available to your patient, but the latter does it in a way that clearly communicates caring.

Avoid Assumptions

Another relevant caring intervention is "avoiding assumptions" from the "Knowing" theme. "Avoiding assumptions" stresses the importance of the nurse not to rely upon another nurse's judgments about the patient, but to make her own assessments by approaching the patient with a "clean slate" (Swanson, 1991). A common example of this in practice is when a nurse gives a "loaded" report filled with judgments about the patient and the kind of shift the next nurse will have. It is imperative to make your own assumptions based on your interaction with the patient. Why is this so important to do? Because when a nurse makes a preconceived judgment, he/she ceases to be able to demonstrate caring.

Develop a "Plan of Caring"

The framework that Swanson identified with five caring processes and related caring interventions provided a valuable guide to situate caring behaviors for my fundamental nursing students. In my clinical setting, I had five clinical weeks, one for each of the five caring themes.

To implement this emphasis on caring, I did the following before the first clinical:

1. Presented a brief overview by PowerPoint of the historical legacy and relevance of caring to the nursing profession.
2. Created a one-page handout that highlighted quotes from Florence Nightingale, Isabel Hampton-Robb, Patricia Benner, and Kristen Swanson on caring.
3. Provided students with an article/interview, "Caring Made Visible," by Swanson that provides an overview and discusses her caring theory so it can be readily understood and applied by students.
4. Created a one-page template for each of the five caring processes (see example).
5. Each clinical week I chose a caring theme to apply for that clinical. BEFORE each clinical, students put in their own words how they would practically implement at least two of the caring interventions of that specific theme. This was the students' "plan of caring" in addition to a traditional "care plan" that required caring nursing interventions and then documenting the effectiveness or evaluation of these caring interventions at the end of clinical.
6. Students submitted this caring tool each week for faculty to note and provide feedback. This tool was not graded, but used to encourage and guide development of caring behaviors and patient-centered care.

I conducted an anonymous survey at the end of clinical. Eighty percent of the students found the application of Swanson's caring framework meaningful to their growth and development of caring behaviors. Eighty-six percent of students reported that they received favorable and positive feedback from their patient when Swanson's caring interventions were implemented.

Developing a Plan of Intentional Caring:
Application of Swanson's Caring Processes
CLINICAL WEEK 2

II. Being With: (Emotionally present) Being emotionally present to the other.

Choose at least 2 to implement	Nursing Caring Interventions	Evaluation (Client Response)
1. Being there		
2. Conveying availability		
3. Sharing feelings		
4. Not Burdening		

The most common theme identified was that patients appreciated the communication of caring that these interventions expressed as well as deepening the nurse-patient trust and connection with the student nurse. Students felt they became more "patient-focused" and not just skill-oriented in their care, and that Swanson's caring theory was an effective, practical tool to teach the "art" of nursing.

Some of the comments students provided at the end of the semester included the following:

"I believe that overall the Swanson caring process really made me 'check myself' before entering the patient's room…Swanson helps me remember to do them each and every time I enter a patient's room."

"I grew a lot professionally—I am so much more comfortable talking with patients and expressing compassion than before."

"I realized that, no matter how defensive or solitary some patients are, they all have a common need to feel truly loved and cared for. I think this applica-

tion of caring is crucial to being an effective and healing nurse."

Though there were numerous caring interventions between the five caring themes, my students identified the following five caring interventions derived from the caring processes to be the most widely used and relevant as a novice nurse:

- Being there (nurse presence)
- Conveying availability
- Centering on the one cared for
- Avoiding assumptions
- Performing competently and skillfully

These top five caring interventions capture the essence of Swanson's caring theory and provide practical caring interventions that students can use while providing patient care. To simplify the application of Swanson's caring theory for advanced students so that it did not need to have a separate caring theme each week, I created a one-page template with these five interventions as an alternate approach to situate this caring theory for students. I provided the same brief overview of caring presentation and handout, and had students put in their own words how they would implement each caring intervention in the clinical before the first clinical. The strength of this approach is that it was much shorter and could be easily covered in clinical orientation.

Though nursing students may feel that they are "caring," they benefit from an evidence-based framework that defines caring from a patient's perspective. Students who are adult learners prefer active learning situations and learn best when they actively integrate new knowledge with existing knowledge (Russell, 2006). The practical application of Swanson's framework was an effective strategy that complements the learning style of adult learners and defines caring behaviors in a way that students can readily apply. The application of Swanson's caring theory in the clinical curriculum can help make caring central and relevant to all that is done by the nurse.

For more information and to download the tools to implement this activity in the clinical setting, go to: KeithRN.com/faculty-resources/teaching-caring/

Additional Ways to Develop Caring

- Additional strategies to help develop caring behaviors in students can include (Shaw, 2017):
- Require students to perform a self-awareness of caring evaluation by answering questions such as:
  - Are you a caring person?
  - What does that mean?
  - Provide examples when you demonstrated caring?
- Have students interview their patient: "What does caring mean and look like to you?"
- Ask students to reflect on three acts of caring/kindness during the clinical day and share this and the patient response during post-conference.
- Clinical faculty can follow up with each patient at the end of clinical by asking, "How did the student make you feel cared for today?"

Strategies to Develop Empathy

The following empathetic caring strategies were derived from Sweeney's research (2012) and patient reflections that students can use to demonstrate sensitivity to the patient's needs and provide empathetic care in the clinical setting.

Entering the Room for the First Time

- Always knock before entering the patient's room. Remember, it's their personal space.
- Tell the patient your name, school where you are a student, and why you are there.
- Ask the patient how they want to be addressed. Be sure to avoid calling the patient "Honey," "Sweetheart," or "Darling."
- Show honor and respect. Address your patient by "Mr.," "Mrs.," or "Ms." during your first encounter and then allow the patient to express their preference regarding how they want to be addressed: by their first name, nickname.
- Before leaving the room, ask if there is anything else the patient needs.
- When you leave the patient's room, always offer to shut the door. Give them the choice.

Beginning of the Clinical Day

- Do not immediately start taking vital signs and doing tasks. Instead, remove the stethoscope from your shoulders, sit at their bedside, and ask them how they are doing today. Engage person to person, not nurse to patient.
- Start your shift by asking your patient about their greatest fear or concern they may have.
- Have your patient identify their greatest hope and goals.
- Encourage the patient to share his or her story. This can involve the number of children, grandchildren, or their interests or hobbies.
- Know what is most important about your patient and give him or her the opportunity to talk about it.

While Providing Care

- Honor and respect patients' privacy and keep them appropriately covered at all times.
- Offer a soapy washcloth to cleanse their hands before eating.
- Keep the patient's room clean. A clean room is a healing environment.
- Anticipate the needs of your patient. This includes the need for water or pain medications.
- Offer a back rub, hair wash, or give a shave to your male patients. They will appreciate this extra effort!

General

- If your patient is from a different culture, ask relevant questions to increase your cultural sensitivity and show that you care.
- Never share your problems with your patient. It's always about them, not you.
- Never tell a patient how tired or busy you are.
- Encourage your patients by letting them know what they are doing well.

Final Takeaways

- Treat each patient as you would a beloved family member.
- Treat your patient the way that you would want to be cared for.
- Be completely engaged and maintain your focus on the patient at all times in the clinical setting.
- Remind yourself that you have been called to do the most important work in the world as a nurse!

Building Block #2: Holistic and Spiritual Care

Spiritual Assessment Questions

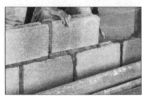 Just as there are a series of questions that students are taught to ask when completing a patient history or nursing assessment, there are also questions that are helpful to perform a spiritual assessment by the nurse when needed. If a patient has a new life-altering diagnosis such as cancer, a need for hospice, or major surgery, students must be prepared to perform a basic spiritual assessment to guide the need for a possible chaplain referral or immediate nursing support. Use these categories to guide what specific questions are most relevant based on the situation.

Meaning and Purpose

- What gives your life purpose?
- What keeps you going in life?
- What meaning do you give to your current situation?
- How has this illness affected the way you view life?

Faith

- Are you connected with a faith community?
- How has your health problem affected your spiritual beliefs?

- What is your source of strength?
- What can I do to support your faith?
- How do your beliefs help you cope with suffering and illness?

Love

- Who do you receive love and support from?
- Are you lonely?

Forgiveness

- Do you feel like God has abandoned you or is punishing you?
- Are you angry with God?
- Do you have any unfinished business? (Wilt & Smucker, 2001, pp. 55–56)

These three strategies in the classroom, clinical, and simulation settings improved student competence and confidence in providing spiritual care for first semester nursing students (Conners, Good, & Gollery, 2017):

1. **Classroom instruction on the topic of spirituality and caring behaviors**. Introduce the concept of caring and spirituality before their first clinical rotation. Students then met in small groups and collaborated to develop therapeutic responses to salient scenarios that contextualized spiritual or emotional distress.

2. **Structured spiritual assessment in the clinical setting.** Students submitted this to the clinical instructor. This emphasis encouraged students to develop a trusting therapeutic relationship.

3. **Simulation that addressed spiritual/holistic care.** Students were required to perform an admission assessment on a patient who recently had a stroke, but a family member was in obvious distress and needed care, too. Caring behaviors and other therapeutic approaches to provide holistic care for the family member were incorporated.

The spiritual assessment questions and Clinical Dilemma case studies could also be adapted with these three practical strategies as well.

Case Studies to Practice the "Art"

Since the ethical comportment of nursing practice can be more difficult to integrate in the curriculum, I created a series of shorter clinical reasoning case studies that integrate the most common dilemmas that students will experience when the psychosocial aspects of patient care become a priority. This formal instruction to help students develop empathy may be helpful. Nurse educators need to identify appropriate teaching strategies to promote empathy development in nursing students (Mennenga, Bassett, & Pasquariello, 2016).

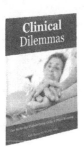 How will the nurse "think in action" when the patient who initially presented with a physical problem, now has psychosocial, emotional, or spiritual priorities because they are depressed, anxious, or in spiritual distress that require the "art" of nursing to be utilized to successfully resolve? "Clinical Dilemmas" are a unique series of case studies that address the unique nursing dilemmas that are most common in clinical practice. Case studies that contextualize these ethical and moral dilemmas and allow students to PRACTICE the ethical aspect of the profession can be an effective tool to teach the importance and relevance of the "art" of nursing to practice.

I have situated the most common themes of dilemmas in real-life scenarios that I have experienced into four general categories:

PATIENT dilemmas. How should the nurse respond when their patient is anxious, has lost hope, has a spiritual crisis or shows possible drug-seeking behavior?

TREATMENT dilemmas. How to support a patient when facing end of life and needs to choose between hospice/comfort care and aggressive medical management.

ETHICAL dilemmas. What to do when family members are in disagreement with code status or concern of medical futility.

NURSE dilemmas. How to address incivility in practice and academia as well as student burnout.

Each study has an emphasis that integrates aspects of caring, spiritual care, nurse engagement/presence, and ethical decision making and its relevance to nursing practice.

Structure

Clinical Dilemmas are brief (two pages) and can be completed in 15-20 minutes. This makes it easy to integrate them as an active learning tool in the classroom or clinical post-conference. Each case study has a blank student version (PDF) that can be posted as well as a fully developed answer key (PDF) for faculty. The activity begins with a scenario and the need to identify what is relevant and why in order to grasp the essence of the current problem.

Sample Scenario: Anxiety or Spiritual Distress?

History of Present Problem:

John James is a 77-year-old man who had coronary artery bypass graft (CABG) x 4 vessels three days ago for multi-vessel coronary artery disease. He lost over 1000 mL of blood shortly after surgery due to a bleeding graft site and almost died as a result. He is currently off all vaso-active drips, his arterial line has been discontinued, and he is clinically stable. John is scheduled to transfer to the cardiac step-down unit later today.

Personal/Social History:

John's wife died six months ago after 50 years of marriage. He lives alone in his own apartment. He has one son who lives in the area and checks in at least once a week to see how he is doing. He is a Vietnam War veteran who has not been active in his church since he returned from the war over 40 years ago.

Current Concern:

John puts on his call light and as you enter the room; he states that he feels short of breath and is visibly anxious. His breath sounds are clear and his O2 saturation is 98% on 2 liters n/c. His respiratory rate is 20/minute and his heart rate is 78/minute-sinus rhythm. He acknowledges that he is anxious and feels like he is having a panic attack and has never felt like this before. When you ask him if there is anything that he may be anxious about, he shares the following: "I used to go to church when I was little, but when I saw so many of my friends die in Vietnam and was helpless to save them, how could I believe in a God who allowed such horrible things to happen? Before the war I could not even kill a cat or dog. In Vietnam, I killed so many people. How can I be forgiven for what I have done?"

Several questions follow that include the following:
- Identify the essence of the dilemma and if additional information is needed

- What additional members of the health care team are needed?
- Identify the current plan of care with most relevant nursing priority and interventions
- Expected response to indicate plan of care was effective or does it need to be adjusted?
- How the nurse can practically demonstrate empathy and engagement?

I have included both the student version and the answer key for this case study as a supplement in the Transformation Toolbox included with this book.

Building Block #3: Professionalism in Practice

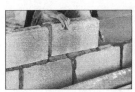 To have a "high bar" of professionalism with students, expectations for professional conduct must be clearly defined. I created a two-page handout titled "Your Professional Responsibilities as a Student Nurse" that is included as a supplement to this book that clearly defines these professional behaviors. I included this handout in my clinical orientation and it is reviewed and signed by each student. This was my way of holding my students accountable to a high standard of professional behavior.

This summary of professional behaviors that I include in my handout for students is derived from my own observations in practice as well as from those who have been my mentors:

1. **Reflect on your practice.**
   - Reflect on what went well/poorly and make needed adjustments to prevent similar problems in the future.
   - Reflection will guide students to learn from their mistakes, receive constructive feedback, and grow as a result.
2. **Be prompt and prepared.**
   - Be on time for clinical, prepare for care in the time allotted, and be ready to receive report on time at the beginning of clinical.
   - Complete treatments, medications in the time frame they are ordered.
   - Complete all clinical documentation in a timely manner.
   - Have all aspects of care completed at the end of shift and be present in post conference before it begins.

3. **Hold yourself to high standards.**
   - Desire to be the best nurse you can be!
   - Resist the natural tendency to do only what is needed to "get by."
4. **Be clinically curious.**
   - Ask questions and desire to know the WHY of what you do not know or understand.
   - Use appropriate resources to accurately obtain the information needed to promote your own learning.
5. **Embrace the responsibility.**
   - You are holding the life of another in your hand. Never take this responsibility lightly!
   - Take initiative, ownership, and responsibility for the care of your patients, but do not hesitate to ask for help or collaborate with your colleagues as needed!
6. **Be caring.**
   - Be truly engaged and empathetic toward those you care for and demonstrate this by your caring presence.
   - Reflect on what you can do to practically demonstrate empathy and show that every patient and family member matters to you.
7. **ZERO tolerance for incivility.**
   - Do NOT talk negatively about any student or faculty to others.
   - Be respectful and direct in all communication with students and faculty. Make a commitment to go to any student or faculty you have a concern about.
   - Stand up for the absent colleague if students are gossiping about another. Encourage the person to go directly to the other person and keep it between them and NOT the group.

ABCDs of Professional Introductions

The first step in effective communication that students must incorporate is a professional introduction when they meet their patient for the first time. One simple strategy is to teach the ABCDs of a professional introduction (Burke, LeBlanc, & Henneman, 2016).

- **Always** introduce yourself to the patient using your first and/or last name.
- **Be** transparent. Tell the patient, family, or nurse your credentials and role in the patient's care.
- **Clarify** how you would prefer to be addressed.

- **Document** your full name and role on the bedside communication whiteboard if present in the patient's room.

Establishing a Therapeutic Relationship

The ABCDs can also teach students the importance of developing a therapeutic relationship with the first contact with the patient (Burke, LeBlanc, & Henneman, 2016):

- **Ask** the patient how they would like to be addressed.
- **Be** culturally sensitive and respectful.
- **Confirm** the patient's answers by restating their name.
- **Document** this information on the patient whiteboard or in the medical record.

Developing a Personal Mission Statement

What do the business you work for, the college you attend, and nursing programs all have in common? They all most likely have a mission statement. A mission statement is used to guide the actions of an organization, spell out its overall goal, provide a path, and guide decision making. For example, the health care organization I work for has the following mission statement: "We serve our communities by providing excellent care as we prevent illness, restore health, and provide comfort to all who entrust us with their care"("Our Mission," 2014). This statement concisely captures its purpose (provide excellent care) as well as the outcome of this purpose (restore health and provide comfort).

What's Your Mission?

If a mission statement is essential for an organization, what about a personal mission statement to concisely capture the purpose and goals that you want to see realized as an educator for each nursing student? This exercise is also relevant for nurse educators to complete as well! Encourage students to reflect on WHY they wanted to become a nurse. Now it is time to take the essence of this motivation and put it into writing. Because of the hard work and stress that most students experience, some students will lose perspective and at times wonder if it is worth it to complete nursing education. .

Principles to incorporate in a personal mission statement should include:

- Vision to be the best

- What is your motivation to serve?
- What do you want to accomplish?
- What is your overriding goal?
- What values will you embody?

Student Examples

I recognized the value of this exercise and had my entire class develop and write their personal mission statements that would define them as student nurses as well as nurses in practice. I encouraged them to write down their personal mission statement and put it in a place such as their smartphone or notebook where they would be able to see it and review it often.

Here are a few of their examples:

"To be a knowledgeable and compassionate professional nurse that truly makes a difference in patients' lives through providing holistic nursing care."

"To integrate critical thinking and the nursing process to serve people in a Christ-like manner."

"To be a competent and lifelong learning nurse while providing empathetic and compassionate care, maintaining honesty and integrity, and being respectful of all cultures and individual choices."

"I will work with an open heart to give the best care possible to every patient I come in contact with. I will remain educated, honest, and professional for the duration of my career as well as in life."

"To provide excellent care for each individual to the best of my ability and to incorporate optimal skill, compassion, and character into every situation I am involved in."

Reflect

1. What strategies could you incorporate in the classroom or clinical setting to develop the "art" of nursing with students?

- Caring & Compassion

- Spirituality

- Professionalism & Reflective Practice

References

Benner, P. (1984). *From novice to expert: Excellence and power in clinical nursing practice.* Upper Saddle River, NJ: Prentice Hall.

Benner, P., & Wrubel, J. (1989). *Primacy of caring: Stress and coping in health and illness.* Menlo Park, CA: Addison-Wesley Publishing Company.

Bevis, E. (1989). Teaching and learning: The key to education and professionalism. In E. Bevis & J. Watson (eds.), *Toward a caring curriculum: A new pedagogy for nursing* (pp. 153–185). New York: National League for Nursing.

Burke, M.E., LeBlanc, R.G., & Henneman, E.A. (2016). ABCDs of professional introductions: Teaching nursing students the most fundamental of all communication skills. *Nurse Educator, 41*(3), 115-116.

Conners, J., Good, P., & Gollery, T. (2017). Using innovative strategies to improve nursing student competence and confidence in providing spiritual care. *Nurse Educator, 42*(2), 62-64.

Cronin, S., & Harrison, B. (1998). Importance of nurse-caring behaviors as perceived by patients after myocardial infarction. *Heart & Lung, 17,* 374–381.

Mennenga, H.A., Bassett, S., & Pasquariello, L. (2016). Empathy development through case study and simulation. *Nurse Educator, 41*(3), 139-142.

Nelms, T. P., Jones, J. M., & Gray, D. P. (1993). Role modeling: A method for teaching caring in nursing education. *Journal of Nursing Education, 32*(1), 18–23.

Ostrogorsky, T.L., Raber, A.M., McKinley Yoder, C., Nielson, A.E., Lutz, K.F., & Wros, P.L. (2015). Becoming a nurse: Role formation among accelerated baccalaureate students. *Nurse Educator, 40*(1), 26-30.

Our Mission (2014). Retrieved from http://www.allina health.org/uploadedFiles/Content/Allina-Health-mission-vision-values-promise.pdf

Serber, S. (2014). Nurses where's the caring? *Nurse Educator, 39*(1), 15-16.

Shaw, P. (2017). Innovative strategies to develop caring nurses. *Nurse Educator, 42*(2).

Simonson, C. L. (1996). Teaching caring to nursing students. *Journal of Nursing Education, 35*(3), 100–104.

Swanson, K. M. (1991). Empirical development of a middle range theory of caring. *Nursing Research, 40*(3), 161–166.

Sweeney, C. (2012). *160 ways to empathize.*

Tanner, C. A. (1990). Caring as a value in nursing education. *Nursing Outlook, 38*(2), 70–72.

Wilt, D.L., & Smucker, C.J. (2001). *Nursing the spirit: The art and science of applying spiritual care.* Washington, D.C.: American Nurses Publishing.

Raising the Walls:
The Applied Sciences of Nursing

Keith Rischer, RN, MA, CEN, CCRN

"U.S. nursing programs are not generally effective in teaching nursing science…
the nursing curriculum is additive; rather than rework the material to reflect
current practice, the faculty simply incorporates more."

—*Educating Nurses: A Call for Radical Transformation,* p. 12

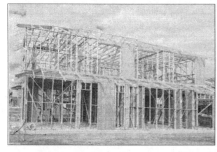

Now that the foundation has been laid by integrating and emphasizing the "art" of nursing, it is time to build and then raise the walls of the "living" house that each student represents. The walls consist of each student mastering and UNDERSTANDING the applied sciences of nursing that include anatomy and physiology, pharmacology, and fluids and electrolytes. These applied sciences must be able to be APPLIED to the bedside. They are foundational for the critical and clinical thinking that is expected and required of the professional nurse.

In nursing education, the historical emphasis has been on knowledge acquisition (Benner, et al., 2010). But this is not enough. Students need to UNDERSTAND what they have learned and USE that knowledge in practice (Eraut, 1994). In this chapter I use my lens of current clinical practice to emphasize the aspects of the applied sciences that promote DEEP learning of what is MOST important so that students can use this knowledge and apply it to the bedside.

In order to establish correct care priorities, recognize the RELEVANCE of clinical data, and understand WHY primary care providers order the treatments and medications that patients receive, students need to understand the applied sciences. To translate and breakdown the knowledge that students need to acquire, the nurse educator must also possess a mastery and deep understanding of this content. The three walls of the applied sciences that lay the foundation for critical/clinical thinking include:

1. Pathophysiology
2. Nursing Pharmacology
3. Fluids & Electrolytes (F&E)

Wall #1: Pathophysiology

A thorough understanding of pathophysiology is foundational for nursing practice and must be deeply understood to provide holistic, patient-centered care. But understanding pathophysiology is difficult for students because it integrates difficult content from anatomy, physiology, biology, and chemistry and requires students to USE this knowledge to understand disease processes and resultant nursing interventions and set priorities in the clinical setting (Van Horn, Hyde, Tesh, & Kautz, 2014).

To strengthen the critical thinking required for practice, pathophysiology must be integrated and CONTEX-

TUALIZED in all aspects of the nursing program. This includes the classroom and clinical settings. Does your classroom lecture include a highlight of the pathophysiology of the disease you are presenting? It should. In the clinical setting, do you have your students apply pathophysiology by helping them understand the mechanism of action of the most important medications used in practice and then concisely state this as part of their required safety checks before they administer? You should, even at the beginning of the program.

Because of their lack of clinical experience, students struggle to recognize clinical relationships and see how data is connected. The thread that ties the connections in clinical practice is understanding and then applying pathophysiology to each patient.

To provide safe patient care, the following connections must be made between the following by understanding the applied sciences:

- Primary problem (understanding pathophysiology of this problem)
- Mechanism of action of medications administered
- Relevant abnormal lab values
- Relevant abnormal vital signs
- Relevant abnormal assessment findings

Let's use a scenario of a patient who is admitted with heart failure exacerbation to see why pathophysiology must be understood. Furosemide, a potent loop diuretic is ordered. The creatinine has increased from the patient's baseline of 1.5 to 2.2, heart rate is 110 irregular, and the rhythm is atrial fibrillation, RR 24. His blood pressure is 166/90. He has bibasilar crackles and 3+ pitting edema in his lower extremities. To tie each of these pieces of clinical data together and recognize how this data is related, the nurse must understand the pathophysiology of right vs. left-sided heart failure.

CO=SVxHR

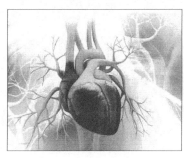

Another reason that pathophysiology must be understood and applied to practice is the formula from A&P that many students are able to recite, but struggle to understand:

CO=SVxHR

Cardiac output is measured by the stroke volume or the amount of blood that the left ventricle pushes out multiplied by the current heart rate. This is the exact measurement of the minute-by-minute cardiac output of the heart. Four to eight liters is normal to maintain adequate perfusion to the entire body.

Whenever cardiac output is decreased due to severe dehydration, heart failure, hypovolemia, or any shock state including sepsis, the FIRST and earliest compensatory response by the heart is to INCREASE the rate to maintain adequate cardiac output. This is why an elevated heart rate without an obvious reason (elevated fever/severe pain) is always a clinical RED FLAG that must be recognized by the nurse. In early shock or hypovolemia, the HR will be elevated, but the BP will be normal or only slightly decreased.

If this early sign of decreased cardiac output goes unrecognized and begins to worsen, the problem will perpetuate. Over time, the blood pressure will begin to significantly drop to a shock state. By then it may be too late, and the patient may have an adverse outcome or even death as a result. When CO=SVxHR is deeply understood by students, the RED FLAG and clinical significance of an elevated HR and normal or dropping BP becomes readily apparent.

To contextualize this aspect of pathophysiology to practice, review and use the following four clinical scenarios to see if your students can determine how CO=SVxHR will help interpret the clinical data in each scenario. When this is done correctly the urgency of the situation and the nursing and clinical priorities become evident.

1. June, a 52-year-old woman who is six hours post-op with a posterior spinal fusion. She is afebrile, but HR and BP pre-op were 78 and 132/80. Since her return to the surgical floor, her HR has been consistently 100-110 with a BP 100/60.
2. James, a 45-year-old man who presented to the ED intoxicated with a large coffee ground emesis. His HR is 130 and BP 80/40.
3. Jennifer, a 68-year-old woman who is post-op day #2 with a hemicolectomy due to a bowel obstruction. Her HR and BP pre-op were 90 and 110/82. She spiked a temp to 101.2 and HR is now 105 and BP 90/50.

4. John, a 68-year-old man admitted with heart failure exacerbation who has ischemic cardiomyopathy and an ejection fraction of 15%. His resting HR is consistently 90-100.

Scenarios Explained

1. Why is there an elevation of heart rate with a lower BP? Though sepsis is possible, it is unlikely because of the short time frame after surgery and the temperature is normal. The most common and likely explanation early post-op is that the patient has a fluid volume deficit and is dehydrated. The nurse must recognize the significance of the clinical data collected and recognize the need to contact the primary care provider. The recommendation should include an IV bolus and reassess the response if successful (decreased HR and increased BP).

2. This patient is intoxicated with a coffee ground emesis. The clinical connection of likely chronic alcohol abuse and a gastrointestinal bleed must be recognized. Combine this with a heart rate that is tachycardic and blood pressure that is too low captures the severity and crisis of an acute GI bleed that requires rapid intervention and rescue.

3. To clinically reason, the nurse must recognize and identify the clinical trend or trajectory of clinical data collected in this scenario. What direction is the TREND going? The temperature is rising and the heart rate is increasing and the blood pressure is decreasing slightly from the most recent. When the nurse deeply understands not only CO=SVxHR, but that sepsis is the most likely complication of any invasive procedure, she/he will realize the inflammatory response causing vasodilation resulting in decreased cardiac output is present. This patient must be recognized as critical with emergent interventions.

4. When the nurse knows that a normal ejection fraction is 60-70%, this patient's strength of cardiac contraction is 1/4 that of a healthy heart. Since stroke volume is the other component in this cardiac output equation, the elevated heart rate is most likely his baseline to maintain adequate CO with his end stage heart failure, but the respiratory system must also be closely assessed for signs of pulmonary edema.

Make it a priority to practice this essential concept through scenarios students may see in the clinical setting or through scenarios that I have developed in my clinical reasoning case studies. By helping students deeply understand CO=SVxHR, you will not only prepare your students for the NCLEX, but more importantly, real-world clinical practice!

Wall #2: Nursing Pharmacology

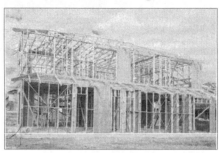

Once in nursing practice, students will likely pass medications every day. Therefore, it is essential that they possess a DEEP UNDERSTANDING of pharmacology. This is more easily said than done. Currently, there are more than 5,000 medications used in practice and most nursing drug manuals are well over 1,000 pages in length. Nursing drug manuals have content areas of the following:

- Indications
- Mechanism of action
- Pharmacologic classification
- Time/action profile
- Contraindications
- Side effects
- Interactions
- Route and dosages
- Nursing implications
- Patient education.

If a student has multiple medications to pass, what should they be able to state and understand before they are considered safe to administer? What content areas of the drug manual are the most important? In order to strengthen student understanding of pharmacology, nurse educators need to identify the MOST important aspects of pharmacology that you want your students to master. Use two filters to guide what to include in all content that is taught.

Filter #1: NEED to Know Content

This information must be DEEPLY understood because it is essential and directly relevant to develop clinical/critical thinking as well as representative of the most common themes seen in practice.

Filter #2: NICE to Know Content

This content is NOT essential or representative of what a student will most likely see in the first year of practice. This content will also be learned over time and with experience. Therefore, let this content go and do NOT weigh students down with content that will keep them from mastering what is most important and NEED to know.

Mechanism of Action=NEED to Know!

Anatomy and Physiology (A&P) is a prerequisite for most nursing programs and is typically taught with little to no contextualization to nursing practice by faculty who are not nurses. Essential content and concepts such as preload, afterload, Starling's law, and the classic formula CO=SVxHR have no clear clinical contextual hook to the bedside for pre-nursing students to understand how relevant or important this is to clinical practice and patient care. Therefore, it is essential for nurse educators to correlate essential A&P content to bedside practice to develop the critical and clinical thinking students require. Never assume that just because A&P was covered previously that they know, understand, and are able to apply it. Repeatedly review all need-to-know concepts of A&P wherever and whenever possible and consistently contextualize it to practice.

CO=SVxHR and Pharmacology

The importance of CO=SVxHR was discussed earlier in the context of pathophysiology, but do your students understand this formula DEEPLY enough so they could describe in their own words how preload, afterload, and contractility influence cardiac output and how each of these determinates of cardiac output are specifically affected by each major pharmacologic classification of cardiac medications? To develop a DEEP understanding of the mechanism of action of diuretics, nitrates, beta blockers, calcium channel blockers, and ACE inhibitors, the pathophysiology situated in the mechanism of action must be UNDERSTOOD as well as the implications of the action to cardiac output. This level of applied understanding should be the bar that is expected for the advanced student.

To see why the wall of pharmacology is essential to safe clinical practice, let's use the common cardiac medications of atenolol and amiodarone and see why both mechanism of action and its impact on determinants of cardiac output are relevant to nursing practice.

Atenolol

This is the mechanism of action for atenolol as stated from Micromedex, an online data base used by many hospitals:

"Atenolol is a synthetic beta (1)-selective adrenoreceptor blocking agent. It inhibits beta (2)-adrenoreceptors primarily found in bronchial and vascular musculature at higher doses" ("Atenolol," 2014)

To understand the physiologic impact of atenolol, students must be able to recognize the differences between beta 1 and beta 2 adrenergic receptors, and the physiologic effects of this beta blockage to the heart and lungs.

Based on the formula CO=SVxHR, would your students be able to readily identify how the mechanism of action of a beta blocker affect the following determinants of cardiac output for atenolol?

- Preload (no effect)
- Afterload (directly impacts by lowering systolic BP)
- Contractility (directly impacts by decreasing contractility)
- Workload of the heart (directly impacts by lowering workload due to reduction of afterload and decrease in contractility)

Amiodarone

This is the mechanism of action for amiodarone as stated from Micromedex:

"Amiodarone is an antiarrhythmic drug with predominant class III effects of lengthening cardiac action potential and blocking myocardial potassium channels leading to slowed conduction and prolonged refractoriness." ("Amiodarone," 2014)

For a student to safely administer amiodarone, students must understand the cardiac electrophysiology concepts of action potential, refractory period, and slowed conduction, and how these physiologic effects will directly affect heart rate and rhythm. This contextualization of A&P needs to be developed in each student.

Based on the formula CO=SVxHR, would your students be able to translate this mechanism of action and how it impacts the following determinants of cardiac output when administering amiodarone?

- Preload (no effect)

- Afterload (little to no effect though in practice, it can lower BP)
- Contractility (no effect)
- Workload of the heart (directly impacts by reducing the HR)

My students struggled with this depth of understanding of cardiac medications. To translate this essential content so it could be deeply understood, I created a handout titled "Comprehending Cardiac Medications." This PDF file is included in the Transformation Toolbox so you can strengthen the knowledge of this difficult content for your students as well.

Putting the Puzzle Together

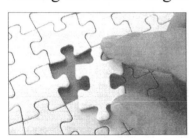 A current weakness of nursing education is the "pedagogies of inquiry." These are the strategies needed to put the clinical puzzle together (Benner, et al., 2010). Students must be encouraged to see that patient care and clinical practice is like putting a puzzle together. This is done by recognizing and identifying clinical relationships. Though there are many pieces of clinical data, most pieces of clinical data do have a relationship and fit together. This is gone into additional detail on this important concept later in the book. But in the context of pharmacology, there are two important clinical relationships that, when recognized and identified by students, will improve their critical and clinical thinking and help them put the clinical puzzle together as they provide care for their patients.

Pharmacology Relationship #1

This is the clinical RELATIONSHIP between the mechanism of action and the nursing assessments required to be safe to administer. When the nurse UNDERSTANDS the pathophysiology of the mechanism of action and how it impacts the body, essential nursing assessments logically follow.

Pharmacology Relationship #2

This is the clinical RELATIONSHIP between the dose of the medication and recognizing if the dose range is low, mid, or high. This relationship will suggest the likely severity of the underlying problem that the medication is treating. The higher the dose range, the more resistive or severe the underlying illness likely has become.

For example, when a student identifies and applies these clinical relationships to practice when administering atenolol 100 mg PO, he understands that this medication is a beta blocker and works by blocking adrenergic (sympathetic nervous system) beta 1 receptors on the heart, which exerts the physiologic effect of lowering heart rate and blood pressure. Therefore, the assessment of heart rate and blood pressure are readily recognized and must be performed before administration to be safe. Recognizing that atenolol 100 mg is in the high dose range, the clinical relationship of the degree of hypertension is identified as likely severe or resistant to treatment.

Five Foundational Pharmacology Questions

I used my lens of clinical practice to determine the sequential and logistical questions that I reflect upon to safely administer medications. I developed the following "foundational five" questions that need to be verbalized and understood for the most common medications administered in the clinical setting. The use of these questions will strengthen student knowledge and mastery of pharmacology. If a student is passing a medication that is not commonly used, I keep it simple, and do not go to this depth of validation, but focus on the indication and safe dose range.

Five Foundational Pharmacologic Questions

1. What is the pharmacologic class? What is it for?
2. Why is your patient receiving it?
3. What is the expected patient response based on the mechanism of action?
4. What assessments do you need to know before you administer and follow up?
5. Is this a safe dose? Is the dose range low–mid–high?

The rationale for these "foundational five" questions include:

What is the pharmacologic class? What is it for?

Students must be able to identify the pharmacologic class

for the most common medications used in practice. This benefits the student by simplifying medication knowledge. Though there are thousands of individual medications used in practice, there are far fewer classifications or families. For example, when a student recognizes that any generic medication ending in "lol" belongs to the beta blocker pharmacologic class, the student understands the mechanism of action, side effects, and nursing assessments needed before or after administration are the same for those medications in this class.

Most medications have one primary indication that must be known. This knowledge allows students to identify the clinical relationship of the medical problem that each medication treats. If there is more than one indication for the medication, this must also be recognized so the student is able to answer the next question!

Here is a scenario that many educators encounter when passing medications that have a common "off-label" use. The medication being administered by the student is gabapentin (Neurontin).

- Teacher: What classification does this drug fit into?
- Student: It is an anticonvulsant.
- Teacher: Does your patient have a diagnosis or history of seizures?
- Student: No.
- Teacher: Then why do you suppose that your patient is taking it?
- Student: I have no idea.

This provides an opportunity to discuss diabetes and the complication of neuropathy, but most students cannot make this connection and require faculty guidance.

Why is your patient receiving it?

Because many medications have more than one indication, students must be able to identify which indication applies to his/her patient. Atenolol is an excellent example of this in practice. Though it is most commonly given to control hypertension, it also is used to control the heart rate in patients with atrial fibrillation or decrease the workload of the heart in patients with heart failure.

What is the expected patient response based on the mechanism of action?

To help students develop this essential critical/clinical thinking skill, I have my students state in their OWN words the mechanism of action and not be allowed to "parrot" it word for word from their nursing drug manual or Micromedex.

Want to make sure your students truly understand the mechanism of action of medications they are administering? Then ask the following questions:

- *"What is a calcium channel blocker blocking?"*
- *"What is an ACE inhibitor inhibiting?"*
- *"What is a beta blocker blocking?"*

Then you will be able to quickly assess how much your students really know and understand!

What assessments do you need to know before you administer and follow up?

This is an essential clinical relationship that should become clear when the mechanism of action is DEEPLY understood. An excellent example of this in practice is when a student can recognize that not all cardiac medications require an assessment of the heart rate and blood pressure. Knowing that the primary physiologic effect of an ACE inhibitor is to cause vasodilation which lowers blood pressure, the heart rate does not need to be assessed to safely administer this drug.

Is this a safe dose? Is the dose range low–mid–high?

Identifying a safe dose of a medication is an essential assessment that must be verbalized, but is best suited for fundamental level students. Build on this basic knowledge by expecting your advanced students to not only determine that it is a safe dose, but use the knowledge of dose ranges to identify if it is a low–mid–high range dose. This will develop an awareness of the clinical relationship of dosage and severity of the underlying problem being treated.

Wall #3: Applying F&E to the Bedside

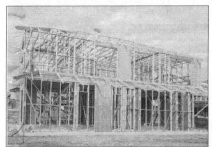

Fluids and Electrolytes (F&E) is challenging to students because it requires application of chemistry, acid/base knowledge, and physiology. It is also relevant and basic to practice and must be DEEPLY understood so this knowledge can be applied to the bedside. The most important objective of this content is NOT to merely memorize the signs and symptoms for the "hypo" and "hyper" of every electrolyte. Just as A&P is essential to understand the mechanism of action, applied A&P must be integrated with F&E for practical application and contextualization to the bedside to be realized.

Danger…TMI in Clinical!

Once students are in the clinical setting, clinical content overload is a given! As novice nurses, they will encounter an overwhelming amount of clinical data in the medical record. Patricia Benner's novice to expert theory identified that because new nurses have a lack of knowledge and clinical salience, they struggle with identifying the most important data in the clinical setting and tend to see EVERYTHING as equally relevant (Benner, 1982)! This includes the numerous lab values found in the most commonly ordered lab panels.

Therefore, filter (remember NEED to know vs. NICE to know!) clinical content by identifying the MOST important labs in your classroom content or clinical setting. Routine laboratory panels are difficult to sort through because of the sheer amount of data. The novice nurse will be unable to identify values that are most important and relevant to the primary problem. This is the responsibility of the nurse educator.

For example, a basic metabolic panel (BMP) has the following ten lab values:

- Sodium
- Potassium
- Chloride
- Carbon dioxide (CO2-bicarb)
- Glucose
- Blood urea nitrogen (BUN)
- Creatinine
- Glomerular filtration rate (GFR)
- BUN/creatinine ratio
- Anion gap

Do EVERY one of these lab values have equal relevance and importance to nursing practice? Not at all. I could easily filter half of these lab values in a BMP as NEED to know and emphasize them as relevant to practice. The other half of these values are NICE to know and will have, at times, situational relevance, but do not need

to be considered for most patients. Decrease clinical content saturation by identifying the specific labs that are most relevant to the nurse.

There are lab values that are ALWAYS relevant because of their physiologic importance and relevance to homeostasis and well-being. Create a SHORT list of lab values that have universal relevance depending on your setting. If they present in the medical record, they MUST be clinically significant and noted even if they are NORMAL. Students tend to think that only the ABNORMAL labs are significant and must be noted. But if a lab is identified as ALWAYS relevant, even if it is normal, it has clinical significance.

I created a list of always-relevant lab values that guided what labs my students addressed. If present in the chart, my students were expected to note these labs and, more importantly, TREND the direction they were going over the last day or two. In the list below the rationale is included as to why they have relevance even if they are normal.

ALWAYS RELEVANT Laboratory Values
(if present in chart)

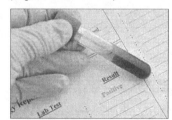 Though a BMP and CBC are the most common lab panels ordered, I have compiled a short list of additional labs, that if present in the chart, are always relevant and must be noted by the nurse because of their clinical significance.

Basic Metabolic Panel (BMP)/Chemistries

- **Potassium (3.5–5.0 mEq/L)** Essential to normal cardiac electrical conduction. If too high or low, can predispose to rhythm changes that can be life-threatening! Potassium tends to deplete more quickly with loop diuretic usage than magnesium. Also needs to be taken into account when giving a bowel prep such as Golytely for a colonoscopy. Potassium can be depleted and needs to be noted before the bowel prep begins.
- **Sodium (135–145 mEq/L)** I consider sodium the fluid balance "Crystal-Light®" electrolyte. Though this is simplistic, it helps to understand in principle how sodium influences fluid balance. For example,

when you add one small packet of Crystal Light to a 16-ounce bottle of water, the concentration is just right. This is where a normal sodium will be (135-145).

- Where free water goes, sodium will follow to a degree. Therefore, if there is a fluid volume deficit due to dehydration, sodium will typically be elevated because it's concentrated (less water in the bottle!). If there is fluid volume excess, sodium will be diluted and will likely be low (too much water in the bottle!).

- **Glucose (Fasting: 70–110 mg/dL)** Required fuel for metabolism for every cell in the human body, especially the brain.
  - Relevant with history of diabetes or stress hyperglycemia due to illness. Elevated levels post-op can increase risk of infection/sepsis.

- **Creatinine (0.6–1.2 mg/dL)/Glomerular Filtration Rate (GFR) (>60 mL/minute)** THE GOLD STANDARD for kidney function and adequacy of renal perfusion. The functioning of the renal system impacts every body system; therefore, it is ALWAYS relevant!
  - When creatinine is elevated, this can be due to damage done to the fragile capillary membrane screen of the glomerulus, which is like a screen door with larger holes that are letting things through that they shouldn't, such as protein and glucose.

Complete Blood Count (CBC)

- **White Blood Cells (WBC) (4500-11,000/mm 3)** ALWAYS RELEVANT based on its correlation to the presence of inflammation or infection. Will usually be increased if infection present, though it may be decreased in the elderly or pediatric patients <3 months.

- **Neutrophils (50–70%)** ALWAYS RELEVANT for the same reason as WBCs. They are the most common leukocyte and their role as a FIRST RESPONDER to any bacterial infection within several hours is always relevant.
  - The more aggressive or systemic the infection, the higher the percentage of neutrophils and WBCs. Immature neutrophils (bands) greater than 8 are also clinically significant and must be

clustered with WBC and neutrophils to determine if sepsis is a clinical concern.

- **Hemoglobin (Male: 13.5–17.5 g/dL, and Female: 12.0-16.0)** THE GOLD STANDARD to determine anemia or acute/chronic blood loss.

- **Platelet count (150–450 x 103/µl)** Relevant whenever there is a concern for anemia or blood loss or a patient is on heparin. If platelets are low, any patient on heparin products must have this noted because of the clinical possibility of heparin-induced thrombocytopenia (HIT), which develops when the immune system forms antibodies against heparin that cause small clots and lower platelet levels.

Cardiac

- **Troponin (<0.4 ng/mL)** It is ALWAYS RELEVANT when ordered to rule out myocardial infarction. It is the most sensitive cardiac marker and will be elevated if there is cardiac muscle damage. Can take up to six hours after chest pain to elevate, so labs are typically ordered every 6-8 hours x 3 and each lab result is carefully trended to the prior to see if trend is increasing and becoming positive.
  - Very sensitive cardiac marker that can be slightly elevated and positive in heart failure and unstable angina.
  - Those with renal disease, usually CKD III-IV, will be unable to clear troponin by the kidneys and may have a baseline that is a low level positive. This is why it is so important to TREND the current level to the most recent in the chart and determine if there is a clinical elevation in this context.

- **CPK-MB (<5%)** Specific iso-enzyme for cardiac muscle. If this is elevated, confirms presence of MI. Because troponin can be sensitive, some physicians order both troponin and CPK-MB to correlate.

- **BNP (B-natriuretic Peptide) (<100 ng/L)** What troponins are to MI, BNP is to heart failure. It is a neurohormone secreted by myocytes in the ventricles. When ventricles are stressed and overloaded, BNP is a compensatory hormone that is a vasodilator and also diuretic to help the body naturally decrease the workload of the heart. It will be elevated in heart failure exacerbation.

Coagulation

- **PT/INR (0.9–1.1 nmol/L)** Measures time required for a firm fibrin clot to form and measures the clotting cascade. It depends on vitamin K synthesis from the liver. Therefore, it will be elevated in liver disease in patients who are not on warfarin. It's a standard anti-coagulant ordered for those on warfarin (Coumadin) to maintain therapeutic goal of INR 2-3.
  - Relevant and must be noted for any patient on warfarin but especially when a bleeding complication secondary to warfarin presents. Warfarin can be reversed quickly if patient is actively bleeding by administering vitamin K IV and/or fresh frozen plasma.

Miscellaneous Chemistries

- **Magnesium (1.6–2.0 mEq/L)** Essential to normal cardiac electrical conduction. If too high or low, can predispose to rhythm changes that can be life threatening!
- **Lactate (0.5–2.2 mmol/L)** Not routinely done, but when present in chart, it is there for a reason! Have students go back to A&P to recognize the relevance of Krebs cycle and lactic acidosis due to anaerobic metabolism. GOLD STANDARD lab to trend with any shock state, especially sepsis! Elevated levels correlate with higher likelihood of dying. For example, in septic shock, a level >4 reflects a 28 percent chance of mortality (Van Leeuwen & Poelhuis–Leth, 2009).

Lab Panel Summaries

In addition to always-relevant labs discussed earlier, there are labs that have situational relevance depending on the primary problem. In the most common lab panels that are ordered, the remaining labs listed below must also be understood by students because of their physiologic significance. The normal ranges are listed for each lab, but note that these ranges can vary slightly between institutions so validate what is normal for your practice setting.

The following lab panels are covered in this section:
- Basic Metabolic Panel (BMP)
- Miscellaneous Chemistries
- Complete Blood Count (CBC)
- Liver Panel (LFT)
- Urinalysis (UA)
- Cardiac Markers
- Coagulation

In addition to identifying labs that have situational relevance, I have included a brief rationale to present the "essence" of this NEED to know content. I have found that as a nurse educator, LESS can be MORE. Though a lab manual goes into needed additional depth, if your students could grasp and understand the essence of the short descriptions of each lab panel described below, they will be well on their way to being prepared for professional practice

One Panel a Week!

One practical way to present this content for your students in the clinical setting is to take one lab panel a week in the basic or advanced med/surg rotation and discuss it in post-conference. Discuss what each lab is testing and why it may be relevant. Use a patient that a student cared for to illustrate the importance of this panel to the primary problem and to contextualize the following labs that have situational relevance.

Basic Metabolic Panel (BMP)

- **Chloride (95–105 mEq/L)** Relevant if NG suction or frequent vomiting is present due to loss of hydrochloric acid. Chloride is the Cl- of hydrochloric acid.
- **CO2 (22–28 mEq/L)** Relevant when there are acid-base concerns. Though it is CO2 on a BMP and students may assume it is carbon dioxide, it actually reflects the amount of HCO3-!
- **Anion Gap (AG) (7–16 mEq/l)** This is the difference between primary measured cations (Na+ and K+) and the primary measured anions (chloride Cl- and bicarbonate HCO3-) in serum. Useful with acid/base concerns typically seen in renal failure.
- **Glucose (Fasting: 70–110 mg/dL)** Relevant with history of diabetes. Elevated levels post-op increase can increase risk of infection/sepsis.
- **Calcium (8.4–10.2 mg/dL)** Relevant with renal failure and ETOH abuse. Low albumin can cause hypocalcemia, while elevated levels can be seen with cancer (with and without bone metastases).
- **BUN** (7–25 mg/dl) I use creatinine/GFR as the most relevant/important lab to determine renal function. I do not consistently use BUN in practice as it can be

elevated for other reasons rather than renal, though it is relevant with renal failure to trend with creatinine and will also be elevated with dehydration.

Miscellaneous Chemistries

- **Phosphorus (2.5–4.5 mg/dl)** 85 percent stored in bones. Primary intracellular anion and responsible for cellular metabolism and formation of bones and teeth. Relevant in renal failure and will be increased due to decreased renal excretion.
- **Ionized Calcium (1.05–1.46 mmol/L)** Represents Ca++ that is metabolically available compared to serum Ca++ that is more generalized. This value is a more accurate determinate of calcium and if low, serum calcium is usually also decreased.
- **Amylase (25–125 U/l)** Digestive enzyme breaks down complex carbohydrates. Primarily formed in pancreas and will "leak" into circulation with pancreatic inflammation.
  - Relevant with pancreatitis/cholecystitis and obstruction of common bile duct that leads to pancreatic inflammation.
- **Lipase (3–73 units/L)** Glycoprotein produced primarily in pancreas to break down fats. Will "leak" into circulation with pancreatic inflammation. Relevant with pancreatitis/cholecystitis and obstruction of common bile duct that leads to pancreatic inflammation.
- **Ammonia (20–100 mcg/dL)** Blood ammonia comes from two sources: deamination of amino acids during protein metabolism, and degradation of proteins by colon bacteria. The liver converts ammonia in the portal blood to urea, which is excreted by the kidneys. When liver function is impaired, ammonia levels rise. Ammonia is potentially toxic to the central nervous system and causes acute confusion and altered mental status. Is a contributing factor to hepatic encephalopathy in end-stage liver disease.

Complete Blood Count (CBC)

- **Hematocrit (male: 39–49 %; female: 35–45 %)** In comparison to hemoglobin, hematocrit is not as relevant, though elevation can be seen to confirm fluid volume deficit. It will be concentrated and elevated in this context.

- **RBCs (male: 4.3–5.7 (x108/µl); female: 3.8–5.1 (x108/ µl)** Identifies the number of RBCs in a cubic millimeter. In anemia or when there has been a significant blood loss, hemoglobin is the GOLD STANDARD that must be noted. I rarely find this value relevant as most practitioners emphasize hemoglobin in practice.
- **Platelet count (150–450 x 103/µl)** Relevant whenever there is a concern for anemia or blood loss or the patient is on heparin. If this is low, it will obviously be significant and must be noted. Any patient on heparin products must also have this noted because of the clinical possibility of heparin-induced thrombocytopenia (HIT), which develops when the immune system forms antibodies against heparin that cause small clots and lower platelet levels.

WBC Differential

- **Band forms (3–5 %)** Immature neutrophils that are elevated in sepsis as the body attempts to fight infection and releases these prematurely. If elevated, it's a clinical RED FLAG in the context of sepsis. If elevated to >8, it is considered a "shift to the left," which indicates impending sepsis.
- **Lymphocytes (23–33%)** Relevant when there is a known or suspected VIRAL infection.
- **Monocytes (3–7%)** Are phagocytes similar to neutrophils, but not as dominant, nor are they as clinically significant and relevant to practice as neutrophils.
- **Eosinophils (1–3 %)** Elevated with parasitic infections or allergic responses.
- **Basophils (0–1%)** Phagocytes, but not as dominant nor are they as clinically significant and rele-vant to practice as neutrophils.

Liver Panel (LFT)

The relevance of this panel will depend on the primary problem and chief complaint, but if patient has a Gastro Intestinal (GI) primary problem, they are ALL relevant!

- **Albumin (3.5–5.5 g/dL)** is a large colloid plasma protein made by the liver. Because it is comprised of protein, it will be decreased in malnutrition. Therefore, it can be a contributing factor to ascites or edema.
- **Total Bilirubin (0.1–1.0 mg/dL // 0.0–0.3 mg/dL)**

Total of both direct/indirect bilirubin. Bilirubin is metabolized by the liver and is broken down by-product of heme protein in RBCs. Relevant in any liver disease.

- **Alkaline Phosphatase (male: 38–126 U/l; female: 70–230 U/l)** Nonspecific hepatic iso-enzyme that has large concentration in liver, but found in other parts of the body. If there is a primary liver disease, focus on ALT, AST as these are much more specific to liver function.

- **ALT (8–20 U/L)** Relevant with any primary liver disease. This enzyme is found in the liver. It's released into circulation when liver cells are damaged. Has a higher specificity to liver than AST.

- **AST (8–20 U/L)** Relevant with any primary liver disease. Found in the liver, this enzyme is released into circulation when liver cells are damaged.

Urinalysis

- **Color (yellow)** Clear to pale yellow is usually seen with aggressive diuresis. Orange color typically due to bilirubin in urine with liver disease. Dark amber is commonly seen with dehydration or fluid volume deficit.

- **Clarity (clear)** Though the context here is a UA, students must recognize the importance of always evaluating the clarity in the tubing of any patient with a Foley catheter. If urine is cloudy or has sediment, this reflects possible urinary tract infection (UTI). UA should be obtained, especially if new finding.

- **Specific Gravity (1.015–1.030)** Measures the kidney's ability to concentrate or dilute urine in relation to plasma. Increased with dehydration and decreased with diuresis.

- **Protein (neg)** Relevant when positive in any patient with renal disease. If kidneys have been damaged or there is a new finding of renal failure, proteins, being a large colloid, should be filtered by glomerulus. If there is damage to the glomeruli, the inability to adequately filter urine will be present and, therefore, will be positive. However, in active young adolescent females there is a phenomenon that produces a higher protein in the urine. A first voiding of the day should be measured with these individuals.

- **Glucose (neg)** Relevant if patient is diabetic. The degree of presence in urine reflects poorly controlled diabetes. Same rationale as protein above. Glucose is also a large particle that should be filtered by glomerulus.

- **Ketones (neg)** Ketones are formed from the metabolism of fatty acids. Relevant and most commonly seen in DKA and dehydration.

- **Bilirubin (neg)** Must be noted and relevant with liver disease. Should be negative, but with liver disease may be positive.

- **Blood (neg)** Will typically be positive if patient has UTI or renal calculi.

- **Nitrite (neg)** To rule out UTI or determine if present, nitrites, LET, and WBC micro must be assessed together. Nitrites are relevant because if positive, they reflect the presence of gram negative bacteria in the urinary tract, the most common being E. coli. By itself is not a predictable indicator of urinary infection.

- **LET (Leukocyte Esterase) (neg)** To rule out UTI or determine if present, nitrites, LET, and WBC micro must be assessed together. LET is relevant. This enzyme is present if WBCs are in the urine. By itself is not a predictable indicator of urinary infection.

UA Micro

- **RBCs (<5)** Must be noted if UTI or renal calculi–this gives amount of RBCs present which can correlate with severity.

- **WBCs (<5)** ALWAYS RELEVANT and GOLD STANDARD. By itself, WBC indicates the presence of UTI if patient has symptoms. Most clinicians will diagnose UTI if >5 WBCs are present in urine and symptomatic. Amount of WBCs present indicates severity. To rule out UTI or determine if present, nitrites, LET, and WBC micro must be clustered and assessed together.

- **Bacteria (neg)** Does not consistently correlate to presence of infection, though it can be clustered with WBC, LET, and nitrites.

- **Epithelial (neg)** Skin cells that are present but not relevant in itself.

Trending to Rescue

Trending ALL RELEVANT clinical data including relevant lab values is foundational to thinking like a nurse in practice. This will be discussed in more depth in the upcoming chapters. Consistent trending and comparison of all relevant clinical data allows the nurse to identify and capture trends that may reflect a concerning change in patient status. Vigilant trending allows the nurse to rescue his/her patient and initiate needed nursing interventions before an adverse outcome occurs. To do this in practice, students need to identify the lab values that are most important and RELEVANT based on the PRIMARY PROBLEM. This is the transfer of knowledge from the classroom to the bedside that needs to take place so students are well prepared for real-world practice.

Reflect

Wall #1: Pathophysiology

1. What applied sciences do you need to deepen your understanding of to be a more effective nurse educator?

2. How do you integrate pathophysiology in your classroom lecture or clinical setting?

Wall #2: Nursing Pharmacology

1. How do you integrate pharmacology and the mechanism of action in your classroom lecture or clinical setting?

2. What do you expect your students to know before they administer medications in the clinical setting? Could this bar be higher?

Wall #3: Fluids & Electrolytes (F&E)

1. How do you integrate F&E and lab values in your classroom lecture or clinical setting?

2. What is your current bar for student knowledge of lab values? Could it be higher?

3. Do you filter for your students the most and least important lab values in your clinical setting or the most commonly used lab panels?

References

Amiodarone. Micromedex. (2014). Retrieved from http://www.micromedexsolutions.com/micromedex2/librarian/ND_T/evidencexpert/ND_PR/evidencexpert/CS/D1F681/ND_AppProduct/evidencexpert/DUPLICATIONSHIELDSYNC/CE977D/ND_PG/evidencexpert/ND_B/evidencexpert/ND_P/evidencexpert/PFActionId/evidencexpert.DisplayDrugpointDocument?docId=025645&contentSetId=100&title=Amiodarone+Hydrochloride&servicesTitle=

Benner, P. (1982). From novice to expert. *American Journal of Nursing, 82*(3), 402–407.

Benner, P., Sutphen, M., Leonard, V., & Day, L. (2010). *Educating nurses: A call for radical transformation.* San Francisco, CA: Jossey-Bass.

Eraut, M. (1994). *Developing professional knowledge and competence.* Washington, DC: Falmer Press.

Van Horn, E, Hyde, Y.M., Tesh, A.S., & Kautz, D.D. (2014). Teaching pathophysiology: strategies to enliven the traditional lecture. *Nurse Educator, 39*(1), 34-37.

Van Leeuwen, A., & Poelhuis-Leth, D. J. (2009). *Davis's comprehensive handbook of laboratory and diagnostic tests with nursing implications.* (3rd ed.). Philadelphia, PA: F.A. Davis Company.

Strategies and Tools to Teach the Applied Sciences

Keith Rischer, RN, MA, CEN, CCRN

"What has been gained by knowledge is too easily forgotten.
Look for the ideal, but put it into the actual."

—Florence Nightingale

Active Learning Strategies for Pathophysiology

Whether your program teaches pathophysiology as a prerequisite by science professors or by nursing faculty, reinforce this essential content in your nursing program with the following active learning strategies to help students apply this essential content to clinical practice (Van Horn, Hyde, Tesh, & Kautz, 2014).

Case Studies

Case studies that emphasize the underlying pathophysiology, clinical manifestations, and rationale can effectively contextualize this content to practice. Emphasize and develop questions related to the pathophysiology with a salient clinical scenario. For example, in a patient with heart failure and hypokalemia, develop questions related to right-sided heart failure vs. left-sided heart failure and biventricular heart failure. If the patient develops runs of ventricular tachycardia, explore the relationship between hypokalemia and cardiac rhythm disturbances.

Visual Demonstrations

Be creative using visual demonstrations or illustrations when teaching pathophysiology. Visual demonstrations can help students make connections that enhance their understanding and retention. This is especially helpful for students who are visual learners.

For example, the Frank-Starling law of the heart can be demonstrated using a rubber band. When the rubber band is at first stretched and released, it responds by flying a significant distance. But when the band is repeatedly stretched it loses its elasticity and recoil and does not go as far. This represents what happens to cardiac muscle fibers when they are overstretched repeatedly in heart failure.

Create an Educational Pamphlet

Instead of relying on the educational pamphlets of the institution where you have clinical, have students create their own. Break students into small groups and review the pathophysiology, clinical manifestations, rationale for treatment, and patient education required for the medical problem that is selected. Students take what they know about this topic and create an educational pamphlet on this topic in lay person terminology that is no higher than a seventh-grade reading level.

This requires students to synthesize large amounts of complex content and break it down to the bare essentials. Once this has been completed, students develop questions to use with the patient to assess knowledge of what has been taught using this pamphlet. Once this project is completed, the pamphlet can be used to educate patients and/or families when students are in the clinical setting.

Tool #1:
Medications to Master Worksheet

A practical strategy to filter pharmacology content and develop mastery of what is most important to clinical practice is to identify the top ten medications used in your clinical setting or related to the topic you are teaching in the classroom. Make a list of the top ten medications or pharmacologic classifications that must be deeply understood because they are most important or most commonly used in their practice setting. Physicians and primary care providers are creatures of habit, and tend to order and use the same medications consistently. Therefore, let your students know that 75–100 medications will make up the majority of the medications used in most clinical areas.

To simplify this process of med knowledge acquisition, I created a blank template titled "Medications That Must Be Mastered Worksheet" that is included in the Transformation Toolbox supplement to this book. It incorporates the "foundational five" questions to DEEPEN student knowledge. Consider having your students complete this worksheet BEFORE the first clinical for the most commonly used medications in the clinical setting where they work.

Make it a goal for each student to internalize the essence of these "foundational five" questions for the most common medications in your clinical setting by the end of the clinical rotation so they can be stated from memory. This knowledge can be carried over into the next clinical experience with another 10–15 medications to master.

If this exercise is done in every clinical rotation of basic med/surg, advanced med/surg, OB, peds, mental health, and capstone or summative clinical experience, your students will have DEEP knowledge of at least 60–100 medications that will prepare them for professional practice as well as the NCLEX. To maximize the effectiveness of this approach, develop a departmental consensus of the overall top 60–100 medications. Once this has been determined, decide which medications will be emphasized for each clinical rotation.

This list of 45 medications are most commonly administered in acute care settings where I practice. Use this list as a starting point to get the ball rolling! Add or subtract from this list depending on the clinical setting that you teach.

Most Common Medications That Must Be Mastered (Generic)		
Antihypertensives B-blockers: Atenolol/Metoprolol ACE-I: Captopril/Lisinopril Ca-channel blockers: Diltiazem	**Respiratory** Albuterol fluticasone/salmeterol (Advair Diskus)	**Non-opioid Analgesics** Ketorolac Acetaminophen Ibuprofen
Antiarrhythmic Amiodarone Digoxin	**GI** H2 blocker: Ranitidine/Famotidine PPI-Pantoprazole/Omeprazole Ondansetron/Metoclopramide Docusate/Senna	**Opioid Analgesics** Hydromorphone Morphine Percocet/Vicodin (trade name)
Diuretics Loop: Furosemide Thiazide: HCTZ K+ sparing: Spironolactone	**Diabetic** All insulins Humalog/Novolog Regular/NPH Lente Glyburide/Metformin	**Antianxiety** Lorazepam/Diazepam **Anti-Infectives** Ciprofloxacin Vancomycin Metronidazole
Lipid lowering Statins (all)	Misc.	Cefazolin piperacillin/tazobactam
Anticoagulants Warfarin Heparin/Enoxaparin	Potassium chloride Levothyroxine Prednisone/Methylprednisolone	

Tool #2:
Lab Planning Worksheet

The need to teach multiple ways of nurse thinking in addition to critical thinking or clinical reasoning is needed to realize change in nursing education (Benner, et al., 2010). Another way of nurse thinking is developing a plan of care based on RELEVANT, abnormal labs for each patient. I call this "lab planning." It is not enough to identify that a lab value is abnormal. The nurse must know the pathophysiology and determine if it is RELEVANT to the primary problem. If the answer is yes, the nurse must be able to identify what to DO about it by determining the assessments and interventions to implement because of this relevant, abnormal lab.

The ability to recognize the relevance of abnormal clinical data including labs requires time and experience to develop in the clinical setting. By putting this content into context in practice, students will identify and recognize the relationship between the primary problem and the most relevant clinical data.

For example, a student is caring for a patient who has been admitted for heart failure exacerbation and collects the following data from the chart:

- Creatinine increased from a baseline of 1.4 and is now 2.5
- B-Natriuretic Peptide (BNP) increased from a baseline of 180 and is now 1255

The nurse can use these relevant, abnormal findings to create a "lab plan of care" that will dovetail with traditional nursing care priorities based on the primary problem. Because creatinine is a key indicator of renal function and kidney perfusion and the BNP represents the degree of ventricular stretch and overload, the student nurse needs to recognize the clinical significance and relationship of these labs to the primary problem. If this is done, the nurse will be able to use this knowledge to develop a "lab plan of care" with needed nursing assessments and interventions. A full page template of this "Lab Planning" activity is included in the Transformation Toolbox in the appendix.

For example:

Relevant Lab:	Nursing Interventions:
Creatinine: 2.5 (0.6-1.2 mg/dL	1. Assess urine output and I&O. Determine if minimum of 30 mL/hour of urine output is present 2. Fluid restriction if ordered 3. Assess for signs of fluid retention/edema 4. Assess daily weight and trend daily

Relevant Lab:	Nursing Interventions:
BNP: 1255 (<100)	1. Assess respiratory status for tachypnea and breath sounds for basilar or scattered crackles (may be fine or course crackles depending on severity) 2. Assess HR and SBP carefully to promote decreased cardiac workload 3. Assess tolerance to activity 4. Assess I&O and urine output 5. Assess daily weight and trend daily 6. Assess lower extremities for pitting edema 7. Assess CMS of extremities

Reflect

Identify Your Top 10 Medications

Identify your top ten medications that your students must know DEEPLY for your classroom content or clinical settings:

1.

2.

3.

4.

5.

6.

7.

8.

9.

10.

Identify Your Top 10 Labs

Identify your top ten labs that your students must know DEEPLY for your classroom content or clinical settings:

1.

2.

3.

4.

5.

6.

7.

8.

9.

10.

References

Van Horn, E.R., Hyde, Y.M., Tesh, A.S., & Kautz, D.D. (2014) Teaching pathophysiology: Strategies to enliven the traditional lecture. *Nurse Educator, 39*(1), 34-37.

Raising the Roof:
Four Trusses of Nurse Thinking

Keith Rischer, RN, MA, CEN, CCRN

*"Are nurses entering practice equipped with the knowledge and skills
for today's practice...we found that, in short, the answer is no."*

—*Educating Nurses: A Call for Radical Transformation,* p. 31

In a home, the roof trusses tie the four walls and the rest of the structure together. The same is true for the "roof" of nurse thinking. It ties the walls of the applied sciences and the foundation of the "art" of nursing together. If the roof of nurse thinking is weak and not well developed, the development of the "living house" is impacted adversely and not as strong in order to be safe in practice. Though the "art" of nursing is foundational to my "living house" metaphor of nursing education, it is the roof of NURSE THINKING, or lack of it, that can make the difference between life and death. This can happen when a student fails to apply content knowledge, think like a nurse, and rescue a patient with a change in status.

Four Trusses of Nurse Thinking

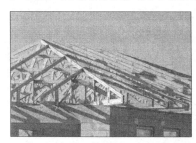
Thinking like a nurse is something that experienced nurses tend to take for granted. But the "roof" of "nurse thinking" must be built from scratch and needs to be developed in students who will continue to progress and strengthen this skill with clinical experience. The goal of nursing education is to provide the framework for each roof truss with relevant content

so it can be strengthened by ongoing clinical experience as a student and then progress once in autonomous practice.

Multiple ways of nurse thinking need to be incorporated into nursing education (Benner, et al., 2010). As I reflect upon my own clinical experience and practice, thinking like a nurse has four distinct constructs or "roof trusses." Each truss of nurse thinking must be DEEPLY understood and then applied to practice.

These roof trusses are:

1. Nursing process
2. Critical thinking
3. Recognizing relationships of clinical data (pattern recognition)
4. Clinical reasoning

In traditional nursing education, the two "roof trusses" of nursing process and critical thinking have been emphasized the most. Identifying and recognizing the relationship of clinical data and clinical reasoning are also essential to thinking like a nurse and need to be addressed to prepare students for professional practice. Clinical reasoning must be emphasized to bring needed transformation to nursing education. As each of these "roof trusses" of nurse thinking is reviewed in depth, carefully reflect and evaluate what needs to be strengthened in your program so that students are able to think more like a nurse and successfully transition to professional practice.

Roof Truss #1: The Nursing Process

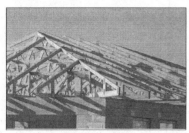 The nursing process has been the bedrock of nursing education for decades. Understanding and then applying the nursing process to the bedside is the essence of thinking like a nurse and typically introduced and taught at the fundamental level. In this brief review, I will share some additional insights on each step:

Assessment

Comprehensive, systematic assessment is the first step in delivering nursing care that includes collecting and recognizing RELEVANT clinical data. This encompasses not only physical assessment data, but also psychological, sociocultural, spiritual, economic, and lifestyle assessment data as well. TRENDING assessment data involves applying critical thinking and interpreting the data obtained from the patient.

Nursing Priority/Diagnosis

This is the priority that is identified once clinical data from the chart as well as data personally collected is assimilated by the nurse. This judgment forms the basis for the plan of care. Critical thinking and clinical reasoning must also be incorporated and are essential skills to recognize the correct nursing priority.

I relate step 2 of the nursing process to clinical practice by emphasizing and establishing a nursing PRIORITY, which is a key component of clinical reasoning and de-emphasizing nursing diagnosis. You cannot have a nursing diagnosis without NANDA. Based on my clinical practice of 35 years, a three-part NANDA nursing diagnostic statement does NOT represent the essence of how nurses think and set priorities once in clinical practice.

The emphasis of NANDA nursing diagnostic NANDA must be de-emphasized and clinical reasoning emphasized by placing the nursing process within this framework of clinical reasoning. By implementing this paradigm shift, students will be well prepared for clinical practice (as well as the NCLEX!).

Outcomes/Planning

Based on the assessment and establishment of nursing priorities, a plan of nursing care is established. The nurse also sets measurable and achievable short and long-range outcomes.

Implementation

Nursing care is implemented according to the care plan, which is specific to the patient and focuses on achievable outcomes.

Evaluation

Both the patient's status and the response to nursing care must be continuously evaluated, and the care plan modified as needed to determine if outcomes have been met (Berman, Snyder, & Frandsen, 2016). Clinical reasoning, with its emphasis of thinking in action, must also be incorporated and applied to this final step.

Clinical Reasoning and Nursing Process

Nursing process and clinical reasoning are two separate constructs but complement one another in practice. Clinical reasoning can be defined as the ability of the nurse to think in action and reason as a situation changes over time by capturing and understanding the significance of clinical trajectories and grasping the essence of the current clinical situation (Benner, et al., 2010). Highlighted below are aspects of clinical reasoning that are clearly situated in nursing process. This emphasis can be incorporated when nursing process is first taught so key components of clinical reasoning can be situated as nursing process is taught to beginning students.

Assessment: Recognizing RELEVANCE

As novice nurses, students see EVERYTHING that is collected in the clinical setting as equally relevant and important (Benner, 1984). They do not have clinical experience to guide them to FILTER clinical data by relevance. Make it a priority throughout each level of your program to APPLY classroom and clinical knowledge students have developed.

When content is contextualized and applied to the bedside, it will help students recognize what is most and least important so they can determine if an actual problem is present (Benner, et al., 2010). Clinical data does NOT need to be abnormal to be RELEVANT. Vital signs are ALWAYS vital, and even when normal, are always relevant.

For example, consider a patient who just arrived to the floor from the OR who has a

- Temperature: 98.6 F (37.0 C)
- HR of 80
- RR of 20
- BP of 120/80
- O2 sat of 95%.

Though this clinical data is normal, it is relevant because it communicates clinical stability. It is not uncommon to have students write N/A when asked the clinical relevance of vital signs within normal range!

Nursing Priority: What Is My PRIORITY?

Assessment must be performed accurately and thoroughly. Only when students can translate classroom theory to the bedside and identify relevant clinical data and INTERPRET its importance will they be able to identify the presence of a possible problem and establish proper nursing priorities. Failure to rescue a patient with a worsening change of status is a failure to apply clinical reasoning to the assessment and nursing priority steps of the nursing process.

Outcomes/Planning: Think in ACTION

Unless the correct nursing priority is identified through assessment of relevant clinical data, identified outcomes and planning will be affected. Assessment is like the first of several dominos set upright. Get it right and the series of dominos will fall correctly and in the right direction. But if the nurse misses relevant data and a problem goes unrecognized, the dominos will also fall, but in the wrong direction! This will ultimately lead to failure to rescue a patient with a change of status by making an incorrect judgment, leading to the wrong nursing priority, which will lead to an incorrect plan and implementation.

Implementation: Failure to Rescue

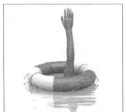

Implementation is only as good as the assessment, correct nursing priority, and resultant plan of care. If clinical reasoning has not been correctly situated, patient outcomes will be impacted by NOT implementing needed interventions. This will ul-

timately lead to failure to rescue. This chain of events can be readily seen during simulation, when students can continue even when essential data is missed and the Sim-Man reflects a status change that can ultimately progress to a full arrest! Unfortunately, this can also happen in practice and can lead to the same outcome!

Evaluation: Think in ACTION

The ability to think in action is a key component of clinical reasoning and the essence of evaluation. Clinical data is continually collected and the patient's response to the plan of care is evaluated by the nurse. But unless the nurse recognizes the relevance and significance of evaluative data that is collected, a change of status, if present, will remain unrecognized. EARLY assessment findings of common complications must be identified so that students will recognize the significance of subtle but significant changes earlier vs. later, when it may be too late.

An excellent example of this principle in practice is when a patient develops sepsis. If early signs of sepsis that include tachycardia but a normal blood pressure are not recognized, when the nurse evaluates the next set of vital signs and finds that the blood pressure has dropped to 78/30, evaluation will identify that a problem is present. Unfortunately, it may be too late to prevent an adverse outcome.

Roof Truss #2: Critical Thinking

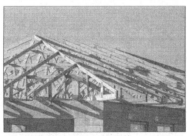

Critical thinking has been emphasized as an essential nurse thinking skill for decades (Dressel & Mayhew, 1954), and is an essential concept that must be applied to practice. But according to Educating Nurses, it must be de-emphasized yet still retained (Benner, et al., 2010).

But critical thinking is NOT the same as clinical thinking. Despite textbooks on the topic, critical thinking does not improve, despite attempts to teach it (Tanner, 2005). Staib (2003) identified that there is no consistent correlation between measures of critical thinking and translation to clinical decision making or clinical judgment.

Although critical thinking has been touted as one of the most important characteristics of a professional nurse, no clear explanation exists to define it (Lassater, 2011)! How can students be expected to "critically think" when there is not an agreed-upon understanding of what it comprises? Alfaro-LeFevre (2013) recognizes this dilemma:

"Critical thinking is a complex process that changes depending on context–what you're trying to accomplish. For this reason there is no one right definition for critical thinking. Many authors [including me] develop their own descriptions to complement and clarify someone else's...to analyze it and decide what it means to you rather than simply memorizing someone else's words." (Alfaro-LeFevre, 2013, p. 7)

But if you are a student, would you be comforted by the ambiguity suggested by this essential concept that must be applied to practice? I don't think so. The following are examples of the numerous definitions to describe critical thinking in the literature:

- Critical thinking is influenced by one's knowledge, experience, and using reflective thinking to identify what is needed and synthesize this into practice (Bittner & Tobin, 1998).
- "The nurses' ability to focus their thinking to achieve timely, quality outcomes" (Alfaro-LeFevre, 2013, p. x).
- "Thinking about your thinking, while you're thinking, to make it better, more clear, accurate, and defensible" (Paul & Elder, 2005).

These accepted definitions used in nursing education have relevance, but are too broad in their scope for an overwhelmed novice nursing student to practically translate these definitions to the bedside. According to Benner's work on clinical progression, students who are novice nurses are concrete learners (Benner, 1982). Therefore, critical thinking must also be defined as simply and concretely as possible.

Essence of Critical Thinking

There is an exception to the ambiguity that can define critical thinking. Potter & Perry (2013) have a practical definition that helps students recognize the importance of this construct of nurse thinking. Critical thinking is a commitment to think:

- Clearly
- Precisely

- Accurately
- ACT on what you know about a situation

This is why nurse educators must make it a priority to decrease content saturation and TMI in their content. To critically think, students must KNOW or have a DEEP knowledge of what is most important in order to ACT on what they know. When students are expected to master a broad body of content, they will acquire a superficial depth of understanding to pass a test, but not the deeper level of knowledge required to UNDERSTAND and USE this knowledge at the bedside. When students have the walls of the applied sciences strongly developed and built in their "living house," they will be able to ACT on what they know and recognize relevant clinical relationships of clinical data in each patient they care for, which is the next level of clinical thinking.

Roof Truss #3: Identify Relationships of Clinical Data

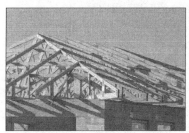

Pattern recognition is the first step of intuitive clinical judgment making that guides advanced nurse thinking. It is the ability of the nurse to recognize relationships of patterned patient responses (Benner & Tanner, 1987). Recognizing clinical relationships is another "way of thinking" (Benner, et al., p. 84) that can help students think more like a nurse. When clinical relationships are recognized and identified by the student, clinical data collected begins to "fit" and the patient puzzle begins to "fit" and come together.

For the puzzle to be CORRECTLY assembled by the nurse, clinical data must be sorted and filtered to determine if it is relevant or most important. The identification of relevant data is needed to make correct clinical judgments that will form the foundation for clinical reasoning in practice. The nurse can ask a series of questions to determine if a relationship of clinical data is present.

The first five relationships address the primary medical problem. The last two questions address the nursing priority in the context of the medical problem and how they are related and intersect, and the relationship of the primary nursing priority to other identified nursing priorities.

SEVEN CLINICAL RELATIONSHIPS OF NURSE THINKING

Medical Problem:
  1. Identify the RELATIONSHIP: What current medications are treating past medical problems?
  2. Is there a RELATIONSHIP between the past medical history and/or psychosocial needs that may have contributed to the development of the current primary problem?
  3. What is the RELATIONSHIP between the primary problem and the current chief complaint?
  4. What is the RELATIONSHIP between relevant clinical data and the primary problem?
  5. What is the RELATIONSHIP between any new orders and the primary problem?

Nursing Priorities:
  6. What is the RELATIONSHIP between the primary medical problem and nursing priority(ies)?
  7. What is the RELATIONSHIP between the primary nursing priority and secondary nursing priorities?

These seven clinical relationships will help the nurse develop the "big picture." Each relationship is further defined and explained below:

1. Identify the RELATIONSHIP: What current medications are treating past medical problems?

This is the most basic clinical relationship that beginning students can be guided to recognize. To identify the clinical relationship between current medications and past medical problems, the nurse must know not only what the medication is for, but based on the patient's history, WHY he is receiving it. For example, if a patient is receiving atenolol, he most likely has a history of hypertension. But if the patient has no history of hypertension but does have atrial fibrillation, would your students be able to identify the clinical relationship between atenolol and atrial fibrillation?

If students DEEPLY understand the mechanism of action of a beta blocker, they will be able to connect this information to atrial fibrillation. Atrial fibrillation can cause a rapid ventricular response or HR>100. Atenolol is indicated to keep the heart rate within normal limits.

Once this clinical relationship is recognized, students will be able to see the "fit" and put these two clinical "puzzle" pieces together. This will build their confidence to help them recognize the significance of the next clinical relationship.

2. Is there a RELATIONSHIP between the past medical history and/or psychosocial needs that may have contributed to the development of the current primary problem?

To recognize this clinical relationship, students must have a strong "wall" built of applied pathophysiology. Pathophysiology must be DEEPLY understood so students can identify the contributing risk factors of the most common disease processes. Another way to view this relationship is the "domino effect." When one domino (problem) begins to fall (develop), it affects the next domino and causes another problem to develop as a consequence.

For example, a student has a patient who is admitted with heart failure exacerbation and has a history of:
  • Hypertension
  • Hyperlipidemia
  • Myocardial infarction (MI)
  • Ischemic cardiomyopathy with ejection fraction of 20%

Would he/she be able to recognize the clinical relationship between any or all of these problems? These problems did NOT develop in isolation, but every one of these illnesses has a relationship to the other. To take this clinical relationship identification one step further, could students list these illnesses that have relationship to one another in the chronological order they most likely occurred from first to last?

In this example, the order of progression with each problem is a domino that caused the next to develop:
  1. Hyperlipidemia as well as hypertension caused underlying damage to the arterial vessels that accelerated the development of atherosclerosis.
  2. This caused the next domino to fall, which is an acute MI.
  3. Because of chronic ischemia secondary to progressive atherosclerosis and MI, the ischemic cardiomyopathy domino has now fallen.
  4. Finally, as the cardiomyopathy progresses, the ejec-

tion fraction domino falls and is reflected by a deterioration of function from a normal range of 60–65% to now only 20%.

Psychosocial Needs

In addition to the physiological problems that may have been influenced by the past medical problem, the patient must be viewed holistically. The relationship of psychosocial needs, including relevant mental health problems, must be identified and addressed by the nurse. If a patient has a history of depression, anxiety, or schizophrenia, these mental health problems can directly or indirectly influence physiologic health.

If a patient is a native of another country, the influence of culture, and the ability to understand English may influence his or her ability to value or understand the plan of care to maintain health. Educational needs, emotional support, current stress level, and recent losses—including the death of a loved one—need to be recognized, identified, and remedied before discharge. These psychosocial needs are not as obvious as the pressing physiologic needs, but when they are intentionally assessed and identified, they will guide the nurse to consistently deliver holistic care.

3. What is the RELATIONSHIP between the primary problem and the current chief complaint?

To recognize this clinical relationship, pathophysiology needs to be understood and applied to the bedside. For example, what if the same patient who was situated in relationship #2 presented to the ED with an exacerbation of heart failure, and had the following presenting symptoms:
- SOB
- Orthopnea
- Decreased tolerance to activity
- 2+ pitting edema in lower legs
- Weight gain of five pounds in the last two days

When the pathophysiology of left- to right-sided heart failure exacerbation is understood, the relationship of these symptoms becomes evident. Shortness of breath and orthopnea are classic signs of left-sided failure, while pitting edema and weight gain reflect right-sided heart failure. When this relationship is recognized, two more pieces of the clinical puzzle for this patient are con-

nected! DEEP understanding of pathophysiology and the ability to think critically in practice will lay the foundation to recognize this relationship in clinical practice.

4. What is the RELATIONSHIP between relevant clinical data and the primary problem?

To recognize this clinical relationship, students must be able to identify the most important clinical data and relate it to the primary medical problem. Relevant clinical data would include physical assessment findings, vital signs, and laboratory values.

Using the same example of a patient with heart failure exacerbation, you have now collected the following relevant clinical data:
- 2+ pitting edema in lower legs
- Coarse crackles half-way up bilaterally
- Respiratory rate 24/minute with O2 sat 88% on room air
- BP: 178/88
- Creatinine: 1.9/last creatinine was 1.1
- BNP: 1125/last BNP was 210

Based on this relevant clinical data and a DEEP understanding of pathophysiology, would your students be able to identify the clinical data that supports right-sided heart failure, and the data that reflects left-sided heart failure? (2+ pitting edema is right-sided failure, while the crackles and low O2 sat reflect left)

Is there a relationship between left-sided failure, crackles, RR 24, and O2 sat of 88%? Is the blood pressure too high? What is the significance of increased afterload for this patient in heart failure? Finally, the laboratory values must be understood and situated with the primary medical problem.

Why would the creatinine be elevated? If students can recognize the relationship between decreased cardiac output from heart failure exacerbation and kidney perfusion, they are on their way to thinking like a nurse! The BNP is also elevated. WHY? The relationship of left ventricular stress and overload and this neurohormone must be recognized. Note the TREND of the BNP. What does this represent clinically?

In addition to recognizing that the BNP is elevated in heart failure exacerbation, could your students state the physiologic effects that BNP has on the body during heart failure? This, too, must be understood. (The body was designed with many compensatory mechanisms, and BNP acts as a vasodilator and has diuretic effects that lower preload as well as afterload and the workload of the heart when it is failing.)

5. What is the RELATIONSHIP between any new orders and the primary problem?

Though the nurse is not a primary care provider, she/he must be able to understand the rationale for everything that is ordered and how these orders relate to the patient's primary medical problem. By questioning an order that does not make sense based on the primary problem and recognizing the importance of this relationship, the nurse can prevent an error that could have devastating consequences when the WHY or rationale of all orders are clearly understood. This is an example of why a nurse must be able to understand the essence of physician practice in order to be a better nurse.

Let's continue with the same patient who has heart failure exacerbation. The primary care provider writes the following orders:

- Furosemide 40 mg IV push
- Nitroglycerin IV gtt-titrate to keep SBP <140

To recognize the clinical relationship of these orders to the medical problem, students must also have a strong "wall" built of applied pharmacology and pathophysiology and understand the mechanism of action for every medication administered. Ask your students, "Why would the primary care provider order these medications for someone with heart failure?" When they UNDERSTAND the mechanism of action for each of these medications, and how they will help resolve the primary problem, this relationship becomes evident.

Furosemide is a loop diuretic that will promote potent diuresis and decrease pre-load. But WHAT IF the patient has 1000 mL of urine output two hours following administration, and the most recent potassium was 3.5? Identifying the relationship of the loss of electrolytes, including potassium, with increased diuresis is essential to safe practice and thinking like a nurse.

The nurse must also recognize that even though the potassium was normal, it was in the low normal range before diuresis. Therefore, the nurse must be able to situate F&E and recall the most common signs and symptoms of hypokalemia, especially if muscle weakness and increased ventricular ectopy are present and then make a correct clinical judgment and use an SBAR to contact the primary care provider to recommend a recheck of the serum potassium.

Why would the primary care provider want the systolic blood pressure (SBP) <140 and how will nitroglycerin IV drip accomplish this objective? Does an elevated SBP and increased afterload increase the workload of the heart? Is this going to help or hurt this patient with heart failure? Nitroglycerin dilates coronary arteries for those with angina, but dilates systemic venous circulation, which will benefit the patient by decreasing preload as well as afterload. This will also decrease the workload of the heart, the primary objective with exacerbation of heart failure.

Another benefit that a DEEP understanding of pharmacology and pathophysiology offers is that it will deepen students' critical thinking. This is done by recognizing any possible implications or contraindications of medications that are ordered. For example, many heart failure patients develop atrial fibrillation. The mechanism of action of medications used to control this rhythm such as diltiazem or metoprolol must be understood.

Do both of these medications have negative inotropic affects that impacts cardiac contractility? (Yes.) Could this be a potential problem with a patient in heart failure? (Absolutely!) Therefore, the effect of these medications could possibly worsen heart failure and the nurse needs to closely assess for this possibility.

6. What is the RELATIONSHIP between the primary medical problem and nursing priority(ies)?

I have addressed five clinical relationships that emphasize a medical problem-based approach to the patient requiring care. But once these first five relationships are deeply understood, the nurse must transition and recognize the relationship of the primary problem to the nursing priority and resultant plan of care.

For example, in this scenario of heart failure, using the ABCs of nursing priority setting, the NANDA nursing diagnostic statement of "impaired gas exchange" or simply stating the nursing priority as "respiratory difficulty" represents the essence of the physiologic changes that are present. The nurse needs to understand the pathophysiology and recognize the relationship between impaired gas exchange (respiratory difficulty) that is caused by fluid in the alveoli secondary to fluid volume overload and biventricular heart failure. Once this relationship is recognized, the nurse will be able to anticipate respiratory improvement as excess volume is removed, pulmonary edema resolves, and oxygenation improves.

7. What is the RELATIONSHIP between the primary nursing priority and secondary nursing priorities?

In addition to the primary nursing priority, every patient has additional or secondary nursing care priorities that also have relationship to one another. When this relationship is recognized and understood, another piece of the clinical puzzle fits and comes together. When the primary nursing priority is resolved and progression of the plan of care is realized, additional nursing problems or diagnostic priorities that are secondary will also likely improve or resolve as well.

For example, in the heart failure scenario, as excess fluid is removed and the secondary nursing priority of fluid volume excess is resolved, the number one nursing priority of improving gas exchange will improve and additional secondary nursing diagnoses/problems will be impacted and resolve. As oxygenation improves, fatigue, activity intolerance, and ineffective tissue perfusion will also improve. These secondary nursing priorities do not exist in isolation but have relationship to each other that the nurse needs to also recognize.

Roof Truss #4: Clinical Reasoning

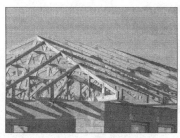

Patients do not stay static. Their condition can gradually improve or it can suddenly change. Therefore, nurses must be able to THINK IN ACTION and be able to transfer classroom learning to the bedside. Students need to be reminded that the most important role of the professional nurse is NOT performing tasks. Nurses are knowledge workers who use the information they have been taught as well as what they have learned from clinical experience and translate this knowledge into action to deliver safe patient care (Porter-O'Grady, 2010). To

think like a nurse, students must understand and then incorporate clinical reasoning into their practice. Clinical reasoning guides a nurse as she or he assesses and collects clinical data. Once data is collected, they need to make a decision if data is relevant, or if it needs to be discarded (Simmons, 2010).

The relevance and understanding of critical thinking in nursing education has been diluted by numerous definitions of the term. Because clinical reasoning is an essential component of the equation to make a correct clinical judgment, it must be succinctly and properly defined. Though there are many definitions of clinical reasoning, the most descriptive and practical working definition of clinical reasoning is found in the work of pre-eminent nurse educator and scholar Patricia Benner (Benner,et al., 2010) and (Benner, Hooper-Kyriakidis, & Stannard, 2011).

CLINICAL REASONING DEFINED

The ability of the nurse to think in action and reason as a situation changes over time by:
1. Identifying the clinical data that is RELEVANT or most and least important
2. Capturing and understanding the significance of TRENDS of collected clinical data
3. Grasping the ESSENCE of the current clinical situation
4. Identifying if an actual problem is present

Defining clinical reasoning is only the beginning. Developing this foundational thinking skill is an ongoing work in progress for every nursing student. Because of clinical inexperience, novice nursing students identify fewer clinical cues and relevant clinical data is often overlooked and not recognized. They are also limited in their ability to cluster data together to recognize clinical relationships and do not reevaluate as often as more experienced nurses (Benner, Tanner, & Chesla, 1992). When relevant data is not recognized by the nurse it can lead to patient deterioration and failure to rescue that can result in patient death (Clarke & Aiken).

Though recognizing and identifying a problem are important aspects of clinical reasoning, the nurse must also be able to think globally and accurately INTERPRET the situation to identify possible reasons WHY the problem is present. For example, when caring for a patient who recently had an open hysterectomy who is beginning to complain of increasing lower abdominal pain, though pain is expected after surgery, what if the pain continues and even gets worse despite opiate narcotics that had controlled the pain earlier?

Is the problem increased pain that needs a higher dose of narcotics, or does the nurse need to investigate and collect additional clinical data? Internal bleeding or ileus are common complications that could be present. If the nurse practices with tunnel vision and does not widen the vision and resultant thinking and use clinical reasoning, increasing the pain medication dosage could lead to failure to rescue.

Attitudes Required to Clinically Reason

In addition to correctly defining and understanding the essence of clinical reasoning, the nurse must bring the right ATTITUDE to the clinical setting to THINK like a nurse. Help students develop these attitudes by having them reflect on the question(s) that follow each attitude listed below (Pesut & Herman, 1999).

1. Intent

Excellent and correct nurse thinking is not random and does not just happen but is intentional. When students are intentional in clinical practice, they understand the rationale of how nursing interventions will advance the plan of care. The nurse has a deliberate plan of thinking and reasons with the end in mind by having a clearly defined purpose or outcome guiding the plan of care.

- *How well do your students understand the rationale and reason for nursing care priorities with each patient?*
- *Do your students have a clearly defined outcome that they work toward with each patient?*

2. Reflection

Everything the nurse does in practice requires reflection to determine if the actions and interventions are effective and working toward the outcome outlined by the plan of care. Clinical reasoning is strengthened and developed when students can reflect on past and current clinical experiences. Reflection is thinking about your thinking and determining what can be learned, affirmed, or done differently to grow and develop as a nurse.

- *How well do your students integrate reflection and*

transfer knowledge from prior clinical experiences to the present?

3. Curiosity

The nurse must ask questions to acquire needed information and knowledge. The origin of curiosity is "cura," which means "to care." Nursing is curiosity or care with a purpose. Reflection and curiosity need to be used together in practice. When the nurse is inquisitive about everything that takes place in the clinical setting, including the ways that the patient acts, thinks, and presents, the greater the level of engagement and caring the nurse will demonstrate in practice.

- *Do your students have a strong desire to deeply understand aspects of patient care that they do not understand? Do they ask why?*

4. Tolerance for ambiguity

This is the ability of the nurse to feel comfortable even when the current situation is unclear and the best outcome is undefined or unknown. Since students are concrete, textbook learners (Benner, 1982), this aspect of practice can be difficult for them to adjust to. The textbook is concrete, while clinical situations are rife with ambiguity, moral and ethical conflict, and family dynamics that are interrelated and contribute at times to ambiguity and volatility in practice.

- *What is your students' comfort level in the clinical setting when ambiguity is present?*

5. Self-confidence

The nurse must possess a certain amount of "mojo" that is balanced and healthy. Encourage your students to believe in themselves and their abilities as nurses even though they are inexperienced. An important aspect of self-confidence is to know your strengths as well as weaknesses, and be willing to do what is needed to turn those weaknesses into a strength.

- *Are your students their own worst enemy or do they have a healthy sense of their abilities as a nurse?*

6. Professional Motivation

The nurse must be committed to the vision, values, and mission of the nursing profession embodied in the code of ethics. These values must be known, assimilated, and lived out by the nurse. Students must choose to act differently and hold themselves to the highest level of moral and ethical practice. This means that they become self-monitoring and will not hesitate to self-report for example if a medication error is made or other deficiency in practice occurs. By using the attitude and skill of reflection, students will learn from any error made and make needed adjustments.

- *Do your students consistently hold themselves to the highest standards of ethical conduct and have a strong desire to be the best nurse possible?*

Components of Clinical Reasoning

Clinical reasoning consists of four components. Just as a roof truss consists of multiple pieces of lumber that provide bracing for strength, the following four components are the pieces of lumber that represent and comprise the essence of clinical reasoning (Benner, et al., 2010):

1. PRIORITY setting
2. RATIONALE for everything
3. Identify and TREND relevant clinical data
4. Grasp the ESSENCE of the situation

1. Priority Setting

For the novice nursing student, the challenge of establishing nursing care priorities is that all tasks and priorities seem to be of equal significance. Knowing which interventions are a priority is not always apparent. A novice nurse has difficulty seeing the big picture and identifying what is clinically significant. Novice nurses are also TASK-oriented and focus on the tasks that need to be done, not necessarily what is most important (Benner, 1982).

Setting priorities is also a key component of Management of Care, the client need category of the NCLEX that comprises the largest percentage of the exam (17–23 percent). To prepare students for professional practice as well as the NCLEX, priority setting must be deeply understood by students. Student nurses require guidance and instruction to identify these priorities in the clinical setting. Clinical faculty need to discuss clinical priorities so students can develop this needed nurse thinking skill. To clinically reason in practice, the nurse must be able to readily identify the following priorities in the clinical setting.

PRIORITY Patient

If a student has more than one patient, who will be seen first as the priority and why? Though students do not consistently have multiple patients in nursing education, they will after they graduate! How to identify the priority patient with a multiple patient assignment will be discussed in depth later in the book.

PRIORITY Assessments

Though a head-to-toe assessment is done on every patient, do your students know when to modify this assessment and identify the priority body system to most thoroughly assess based on the patient's primary problem? For example, a patient admitted with a COPD exacerbation will require a much more thorough and detailed respiratory assessment. Less attention can be paid to the GI system.

Nursing PRIORITY

The ABCs of priority setting are always relevant and must remain in this order. If a patient has airway, breathing, or circulatory priorities, the nurse will set priorities in the sequence of alphabetical order! Encourage nurse vigilance with an awareness of the most likely or worst possible complication for their patient as a means to establish a care priority. This will be discussed in more detail later in this chapter.

PRIORITY Interventions

Priority interventions are implemented once the nursing process has been completed by identifying correct priority assessments, nursing priority, and then determining the interventions needed. If the nursing priority is NOT correctly identified, the interventions that follow will not benefit the patient and advance the plan of care.

2. Rationale for Everything

Students must be able to understand and answer the rationale or WHY of everything that is done in the clinical setting. As a clinical instructor, I have felt at times like a two-year-old asking the following "whys" of my students:

- WHY are you giving these medications?
- WHY will these nursing interventions advance the plan of care?
- WHY did the primary care provider order these labs, treatments, or medications?

Understanding the WHY is the foundation for SAFE

patient care. It is only when a student has a DEEP UNDER-STANDING of the rationale for everything done in practice that the student is SAFE. If a new order or medication does not make sense based on the student's understanding or rationale, it must be questioned and not followed blindly. The ability to apply classroom theory to the bedside is also the essence of critical thinking. Encourage your students to make the most of any down time in clinical to expand and develop their knowledge base so that they can build on their ability to DEEPLY understand the rationale for everything that is done in clinical practice.

3. Identify and Trend Relevant Clinical Data

Identifying the MOST important clinical data and trending it by comparing it to the most recent, is an essential component of clinical reasoning and thinking like a nurse in practice. But since students tend to see ALL clinical data as relevant, they will have difficulty sorting out the least from the most important (Benner, 1984). To "rescue" a patient with a change in status, the nurse must be able to recognize SUBTLE changes in a patient's condition over time. Because students have limited clinical experience, they are unable to grasp the essence of the clinical scenario without guidance from the instructor. It is the EARLY changes in a patient's status that are subtle and, therefore, must be recognized before a problem progresses and an adverse outcome results. In addition to trending vital signs and nursing assessment data, evaluation of nursing interventions and laboratory values must also be consistently compared and trended.

Nurse Collected Data that Must Be TRENDED

What clinical data needs to be trended by students? The short answer is just about everything! The following is a summary of the clinical data that must always be compared and trended with the most recent data in the chart.

Vital Signs

- Temperature
- Heart rate
- Respiratory rate
- Blood pressure
- O2 saturation
- Pain

Nursing Assessment

Respiratory

- Breath sounds
- Rhythm/character
- O2 amount/delivery (if applicable)

Cardiac

- Heart sounds
- Strength/regularity of peripheral pulses
- Cap refill
- Color/temperature extremities
- Telemetry rhythm (if applicable)
- Edema—location/amount/pitting vs. non-pitting
- Breath sounds
- Rhythm/character

Neuro

- Alert/oriented x 4 (person-place-time-situation)
- Level of consciousness (LOC)
- Movement/sensation in extremities

GI

- Appearance of abdomen
- Tenderness w/palpation
- Bowel sounds/flatus/LBM (last bowel movement)

GU

- Urine amount/color/clarity
- Foley—secured/urethral drainage?

Skin

- Color/temperature
- Skin integrity—redness/blanchable over pressure points if present

Psychosocial

- Emotional support/needs
- Spiritual care/needs
- Educational priorities

I&O

- Shift and 24-hour trends if relevant
- Daily weights. Remind students that for every 1 kg. of weight loss/gain, this represents 1000 mL of volume.

4. Grasp the Essence of the Situation

Essence is being able to identify the most significant aspect of the current clinical situation. It is also the ability to break down the patient's current needs to the lowest common denominator of what is needed and what must be done to advance the plan of care. Essence is closely related to priority setting.

As I look back at my own professional development, being able to grasp the "essence" of a clinical situation is the skill that took the most time to develop. This takes months and typically more than a year of clinical experience in the same practice setting. The ability to see the whole of patient care and grasp the essence is a characteristic of proficiency, the fourth stage of clinical competence (Benner, 1984). Essence is developed by seeing patients with similar problems and the patterns that present with the typical chief complaint, nursing assessments, vital signs, lab values, and expected medical treatment. It is not going to be strongly developed in a typical five- to ten-week clinical rotation. Encourage the development of essence by asking students to consistently identify clinical priorities that capture the essence of their current clinical status.

Determining Acceptable Ambiguity

Another nurse thinking skill that students struggle to acquire because of a lack of clinical experience and being concrete textbook learners is developing the degree of acceptable ambiguity of clinical data for their patient. Not all patients have textbook norms of clinical data. Depending on the patient's past medical history or current illness, the patient may have elevated heart rate, respiratory rate or high blood pressure. This may be "normal" for this patient even though it is abnormal by textbook norms.

For example, a patient with chronic COPD will have a lower than normal oxygen saturation and may be slightly tachypneic. The nurse must identify the normal baseline of all clinical data that is collected and determine the significance of any changes based not on textbook norms, but on the norm for this patient.

To determine acceptable ambiguity, teach your students to go back 24 to 48 hours in the medical record and compare and contrast textbook norms for vital signs and assessment parameters with this patient. Then ask the following questions:
- What degree of ambiguity is present between textbook norms and your patient?
- What degree of ambiguity is expected and would be acceptable?
- When would you become concerned? (Koharchik, Caputi, Robb, & Culleiton, 2015)

If ambiguity is present, it is important to determine the clinical significance for the variations that are present and what is responsible for the ambiguity. The following are the most common reasons for abnormal clinical data:
- Past medical history
- Current problem
- Medications
- Abnormal lab findings

The most difficult aspect of accurately interpreting the significance of clinical data when ambiguity is present is that a deviation from what is normal is already present, when should the nurse become concerned and decide to intervene? For example, if the patient with COPD has a baseline respiratory rate of 22 and oxygen saturation of 88–90%, when the respiratory rate increases to 28 and his oxygen saturation drops to 84% with activity, is this expected, or a cause for clinical concern? It depends.

By completing a thorough physical assessment, if the patient is in distress and appears anxious with increased wheezing, the nurse must intervene. But if the patient is in no distress and there is no change in breath sounds, this may be his normal response to activity due to lowered pulmonary reserves. Closely assess to determine if O2 sat increases to prior baseline after rest to determine resultant interventions.

"Five Rights" of Clinical Reasoning

Though nursing education has five to ten rights of safe medication administration that students must memorize to safely administer medications, there are "five rights" of clinical reasoning (Levett-Jones, et al., 2010). These five rights are not widely known to educators but must be seen just as important as the rights of safe medication administration, to promote patient safety.

Familiarize yourself with these five rights, then integrate them in your classroom or clinical settings. Expect students to incorporate and recite these just as fluently as medication rights that your program emphasizes! Knowledge of these five rights will deepen student understanding of applied clinical reasoning to practice. These five rights are another way to teach the essence of clinical reasoning and are an easy acronym to guide nurse thinking in the clinical setting!

1. RIGHT Cues

This is the clinical data that is collected and clustered by the nurse. Recognizing the RELEVANCE and RELATIONSHIP of clinical data and contextualizing it to each patient is the essence of this "right." EARLY cues that are missed or not identified and allow a complication to progress is a classic example of "failure to rescue" by the nurse when this "right" is not applied to practice.

2. RIGHT Patient

This "right" is not about checking the name and date of birth of the patient, but the ability of the nurse to identify a patient who is high risk for developing a potential complication. An 18-year-old with an appendectomy is not as likely to develop a complication as a patient with the same problem who is 88! Patients who are susceptible hosts due to chemotherapy, radiation, or medications such as prednisone also fall under this "right" as patients at risk.

3. RIGHT Time

This refers to the timeliness of identifying a change of status. Recognizing EARLY signs of a complication and then initiating nursing interventions at the RIGHT time and in the RIGHT sequence is imperative to prevent a bad outcome. Remember that "failure to rescue" occurs not only by missing a complication that develops, but also when nursing/medical interventions are implemented too late.

4. RIGHT Action

Once a problem is recognized, the right action or intervention must be initiated. Clinical data that suggest a potential complication must be acted upon. The consequences of an incorrect clinical judgment can make the difference between life and death. In one study, 50 percent of patients who had cardiac arrests on the hospital floor had clinical signs of deterioration 24 hours before the arrest. These early signs were not recognized and acted upon by the nurse (Thompson, et al., 2008).

5. RIGHT Reason

The right reason is understanding the RATIONALE or WHY of everything that is done in practice. To do this consistently, the nurse must be able to apply key aspects of clinical reasoning, which include grasping the essence of the current situation to put the clinical puzzle together.

Clinical Example

To see the relevance of these five rights to clinical practice, I will use the clinical scenario I used in the introduction. Ken was an elderly male patient who had a perforated appendix and was post-operative day #2. Ken was a RIGHT PATIENT who was at high risk for a possible change of status because he was elderly, had an invasive procedure, and his ruptured appendix spilled bacteria into a sterile peritoneum.

Ken developed the RIGHT CUES. He became restless for no apparent reason; his initial BP was normal but his HR was in the 100s at rest. Tachycardia with a normal BP is a classic presentation of EARLY shock as the body compensates for a low output state by increasing heart rate.

If the nurse had correctly interpreted these clinical cues, she would have recognized the possibility of sepsis in the RIGHT TIME and contacted the primary care provider as a RIGHT ACTION to address this concern.

Instead, Ken was given pain medication for restlessness, albuterol neb for tachypnea, and the RIGHT ACTION for the RIGHT REASON did not take place. Had these five rights been correctly acted upon in this scenario, Ken would likely still be alive today.

Nurse as Lifeguard

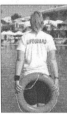 Have you ever thought of the similarities that a nurse has to a lifeguard? This is a metaphor that will help students grasp the essence of the responsibility of being a professional nurse. Just as a lifeguard continually and vigilantly scans the water for signs of a struggling swimmer, the nurse must also look vigilantly over his/her patient to assess for a deteriorating change of status, in order to rescue a patient who may be experiencing a complication. TRENDING all clinical data and assessing EARLY signs and symptoms must be done so that a complication is not allowed to needlessly progress. There is a short distance and time frame be-

tween the body's ability to compensate and the "swirl" of decompensation (Scott, 2009).

For example, in sepsis that progresses to septic shock, the body can briefly compensate by elevating heart rate and maintaining blood pressure—but not for long before the bottom literally falls out!

One distinction between a novice and more experienced nurse is that a more experienced nurse anticipates potential problems, recognizes the significance of clinical cues, and practices PROACTIVELY to PREVENT a possible patient complication (Levett-Jones, et al., 2010). Novice nursing students tend to practice REACTIVELY. They don't anticipate potential problems, and react to them after they have already developed (Levett-Jones, et al., 2010).

When analyzing a new graduate's ability to think critically, especially in the context of a change of status, del Bueno (2005) identified four questions that help a nurse anticipate a change of status. Use these questions in the clinical setting to help develop proactive clinical reasoning skills with your students.

1. Can the nurse recognize a problem is present?

Until the problem is recognized, no action will be taken by the nurse. To recognize a problem, the nurse must do the following:

- Recognize RELEVANT clinical data.
- INTERPRET clinical data correctly (Tanner, 2006).
- Identify medical/nursing PRIORITY.
- Identify the most likely WORST POSSIBLE COMPLICATION for your patient.
- Maintain intentional vigilance. LOOKING for this complication, trending all RELEVANT clinical data and required assessments over time.

2. Can the nurse manage the problem safely and effectively?

- Proper nursing interventions initiated based on current problem once identified.

3. Does the nurse have a relative sense of URGENCY?

- Lack of clinical experience often causes a lack of urgency when RED FLAG clinical data is present. I have seen new nurses have no sense of urgency when a patient at risk for sepsis drops his BP to 70/30!

4. Does the nurse take the right action for the right reason?

- Once the problem is identified, does the nurse take the priority action for the right reason by understanding the rationale?
- Does the nurse contact the physician promptly to initiate needed interventions?

del Bueno's research identified the importance of a nurse's ability to RECOGNIZE a problem before rescue can take place. It is only when a problem is recognized that the nurse will intervene and do something about it. This is closely related to correctly interpreting clinical data to make a correct clinical judgment (Tanner, 2006).

Clinical Reasoning Step-by-Step

As a new fundamental instructor I had no idea how complicated it was to wash my hands! A skill that I performed intuitively because of clinical experience had over ten sequential steps that needed to be followed in the correct order! For inexperienced nursing students any new clinical skill must be broken down step-by-step so they can identify each step and ensure that it is done correctly and in the right sequence. Thinking like a nurse using clinical reasoning is also a skill that needs to be broken down step-by-step so students can identify each step and incorporate it into their practice.

As I reflected on how I prepared to care for any patient over my 35 years of clinical practice while collecting data from the chart and receiving report, what were my priorities and internalized sequence I used when I was assuming care of a patient for the first time? From my lens of clinical practice and drawing from the nursing literature, I created a handout (found in the Transformation Toolbox that comes with this book) "Clinical Reasoning Questions that Develop Nurse Thinking" that deconstructs clinical reasoning by breaking it down, step-by-step. It identifies how a nurse systematically sets and establishes care priorities when preparing for patient care as well as throughout the shift.

These twelve clinical reasoning questions have been derived and adapted from the work of leading nurse educators including Patricia Benner, Chris Tanner, and Linda Caputi. I have filtered their work through my lens of clinical practice to develop this unique practice based model of clinical reasoning. This template of clinical reasoning questions is not unique to how I approach professional practice, but represents the essence of how a nurse thinks and sets priorities in the clinical setting.

This template is divided into two sections. First, there is a series of eight questions that represent the sequential thinking that is required BEFORE a patient is seen by the nurse. As the nurse reviews the chart and obtains report, these eight questions must be reflected upon then answered. These first eight questions emphasize:

- RELEVANT data collection
- Care planning PRIORITIES/interventions
- Nurse vigilance by identifying the worst possible or most likely COMPLICATION and what to do if it presents

The second half of my template has four questions to guide nurse thinking, AFTER the patient is seen for the first time and the nurse has collected clinical assessment data firsthand. These four questions emphasize the following aspects of clinical reasoning:

- RELEVANCE of VITAL SIGNS, assessment data collected, how collected data trends with existing data
- Nursing PRIORITY…possible changes

- PRIORITY educational needs to address
- RATIONALE of primary care provider's plan of care

To deepen student understanding of this template of clinical reasoning and thinking like a nurse in practice, background is provided and what is most important and relevant for each of these questions. Students will then be able to incorporate this information into their practice as they prepare and then provide patient care. These clinical reasoning questions can also be used to replace the traditional care plan (I recommend at an advanced level) because it combines care planning, nursing process, and clinical reasoning in a single practice-based construct. Faculty around the country have successfully transitioned to this template in the clinical setting and eliminated the traditional written care plan. I encourage you to do the same.

Part I: Reflect on the Following BEFORE Providing Care:

1. What is the primary problem and what is its underlying cause or pathophysiology?

This is the admission medical problem or diagnosis. The most important aspect of this question is student

---

Clinical Reasoning Questions to Develop Nurse Thinking

Formulate and reflect on the following BEFORE providing care:

1. What is the primary problem and what is its underlying cause or pathophysiology?
2. What clinical data from the chart is RELEVANT, clinically significant, and needs to be trended?
3. List all relevant nursing priorities. Which nursing priority captures the "essence" of your patient's current status and will guide your plan of care?
4. What nursing interventions will you initiate based on this priority and what are the desired outcomes?
5. What body system(s), key assessments, and psychosocial needs will you focus on based on your patient's primary problem or nursing care priority?
6. What is the worst possible/most likely complication(s) to anticipate based on the primary problem?
7. What nursing assessments will identify this complication EARLY if it develops?
8. What nursing interventions will you initiate if this complication develops?

Formulate and reflect on the following WHILE providing care:

1. What clinical assessment data did you just collect that is RELEVANT and needs to be TRENDED because it is clinically significant to detect a change in status?
2. Does your nursing priority or plan of care need to be modified in any way after assessing your patient (include psychosocial priorities)?
3. After reviewing the primary care provider's note, what is the rationale for any new orders or changes made?
4. What educational priorities have you identified and how will you address them?

ability to UNDERSTAND the pathophysiology of the illness causing the primary problem. This understanding will lay the foundation for critical thinking by recognizing clinical relationships and establishing correct nursing care priorities.

Once a student is in practice, they will routinely encounter diseases they barely remember covering in school. Treating the clinical experience as a puzzle that needs to be solved or viewing the nurse as a detective who needs to understand and uncover the clinical mystery will encourage "clinical curiosity" that must be a central part of every student's practice. Make it a priority to promote student learning by using available resources or the Internet to research what students do not know or understand about the patient's primary problem. (emedicine.medscape.com/ is an excellent website resource for this purpose).

2. What clinical data from the chart is RELEVANT, clinically significant, and needs to be trended?

This was addressed at length earlier. But one observation I have made as an educator is that students will take as much time as you give them in the clinical setting to collect data on their patient from the medical record. As novice nurses, students do not have an experiential base to recognize relevant clinical data and, therefore, will tend to write down EVERYTHING that is present in the medical record. The ability to filter clinical data and focus on what is RELEVANT takes time and clinical experience to develop. That is why it is so important to DECREASE the amount of information and filter all content in class and clinical so students can focus on what is MOST important. This question is also one of the five "rights" of clinical reasoning, the importance of the nurse to recognize the right cues or what clinical data is relevant (Levett-Jones, et al., 2010).

3. List all relevant nursing priorities. What nursing priority captures the "essence" of your patient's current status and will guide your plan of care?

Have students make a list of all relevant nursing care priorities based on their patient's primary medical problem. With most patients, they should be able to identify at least three to five relevant care priorities. For example,

a patient admitted to the med/surg floor with an acute COPD exacerbation would likely have the following nursing priorities:

- Fatigue
- Anxiety
- Activity intolerance
- Impaired gas exchange
- Self-care deficit
- Risk for impaired skin integrity

Once students have made a list of all relevant nursing care priorities, which one captures the essence of the current medical problem and is also the PRIORITY? Students can use two approaches to make this determination.

Identify a nursing priority/diagnostic statement that is related to an ABC priority. When the primary medical problem is understood, and resultant relationship of the nursing diagnosis of impaired gas exchange is interpreted as a clear "B" breathing priority, this is also the nursing PRIORITY because the other nursing priorities are NOT "B" or even "C" priorities. Though not clearly stated in this question, the nurse addresses not only the primary priority and resultant plan of care, but other nursing care priorities remain relevant and must be included in the plan of care for that day.

I have seen my students struggle with establishing appropriate care priorities in the clinical setting when NANDA has been the only way taught to establish nursing priorities. There are some NANDA statements that do capture the essence of the nursing priority such as "acute/chronic pain" or "fluid volume excess/deficit." Nurses in practice don't think this way exclusively and neither should your students! There are numerous clinical situations where NANDA does not "fit" or even come close to describe the care priority!

Instead, use the essence of clinical reasoning and apply this to practice. I allowed my students to use a concise statement that captures "the essence of the current clinical situation" (Benner, Hooper-Kyriakidis, & Stannard, 2011) that may or may not be a NANDA nursing diagnostic statement. I encourage you to do the same.

4. What nursing interventions will you initiate based on this priority and what are the desired outcomes?

Questions 2–4 integrate the essence of nursing process by expecting the student to:

- Identify relevant assessment data (assessment)
- Identify correct nursing priority (nursing diagnosis/priority)
- Initiate nursing interventions (implementation)
- Identify desired or expected outcomes

This is the essence of the nursing care plan, but it is positioned within the framework of applied clinical reasoning. Another aspect of clinical reasoning that is inferred but not clearly specified is the importance and expectation that students can identify the RATIONALE for every intervention that is implemented. Correctly stating the rationale ensures safe practice. Make it a priority as a clinical instructor to ask students "WHY" regarding all aspects of patient care.

5. What body system(s), key assessments, and psychosocial needs will you focus on based on your patient's primary problem or nursing care priority?

Though students are taught to perform a systematic head-to-toe assessment for every patient they care for, they must also be able to identify the PRIORITY body system as well as psychosocial needs that must be more thoroughly assessed, based on the patient's primary problem or nursing care priority. This is the first step of a two-step process.

Once the priority body system(s) have been identified, the second step is to identify the specific key assessments. This is an essential skill that experienced nurses use. For example, when a patient who has heart failure exacerbation is anxious, the nurse would identify the following priority body systems and perform these key assessments:

Respiratory
- Anterior/posterior breath sounds
- Work of breathing/presence of retractions
- RR/O2 sat

Cardiovascular
- Cardiac rhythm
- BP/HR
- Color
- Cap refill/strength of peripheral pulses
- Edema

Holistic care is the hallmark of nursing practice. Psychosocial needs, including emotional as well as spiritual needs, must be considered as no less significant than the physical needs that demand immediate attention. Any physiologic problem can cause anxiety, fear, and stress. How is your patient coping? This must also be considered and assessed.

6. What is the worst possible/most likely complication(s) to anticipate based on the primary problem?

Identifying the most likely or worst possible complication BEFORE patient care is assumed is an essential critical thinking skill applied to practice. This illustrates the importance of being PROACTIVE vs. REACTIVE, and it can make a difference in improving patient outcomes. When a problem is anticipated and identified EARLY, the nurse is one step ahead. But when the nurse is caught completely off-guard by a sudden change of status, they are one step behind. The problem will likely be more serious because it has been recognized LATER. Sepsis that progresses to septic shock is a common clinical occurrence, with potential life-threatening consequences, if treatment is delayed.

7. What nursing assessments will identify this complication EARLY if it develops?

Once the worst possible/most likely complication is identified, the specific assessments to recognize it must be identified. EARLY recognition of any complication is essential to good patient outcomes. If sepsis progressing to septic shock goes unrecognized until the BP dramatically decreases and is now 70/30, if early signs such as tachycardia that tend to be more subtle go unrecognized, an adverse outcome, and even death, is possible.

For example, if sepsis/septic shock is the most likely complication, the EARLY assessments that the nurse needs to cluster to confirm its presence and then initiate "rescue" are:
- Temperature: fever >100.8 or <96.8
- HR: >90
- BP: downward trend with mean arterial pressure (MAP) <65
- WBC <4,000 or > 12,000

8. What nursing interventions will you initiate if this complication develops?

If you look at these last three questions (6–8), they follow the pattern of putting nursing process and nursing plan of care in the context of the most likely/worst possible complication. This provides a SECONDARY plan of care that experienced nurses follow intuitively, but must be made intentional for students. The potential PRIORITY complication is identified, assessments to conclusively recognize are listed, and nursing interventions to initiate "rescue" can be implemented if needed. This is another "nurse thinking" skill that is not typically taught in nursing education, yet it captures the essence of how nurses in practice prioritize and provide safe care.

To help students DEEPLY understand the importance of early identification of a complication and initiate "rescue" if needed, I have created a metaphor of "Jason," the serial killer from the "Friday the 13th" horror movie series. Remind your students that "Jason is still out there…"

Looking for "Jason"…the Worst Possible Complication

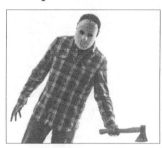
Do you remember "Jason" from the original Friday the 13th slasher/horror movies from the 1980s? Teenagers are murdered one by one as they attempt to reopen an abandoned campground. Since I graduated from high school in 1981, and the first of many in this series started in 1980, I remember all too well the classic ending from the original when it first came out.

Only Alice survived the terrifying night at Camp Crystal Lake. As morning came, she was on a small boat in the middle of the lake. All is calm and quiet, the birds are singing and she has no reason to be concerned. Out of nowhere, Jason leaps out of the water and grabs Alice and takes her down and brings her under the water…but it was only a dream and a movie.

No reason to fear and look for Jason any longer, right? WRONG! Jason is still out there and lurks around the corner of every clinical setting! Who is "Jason"? He is a metaphor for the worst possible/most likely complication any patient may experience. "Jason" is still very deadly, and he has new identities such as sepsis, septic shock, post-op bleed, pulmonary embolism, and cardiac arrest, to name only a few.

Clinical vigilance is required to keep "Jason" from harming the patients in the students' care. If students are looking for him, they will recognize the "Jason" of the worst possible complications before it is too late! It is only when the nurse loses this sense of vigilance and forgets that "Jason" is still out there that complications go unnoticed until it is often too late.

Even if everything appears uneventful and the patient appears stable, just like Alice on the boat, things can change quickly. That is why nurse vigilance is always required in practice. Sepsis is the most common "Jason" and hides early with subtle changes such as a low-grade temperature, slight hypotension, and tachycardia. When the nurse does not recognize the significance of these findings, tachycardia will persist as "Jason" continues to have his way and sepsis progresses to septic shock. It is only when "Jason" is RECOGNIZED that his power to destroy is broken and the patient can be RESCUED from an adverse outcome.

Most Common "Jasons"

At the large metropolitan hospital where I practice, there is a "Rapid Response Team" (RRT) that rounds the hospital 24/7, circulating and responding to calls from nurses who identify a possible change in status that may indicate a need to rescue. Based on statistical data compiled where I practice as to why a RRT is paged, students can anticipate these most common changes of status in the acute care setting (see table below).

In addition to discussing the implications for each of these most common changes in patient status listed in order of frequency, I will highlight the most important assessments that students can use to quickly identify the scope of a potential problem if Jason gets too close.

Most Common Patient Complications
1. Chest pain
2. Increased respiratory distress
3. Hypotension
4. Change in level of consciousness (LOC) or neurologic status
5. Falls

Top Five Patient Change of Status
1. Chest Pain

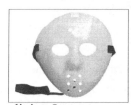

Regardless of the practice setting, the nurse needs to evaluate and assess chest pain in such diverse settings as phone triage, outpatient clinics, and community health clinics. In acute care, this is the most common reason an RRT is paged. Most chest pain is NOT cardiac, but it can still be a potential problem because pneumonia and a pulmonary embolus can also cause this complaint. I encourage the use of mnemonics such as W-I-L-D-A or P-Q-R-S-T to help students concisely and systematically assess and document any complaint of pain.

If a patient has a complaint of chest pain, it is essential to perform the following assessments to differentiate cardiac vs. non-cardiac chest pain. If available in your practice setting, a 12-lead EKG is a standard tool to determine if there are new changes consistent with ischemia. What are these changes? In early ischemia, the T waves that are normally rounded and upright may be flattened or inverted. The ST segment after the QRS complex may be elevated or depressed more than 1 mm.

In addition to the EKG, teach students to do a quick assessment by simply looking at the patient. Does he look as if he is in distress? Has his color changed from pink, warm, and dry to pale, cool, and diaphoretic? Is he anxious, restless? Are other subtle but apparent changes present? If present, this validates that his current complaint is likely more serious. In addition to an EKG, the following nursing assessments must be implemented to put this clinical puzzle together and differentiate the primary problem.

Take a deep breath

- If taking a deep breath causes the pain to dramatically increase, chest pain is most likely non-cardiac. Pleurisy, pneumonia, and a pulmonary embolus also cause pleuritic chest pain. The next assessment to help clarify the cause of this chest pain is palpation.

Palpate the area of pain for reproducible tenderness

- Gently but firmly palpate the location of where the pain is present. If the pain is reproducible with palpation, this is most likely noncardiac and is likely pleurisy, an inflammation of the pleura that is non-emergent.

Location of the pain

- There are gender differences of cardiac chest pain. For example, women tend to have a higher likelihood of nonclassic symptoms that include epigastric pain as well as referred pain with no anterior chest pain. For most patients though, cardiac chest pain will be anterior chest pain in a large, general area of the chest. If the pain is localized to a very small area that the patient can point to, this is unlikely to be angina.

Presence of other complaints consistent with cardiac ischemia

- In addition to the location of chest pain, cardiac chest pain may refer pain to the neck, back, jaw, or arms. Is referred pain or shortness of breath (SOB) present? SOB is also a common component of cardiac chest pain related to coronary artery disease, myocardial ischemia, or pulmonary embolus.

Length of pain

- Angina will typically last longer than five minutes. If the patient reports that her pain lasts for just a few seconds at a time, or less than a minute, this pain is likely noncardiac.

Character of pain

- Determine if this pain is similar to any pain in the past or prior history of heartburn or GERD. If it is, this again is likely noncardiac. Cardiac chest pain is most commonly a diffuse pressure, tightness, squeezing, or achiness.

2. Increased Respiratory Distress/O2 sat <90%

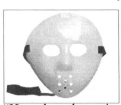

If a patient complains of shortness of breath and/or has decreased oxygenation, immediate intervention and relevant assessments are required. Use the same principle of "How does the patient look?" If he looks like he is in distress, he most likely is! In addition to general appearance, the following are the most relevant assessments that must be closely trended over time by the nurse to recognize if "Jason" is present:

Respiratory rate

- Rate > 20 is a clinical RED FLAG and likely represents distress, anxiety, or both.

Heart rate

- Rate >100 is a clinical RED FLAG due to physiologic distress and sympathetic nervous system stimulation. The nurse must be able to situate knowledge and determine the most likely reason WHY!

O2 saturation

- Saturation <90% is a clinical RED FLAG that reflects hypoxia in a non-COPD patient. With any complaint of SOB, immediately obtain the oxygen saturation to determine the baseline with this change of status, and then administer supplemental oxygenation and titrate to oxygen saturation greater than 92%.

Breath sounds

- Posterior auscultation FIRST if possible, then anterior. There is less subcutaneous fat posterior and the nurse will be able to detect adventitious breath sounds more readily. Listen carefully to all lobes, especially the bases. Compare each lobe right to left.
- Rales or crackles typically represent fluid in the alveoli with heart failure. Rhonchi is most commonly seen with pneumonia. Wheezing or very-diminished aeration is typical with asthmatic or COPD exacerbation. However, an audible wheeze may be present in heart failure due to fluid in the alveoli causing bronchial constriction. This is referred to as cardiac asthma.

3. Hypotension

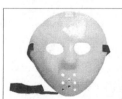 This has many sources, but the most common is fluid volume loss/deficit related to bleeding, dehydration, or sepsis. If the nurse has been carefully trending the systolic blood pressure and it is running 30+ points lower than baseline, or if the systolic blood pressure is less than 100, this is a clinical RED FLAG. If the systolic blood pressure has been trending 130–140 consistently and now it is 100–110, though not less than 100, this is still a RED FLAG. The nurse must step back and ask WHY?

Remember the relevance of this formula of cardiac output to clinical practice:

$$CO=SV \times HR$$

With any shock or volume-depleted state, the earliest compensatory response by the body is to INCREASE heart rate in response to DECREASED cardiac output. The finding of low blood pressure with tachycardia demands an immediate response. When a low blood pressure trend is identified, the following priority assessments must be clustered and trended with the current blood pressure to determine most likely complication that may beginning to manifest.

General appearance

- Does he appear in distress or is the patient tolerating hypotension? The nurse needs to make a clinical judgment if the patient is unstable. This finding will help determine the urgency needed in this clinical situation.

Skin

- If he is in distress with sympathetic nervous system stimulation, he will likely be pale, cool, and diaphoretic. In early shock, his extremities will be cooler when compared centrally by touching his forehead. If a patient is cool centrally and this is a new finding, this is an urgent situation and must be recognized as such.

Pulses

- The pulses must be taken while assessing the coolness or warmth of the extremities. If the pulses are already more difficult to palpate than a prior assessment, this is a critical RED FLAG. It most likely represents a shock state as the body shunts volume centrally from the periphery. Palpate pulses together at the same time to assess any significant differences. If radial pulses can be palpated, the patient has a systolic BP of at least 80 mmHg.

Temperature

A complete set of vital signs, including temperature, is required with a low blood pressure. The most common complication that must be ruled out is SEPSIS. An elevated temperature with tachycardia and a low blood pressure is a classic finding with sepsis. With the elderly, it is not uncommon to have a temperature less than 96.8 when septic. This is a clinical RED FLAG that must be recognized.

Heart rate

- The expected physiologic response to volume depletion and a low blood pressure is tachycardia. If the patient is NOT tachycardic with a low blood pressure, assess his current medications for beta blockers that will prevent the heart rate from being elevated, even when the sympathetic nervous system is activated.

Respiratory rate

- Note the respiratory rate because of its relationship to shock. If progressive shock state is present, he will likely be tachypneic.

Blood pressure

- TREND the BP and its direction. Remember that even if the SBP is >100 but has dropped by 30+ mm/Hg recently from prior assessments, the nurse should recognize this as a clinical RED FLAG.

4. Change in LOC or Neurologic Status

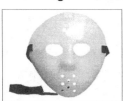 If a change in neurologic status is present, the nurse needs to determine the most obvious reason. For example, if a patient just received a dose of IV hydromorphone and now is more lethargic and difficult to arouse, narcotic over-sedation is the most likely cause. Instead of beginning with the assumption that this is a stroke, begin with this obvious assumption and cluster clinical data. Since the brain is dependent on adequate blood pressure for optimal function, a change in level of consciousness (LOC) and even confusion can result from a sudden decrease in blood pressure from the patient's norm or low blood glucose.

Though narcotic over-sedation is the most common reason for a clinical change and altered level of consciousness, the nurse must also be vigilant for the possibility of a stroke with any of the following NEW assessment findings:

Facial droop

- This is always a clinical RED FLAG. If facial droop is present, a complete neuro assessment must be immediately initiated. This finding can be subtle; just the corner of the mouth may be level while the other side moves or is elevated in comparison. If the nurse

is suspicious that this is present, simply have the patient smile BIG and show their teeth. It will be obvious if a droop is present.

Hemiparesis

- Weakness on either side of the body that may or may not involve both upper and lower extremities is also a clinical RED FLAG. It is not uncommon for an upper extremity to have weakness, but the lower extremity of the impaired side to have normal strength with a stroke.

Slurred speech

- If the patient has slurred speech or expressive or receptive aphasia, this is a clinical RED FLAG that is consistent with a stroke. The nurse must recognize the significance and the need to make this patient NPO until this has been ruled out.

Confusion or disorientation

- This finding can be generalized to other problems besides a stroke. Confusion can be caused by narcotic medications and is also an early sign of ETOH withdrawal.

Cincinnati Pre-Hospital Stroke Scale

A simple, focused neurologic assessment that students should be taught to quickly determine the possibility of a stroke is called the "Cincinnati Pre-Hospital Stroke Scale" (Kothari, Pancioli, Liu, Brott, & Broderick, 1999). It consists of three assessments that may indicate a patient is having a stroke. Though designed for emergency medical staff in pre-hospital care, it can guide nurses in any clinical setting if there is cause for concern with any new neurologic changes.

Patients with one of these three findings as a new event have a 72 percent probability of an ischemic stroke. If all three findings are present, the probability of an acute stroke is more than 85 percent. Even if students may not be confident in their comprehensive neuro-assessment skills, this will simplify what is NEED TO KNOW in this context of a change in neurological status.

Three Essential Neuro Assessments

1. **Facial droop:** Have the patient smile or show his or her teeth. If one side doesn't move as well as the

other or it seems to droop, this is clinically significant and a possible stroke.

2. **Arm drift:** Have the patient close his or her eyes and hold his or her arms straight out in front, for ten seconds. If one arm does not move, or one arm drifts down more than the other, this is clinically significant and a possible stroke.

3. **Speech:** Have the patient say, "You can't teach an old dog new tricks," or some other simple, familiar saying. If the person slurs the words, gets some words wrong, or is unable to speak, this is clinically significant and a possible stroke.

5. Falls

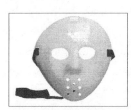

The most important nursing PRIORITY is to determine the MECHANISM OF INJURY related to the fall. If the patient fell in such a way that he has complaints of pain, or may have hit his head, he may require cervical spine immobilization by the RRT nurse. He must be kept perfectly still until this immobilization takes place and a cervical spine injury is ruled out. Additional relevant neurologic assessments include:

- Level of consciousness (LOC)
- Movement of all extremities
- Numbness, weakness, tingling in any extremity

Part II: Reflect on the Following WHILE Providing Care:

1. What clinical assessment data did you just collect that is RELEVANT and need to be TRENDED because it is clinically significant to detect a change in status?

As novice nurses, students consistently struggle with recognizing what is clinically relevant or MOST important. In addition to recognizing relevant data, the student must also consistently compare or TREND the data that was collected and put it side by side with data received in report or last recorded in the chart. Has anything changed? Were any of the findings unexpected? Do they require further assessment or an SBAR to the physician? Because patients rarely stay static but can change quickly, trending all clinical data will encourage nurse vigilance and trigger the need to "rescue" if there is a concerning TREND that may represent a change in status.

2. Does your nursing priority or plan of care need to be modified in any way after assessing your patient (include psychosocial priorities)?

Encourage students to continually reevaluate the nursing priority and plan of care based on the data that was most recently collected. Vital signs and nursing assessment must never be seen as a TASK to check off a list, but an opportunity to THINK in action and make a nursing judgment regarding the CURRENT status of the patient. To advance the plan of care, the nurse must know the desired outcome(s). Once the desired outcome from the nursing priority is identified, the nurse must compare and contrast this desired outcome with clinical data that is assessed to determine clinical progression.

3. After reviewing the primary care provider's note, what is the rationale for any new orders or changes made?

Though the student nurse is not the primary care provider, the nurse needs to understand the primary care provider's plan of care and the rationale for any changes in orders that have been made. The daily progress note or most recent documentation by the primary care provider is a must-read for the nurse to clearly understand these priorities and benefit from the primary care provider's perspective on the patient. When the primary care provider note is understood, the clinical puzzle begins to come together. Make it a priority as a clinical instructor to take at least five minutes with each student to do this needed review in the chart to develop these nurse thinking skills.

4. What educational priorities have you identified and how will you address them?

The professional nurse is also an educator. Encourage students to embrace the responsibility of this role. This is NOT just another task to perform. When teaching is done well it promotes patient learning and understanding, improves patient outcomes, and even prevents hospital readmissions. Students cannot teach what they do not fully understand. Make this an incentive for students to deeply learn content so it can be taught effectively to their patients.

Every patient has a need for education to promote his/her health and care. A practical approach to assess patient knowledge of their health and illnesses that are being managed by medications is to ask when administering medications, "Do you know what this is for?" If the patient is unable to answer this question correctly, students can reinforce or choose to address any knowledge deficits another time during that clinical.

Clinical Judgment: End Result of Nurse Thinking

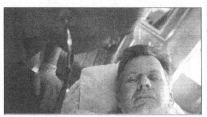

Making a correct clinical judgment is a complex process that is directly influenced by the clinical experience of the nurse and by what the nurse brings to the patient care scenario. This includes the ability of the nurse to use knowledge and grasp the essence of the current clinical scenario by using the skill of clinical reasoning. Clinical judgment is also influenced by how well the nurse knows the patient based on prior clinical experience and the level of engagement that leads to recognizing subtle differences that are clinically significant (Cappelletti, Engel, & Prentice, 2014).

del Bueno (2005) identified that two thirds of new nurses were unable to exercise correct clinical judgment at a basic level to "rescue" (identify the problem and then intervene) their patient in a simulated scenario. del Bueno's research validates why "NCLEX success" must take a back seat to an emphasis that prepares students for practice. If two-thirds of graduate nurses fail the NCLEX, a nursing program would be put on immediate probation. Something is wrong when nursing programs graduate students who pass the NCLEX, but are not able to practically think like a nurse.

The progression of the development of clinical decision making can be observed as students move through nursing education. In one study, traits of first-year students included the ability to interpret and take action independently but needed reassurance. Second-year students were at risk to make inaccurate clinical decisions because of misplaced confidence, but before graduation they were more comfortable anticipating and managing complications (Ostrogorsky, T.L., et al., 2015).

Though clinical reasoning has been emphasized in this chapter so it can be incorporated into student prac-

tice, it is NOT the end point of nurse thinking. The ultimate objective of thinking like a nurse is making a correct clinical judgment. What do students decide to do with the data they have collected? Will they do nothing, act now, or wait? The decision the nurse makes when interpreting clinical data is the essence of making a clinical judgment.

The following summarizes the equation of nurse thinking that is required for safe clinical practice (Alfaro-LeFevre, 2013):

> **Critical Thinking + Clinical Reasoning = Correct Clinical Judgment**

Because clinical judgment is the end result and hallmark of professional practice, it must be properly defined and understood. Tanner (2006) defines clinical judgment as an interpretation or conclusion about what a patient needs and/or the decision to take action or not. Good clinical judgment requires the nurse to be flexible, recognize what is MOST important, INTERPRET the meaning of this clinical data, and respond appropriately.

To make a correct clinical judgment, clinical reasoning selects from all alternatives, understands the rationale for each alternative, collects and recognizes the significance of clinical data, processes this information to understand the current problem, and identifies the current care priority and plan of care (Levett-Jones, et al., 2010). Clinical judgments are made on a continual and ongoing basis in practice. In one study, on a typical med/surg floor over an eight-hour shift, the nurse engaged in an average of 50 significant clinical reasoning concerns that required a clinical judgment (Thompson, Cullum, McCaughan, Sheldon, & Raynor, 2004).

Clinical Judgment Step-by-Step

Tanner (2006) developed a model that breaks down clinical judgment into four steps. This can help students strengthen their ability to make correct judgments by identifying breakdowns and using reflection to identify areas of growth.

The four steps Tanner identified are:

1. Noticing

Can the nurse identify the most relevant clinical data and why is it relevant? This is also a component of clinical reasoning. If the patient presents in a way that is expected or unexpected, a decision can be made based on the nurse's textbook knowledge that is used and applied, as well as prior clinical experience. When the nurse contrasts and juxtaposes the desired outcome with the present status, this will facilitate recognizing relevant clinical data (Pesut & Herman, 1998).

2. Interpreting

Once the essence of the current clinical situation is grasped and relevant clinical data identified, this data must now be interpreted. What does this data mean and what is its significance? Unless a nurse has a deep understanding of the applied sciences, especially pathophysiology, the ability to correctly interpret data will be impacted.

3. Responding

Based on the correct interpretation of clinical data, does the nurse need to ACT or rescue, or is further monitoring warranted?

4. Reflecting

A nurse needs to develop two aspects of reflection. Reflection-IN-action is the ability of the nurse to "read" the patient and her response to CURRENT nursing interventions and adjust what is done based on the patient's response. Reflection-ON-action is done AFTERward. It completes the four-step cycle by determining what can be learned from what was just experienced and how that experience will contribute to ongoing clinical knowledge development. This is especially important if an error in judgment occurred. The nurse needs to learn and grow from errors or incorrect judgments made in practice.

Breaking it down and Putting it all Together

A patient I cared for in the critical setting illustrated how each of the four constructs of nurse thinking addressed in this chapter culminate in making correct clinical judgments. To separate the elements of nurse thinking in this clinical scenario, I will use the following abbreviations:
- NP: Nursing process
- CT: Critical thinking
- PR: Pattern recognition

- CR: Clinical reasoning
- CJ: Clinical judgment

My patient was an elderly woman named Josephine who was in the ICU for close observation post-op day #1 for right femoral-popliteal bypass. But before providing care, the nurse collected the following:

Initial Presentation: Progressive right lower leg pain the past two weeks. Prior history of diabetes type II, hypertension, coronary artery disease, and dementia. Day of admission the nurse at the skilled care facility was unable to find a pulse in the right foot. Ultrasound revealed occluded posterior and anterior tibial arteries. Her right leg was pale, cool, and mottled from the knee down.
- **CT:** Understand the pathophysiology to be able to cluster clinical data
- **PR:** Recognize the pattern or cluster of data that represents a problem as a result of a lack of perfusion and blood flow as well as relationship or pattern between diabetes, coronary artery disease, hypertension, and current problem of peripheral arterial disease
- **CR:** Recognize what clinical data is relevant and why

Shift begins-post-op day #1: Nurse report: Stable, tolerating small amounts of clear liquids. Received hydromorphone 0.3 mg IV PRN for pain. Last dose three hours ago. No current complaint of pain. Incision dry and intact with no drainage, abdomen soft with hypoactive bowel sounds. Unable to use incentive spirometer.
- **CR:** What are the most likely complication (s)?

Fifteen minutes after shift report: Josephine has a sudden large emesis that is dark brown. She is not currently nauseated and apologizes for the mess she made. Resp. rate 16/minute, O2 sat 87% on 2 liters n/c, was 94% last recorded 1 hour ago. Breath sounds clear, diminished in the bases
- **CT:** Recognize risk of aspiration with any emesis
- **NP/CR:** Assesses and recognizes relevant data. O2 sat low, TREND has decreased, breath sounds normal/expected in first day post-op.
- **CJ:** Increase O2 to 4 liters n/c
- **NP/CR:** Assesses and recognize 94% O2 sat increases one minute later

- **NP/CR**: Focused assessment and recognize relevant data. Abdomen rounded-firm, hypoactive bowel sounds.
- **NP/CJ/CT**: Administer Ondansetron 4 mg IV PRN. Use knowledge of how this medication works, time to administer IV push, compatibility with IV solution
- **CJ**: Decision made to contact physician with recommendation to obtain abdomen x-ray to rule out ileus
- **CR**: Recognize relevance. Abd xray-ilieus, stomach distended, large amount of air in colon and small intestine
- **CJ**: Decision made to contact physician for update. Nurse recommends nasogastric tube to low intermittent suction. Received orders for nasogastric tube to low intermittent suction, NPO

Pre-nasogastric tube insertion

- **CT**: Hydromorphone 0.3 mg IV PRN every 3 hours. Has not had. Need to know onset, peak duration, so allow adequate time to take effect before placing NG.
- **CJ**: Decision made to administer hydromorphone before inserting NG
- **CT**: Has dementia, will not be able to cooperate to keep NG in place so…
- **CJ**: Decision made to obtain bilateral mitt restraints so can place at time of insertion

Nasogastric tube insertion

- **NP**: Patient actively resisting placement, swearing, attempted to place in right nare, met obstruction, unable to pass (assessment/intervention)
- **CJ**: Decision made to stop. Reattempt insertion in left nare
- **NP/CR-** Reattempted NG in left nare. Able to place, but no NG returns when connected to suction. Could hear suction sound very loudly. Looked closely in mouth had coiled in mouth (assessment/intervention)
- **CJ**: Incorrectly placed, remove NG
- **CT**: Reattempt NG insertion despite patient resistive, sat patient upright, unable to cooperate with swallowing, second nurse moving chin down once placed through nasopharynx.
- **NP**: Intervention/assessment. Placed to 60 cm, at-

tached to suction, 100 mL of dark brown secretions, NG secured, mitt restraints remain in place.

Post-nasogastric tube insertion

- **NP**: Reassess abdomen. Soft. Hypoactive BS. Resting comfortably. BP 110/60, O2 sat 98% at 4 liters nasal cannula
- **CJ**: Decrease O2 from 4 to 2 liters nasal cannula
- **NP/CJ**: Five minutes later, O2 sat 94% (assessment). Keep O2 at 2 liters.
- **CJ/NP**: Condition is currently stable. Continue to assess

In this practice-based scenario, ten clinical judgments were made in less than an hour! In order to make correct clinical judgments, nursing process, critical thinking, pattern recognition, and clinical reasoning need to be utilized. To demonstrate the importance of clinical reasoning in this scenario, what would have been the consequence if relevant clinical data, including the large emesis and firm abdomen at the beginning of this scenario had not been recognized or interpreted correctly? The ileus would have progressed, resulting in patient distress and another emesis that could have resulted in aspiration.

Thinking like a nurse is complex. In order to prepare students for practice, each of these constructs need to be understood and applied to the bedside. How to provide practice of this essential nurse thinking skill in the classroom and clinical settings will be emphasized in upcoming chapters.

Reflect

Roof Truss #1: Nursing Process

1. Do you integrate clinical reasoning and nursing process together when this content is taught?

2. How could you teach this content differently to address clinical reasoning?

Roof Truss #2: Critical Thinking

3. How do you define the essence of critical thinking?

Roof Truss #3: Identify Relationships of Clinical Data

4. Do you currently emphasize the importance of clinical relationships to guide students in putting the clinical puzzle together?

5. Which clinical relationships could you incorporate to strengthen this aspect of how a nurse thinks in your program?

Roof Truss #4: DEEP Understanding of Clinical Reasoning

6. How do you define and emphasize clinical reasoning in the class or clinical settings?

7. Do your students have a deep knowledge and understanding of clinical reasoning and how to apply this to patient care?

8. Does your program prepare students to think like a nurse in other ways than a traditional care plan and NANDA nursing diagnostic priorities?

9. What aspects of nurse thinking are currently the weakest/strongest in your program?
   - Nursing process

   - Critical thinking

   - Clinical relationships?

   - Clinical reasoning?

10. What is ONE thing you can do to make this current weakness a strength in your program?

References

Alfaro-LeFevre, R. (2013). *Critical thinking, clinical reasoning, and clinical judgment: A practical approach.* (5th ed.). St. Louis, MO: Elsevier–Saunders.

Benner, P. (1982). From novice to expert. *American Journal of Nursing, 82*(3), 402–407.

Benner, P. (1984). *From novice to expert: Excellence and power in clinical nursing practice.* Upper Saddle River, NJ: Prentice Hall.

Benner, P., & Tanner, C. (1987). Clinical judgment: How expert nurses use intuition. *American Journal of Nursing, 87*(1), 23-31.

Benner, P., Tanner, C., & Chesla, C. (1992). From beginner to expert: gaining a differentiated clinical world in critical care nursing. *Advances in Nursing Science 14*(3), 13–28.

Benner, P., Tanner, C. A., & Chesla, C. A. (1996). *Expertise in nursing practice: Caring, clinical judgment, and ethics.* New York, NY: Springer.

Benner, P., Hooper-Kyriakidis, P., & Stannard, D. (2011). *Clinical wisdom and interventions in acute and critical care: A thinking-in-action approach.* (2nd ed.). New York, NY: Springer.

Benner, P., Sutphen, M., Leonard, V., & Day, L. (2010). *Educating nurses: A call for radical transformation.* San Francisco, CA: Jossey-Bass.

Berman, A., Snyder, S., & Frandsen, G. (2016). *Fundamentals of nursing.* (9th ed.). Upper Saddle River, NJ: Prentice Hall.

Bittner, N., & Tobin, E. (1998). Critical thinking: Strategies for clinical practice. *Journal for Nurses in Staff Development, 14*, 267–72.

Cappelletti, A., Engel, J.C., & Prentice, D. (2014). Systematic review of clinical judgment and reasoning in nursing. *Journal of Nursing Education, (53)*8, 458.

del Bueno, D. (2005). A crisis in critical thinking. *Nurs-*

ing Education Perspectives, 26(5), 278–282. Clarke, S.P., & Aiken, L.H. (2003). Failure to rescue. *American Journal of Nursing, 103,* 42-47.

Dressel, P., & Mayhew, L. (1954). *General education exploration in evaluation.* Washington, DC: American Council on Education.

Kautz, D.D., Kuiper, R., Pesut, D.J., & Williams, R.L. (2006). Using NANDA, NIC, and NOC (NNN) language for clinical reasoning with the outcome-present state-test (OPT) model. *International Journal of Nursing Terminologies and Classifications, (17)*3, 129-138.

Koharchik, L., Caputi, L., Robb, M., & Culleiton, A.L. (2015). Fostering clinical reasoning in nursing students. *American Journal of Nursing, (115)*1, 58-61.

Kothari, R. U., Pancioli, A., Liu, T., Brott, T., & Brodeick, J. (1999) Cincinnati prehospital stroke scale: Reproducibility and validity. *Annals of Emergency Medicine, 33,* 373–378.

Lasater, K. (2011). Clinical judgment: The last frontier for evaluation. N*urse Education in Practice, 11*(2), 86-92.

Levett-Jones, T., Hoffman, K., Dempsey, J., Yeun-Sim Jeong, S., Noble, D., Norton, C., & Hickey, N. (2010). The 'five rights' of clinical reasoning: An educational model to enhance nursing students' ability to identify and manage clinically 'at risk' patients. *Nurse Education Today, 30,* 515–520.

Ostrogorsky, T.L., Raber, A.M., McKinley Yoder, C., Nielson, A.E., Lutz, K.F., & Wros, P.L. (2015). Becoming a nurse: Role formation among accelerated baccalaureate students. *Nurse Educator, 40*(1), 26-30.

Paul, R., & Elder, L. (2005). *Critical thinking: Tools for taking charge of your learning and your life* (2nd ed.) Upper Saddle River, NJ: Prentice Hall.

Pesut, D.J., & Herman, J. (1998). OPT: Transformation of nursing process for contemporary practice. *Nursing Outlook, 46,* 29-36.

Pesut, D.J., & Herman, J. (1999). Clinical reasoning: The art and science of critical & creative thinking. Albany, NY: Delmar Publishers.

Porter-O'Grady, T. (2010). Nurses as knowledge workers. In L. Caputi, *Teaching nursing: The art and science,* Vol.2. Glen Ellyn, IL: College of DuPage Press.

Potter, P. A., & Perry, A. G. (2012). *Fundamentals of nursing.* (8th ed.). St. Louis, MO: Mosby–Elsevier.

Simmons, B. (2010). Clinical reasoning: Concept analysis. *Journal of Advanced Nursing, 66*(5), 1151-1158.

Spot a Stroke. American Stroke Association. Retrieved from http://strokeassociation.org/STROKEORG/

Staub, S. (2003). Teaching and measuring critical thinking. *Journal of Nursing Education, 42,* 498–508.

Tanner, C. A. (2005). What have we learned about critical thinking in nursing? *Journal of Nursing Education, 44*(2), 47–48.

Tanner, C. A. (2006a). Thinking like a nurse: A research-based model of clinical judgment in nursing. *Journal of Nursing Education, 45*(6), 204–211.

Thompson, C., Cullum, N., McCaughan, D., Sheldon, T., & Raynor, P. (2004). Nurses, information use, and clinical decision making: The real potential for evidence-based decisions in nursing. *Evidence-Based Nursing, 7*(3), 69–72.

11

Strategies and Tools to Teach Nurse Thinking

Keith Rischer, RN, MA, CEN, CCRN

"Nurse educators focus on their students' acquisition of knowledge; however, nurses must know how to use knowledge in practice."

—*Educating Nurses: A Call for Radical Transformation*, p. 31

Though clinical reasoning is essential to THINK more like a nurse, it is not the end product of nurse thinking. A correct clinical judgment is the end result of how a nurse thinks and both critical thinking and clinical reasoning must be utilized by the nurse. That is why clinical reasoning must be emphasized in nursing education.

Nurse educators require tools to develop clinical reasoning in students (Russell, Geist, & House Maffett, 2013). When educators use strategies and tools that emphasize concrete application of the concept of clinical reasoning to practice, clinical reasoning can be strengthened (Murphy, 2004). In order to strengthen clinical reasoning that will lead to a correct clinical judgment in practice, I will share the ONE tool that will help develop and strengthen the ability of your students to think more like a nurse in your program. It is also included in the Transformation Toolbox in the appendix.

"Clinical Reasoning Questions to Develop Nurse Thinking" Handout

As a newer nurse educator in the clinical setting, I reflected how I used a methodical, sequential approach of applied clinical reasoning to grasp the essence and establish care priorities for each patient in my care.

As I shared at length in the prior chapter, I developed a clinical reasoning tool that is a template of 12 sequential questions on a single page that deconstructs clinical reasoning by identifying the sequential steps a nurse in practice uses to clinically reason from the time they prepare to assume care when reviewing the chart, to when the patient is seen for the first time, and then throughout the shift.

This template of clinical reasoning questions can also be used to replace the traditional care plan (I recommend this for advanced level students) because it combines care planning, nursing process, and clinical reasoning in one construct that closely mirrors how a nurse thinks in practice.

Additional Strategies to Develop Clinical Judgment

Just as it takes time and clinical experience to develop and progress from a novice to the next stage of professional development as a nurse, the same is true with each student's ability to develop and make correct clinical judgments (Alfero-LeFevre, 2013). Encourage students to be fully engaged in the clinical setting to maximize their learning and think more like a nurse. The following are some practical strategies to help students develop and make correct clinical judgments:

- **Become familiar with what is "normal" so the abnormal becomes readily apparent.** This principle is not only true for nurses but also for bank tellers! One effective strategy bank tellers are taught to identify counterfeit bills is to handle the original bills that represent what is authentic and normal. Once they become familiar with the feel and appearance of a normal bill, the abnormal counterfeit is easily recognized.

In the same way in the clinical setting, guide students to make it a priority to establish and compare normal lab values, vital sign parameters, and assessment findings so that abnormal data collected in practice is immediately recognized. For example, once students know and understand the normal heart tones of S1S2; this normal baseline is the standard that every set of heart tones are compared to with patients in the future. Abnormal heart sounds such as murmurs and S3 and S4 gallops are readily recognized when compared to a normal S1S2.

- **Know pathophysiology.** Once the pathophysiology of a problem is deeply understood, clinical data is correctly interpreted and signs and symptoms of a worsening progression or improvement become clear. Once the pathophysiology of sepsis is understood, the significance of an elevated temperature, tachycardia, and elevated WBC and neutrophils are recognized as clinical concerns. Conversely, when the temperature, WBC, and tachycardia return to normal ranges, this clinical data can be correctly interpreted for the clinical improvement that this data represents.
- **Reflect on all clinical data collected and recorded.** Encourage students to resist the temptation to see vital signs and nursing assessments as just another task to complete and document in the chart. Have them REFLECT on what they have collected and compare it to the most recent data to establish TRENDS. Is the data collected expected or unexpected based on report and the primary problem? By taking the time to REFLECT, students will be much more likely to accurately INTERPRET the data, which will lead to a correct clinical judgment.
- **Authentically care.** When the nurse is engaged and empathetically cares, this personal/professional engagement results in heightened vigilance or attentiveness that will lead to better patient outcomes.

Reflect

1. How could this template of clinical reasoning questions be incorporated into your clinical setting to develop nurse thinking in your students?

2. Are your students prepared to identify the worst possible/most likely "Jasons" from harming their patients in the clinical setting?

3. What strategies could you implement to strengthen the ability of students to think more like a nurse?

References

Alfaro-LeFevre, R. (2013). *Critical thinking, clinical reasoning, and clinical judgment: A practical approach.* (5th ed.). St. Louis, MO: Elsevier–Saunders.

Cappelletti, A., Engel, J.C., & Prentice, D. (2014). Systematic review of clinical judgment and reasoning in nursing. *Journal of Nursing Education, (53)*8, 458.

Murphy, J.I. (2004). Using focused reflection and articulation to promote clinical reasoning: An evidence-based approach. *Nurse Education Perspectives, 25*(5), 226-231.

Tanner, C. A. (2006). Thinking like a nurse: A research-based model of clinical judgment in nursing. *Journal of Nursing Education, 45*(6), 204–211.

12

Preparing the Way for Transformation: Taking Down the Golden Calves

Keith Rischer, RN, MA, CEN, CCRN
Patricia Pence, EdD, MSN, RN

As a new nurse educator entering academia after more than 20 years in clinical practice, I (Keith) quickly realized that change does not come quickly or easily in nursing education. I discovered that some things that had to change were now entrenched "sacred" traditions. Just like the idolatrous golden calf that Moses encountered coming down the mountain after receiving the law, long held traditions and ways of doing things need to be carefully examined to determine if they are false objects of adoration in nursing education and if found wanting, they need to be taken down.

The following are the "golden calves" that need to be taken down once and for all so needed transformational change can be realized in nursing education.

1. NANDA nursing diagnostic statements (why NANDA is a NO-NO)
2. Emphasis on "NCLEX Success"
3. Emphasis on "Student Success"
4. Make learning fun"
5. Overreliance on technology
6. Overreliance on PowerPoint lecture

Why NANDA Is a NO-NO

NANDA would be my (Keith) first choice of a golden calf that needs to be taken down. When I graduated from nursing school in 1983, NANDA was in its infancy as a taxonomy for the language of the nursing profession. I remember how awkward I found NANDA nursing diagnostic statements to use as a nursing priority and how challenging it was to write a correctly worded three-part statement in my care plan. After I graduated, I did not think in three-part NANDA statements and intuitively began using the essence of clinical reasoning by identifying relevant clinical data and the nursing priority.

Imagine my horror when I re-entered nursing education 25 years later as a new nurse educator and found that NANDA was still there! In fact, in the program I taught, it was the ONLY way that students were allowed to identify the nursing priority. I was torn. How could I support my students who were repeating the same struggles I had as a student nurse 25 years earlier? It was painful and hard to watch this clinical drama unfold every week as clinical students took their NANDA summary card of all 200+ nursing diagnostic statements and reviewed it over and over to find a statement that would "fit" as a nursing priority for their written care plan.

NANDA has minimal relevance to bedside nursing practice but can be used to establish basic/fundamental nursing priorities. Fundamental content always remains relevant to the practicing nurse. Advanced skills are built upon this foundation in the second level of nursing education. In the same way, once NANDA and nursing process is presented and situated in fundamentals, priority setting (with or without NANDA) and thinking like a nurse using all aspects of clinical reasoning must be incorporated in the second level of nursing education to teach students to think like a nurse and transition successfully to real-world professional practice.

One educator shared how she flips this paradigm in her fundamental classroom when she teaches nursing process. Instead of teaching NANDA nursing diagnostic statements FIRST as a way to situate nursing care priorities, she emphasizes the broad priority FIRST and then the NANDA statement that is most relevant to this priority. For example, a patient with respiratory distress because of pneumonia would have a nursing priority of "respiratory difficulty/problem." The NANDA statement that was closest to the actual problem, which in this scenario would be "impaired gas exchange." This is an excellent approach because it teaches general problem identification FIRST, just as a nurse does in practice and de-emphasizes the need to find a NANDA statement that "fits."

Other Perspectives

Any discussion to remove NANDA from the second step of nursing process remains a polarizing topic in nursing education. Though I have obvious concerns about the relevance of NANDA as a practicing nurse, when I share my perspectives openly, based on the response of my audience, many educators also no longer see its relevance to practice and question if and how it should be taught. I have even had audiences break out in applause when I verbalize my critique of NANDA and its validity to bedside practice! I feel I am communicating openly what many of them are thinking privately.

Two experienced nurse educators recently wrote me to share their reflections on NANDA that need to be considered:

"I find nursing diagnoses ineffective/irrelevant in practice because they 'dumb down' the role of the nurse. When I shared this opinion with colleagues early in my teaching career, I was chastised for my blasphemy and learned to keep my mouth shut. But if we're going to transform nursing education and contextualize nursing practice to active learning environments, these golden calves have to move out to pasture."
—Peggy Hernandez, EdD, APRN, PMHCNS-BC, CNE
Assistant Professor
Wichita State University
Wichita, Kansas

"We need to lose the 'nursing diagnosis' piece from nursing process, and take the valuable time we spend confusing students early on and instead immerse them in activities that require 'thinking like a nurse.' In my opinion nursing diagnosis is archaic, linear, and inhibits the type of thinking we need our students to develop as intellectual habits of mind that are critical to the profession."
—Joanne McDermott, RN, PhD
Associate Professor
MidAmerica Nazarene University
Olathe, Kansas

The Power of Five Smooth Stones

The number of NANDA nursing diagnostic statements, like the size of textbooks, continues to grow. There are currently 216 NANDA statements. As I reviewed the current list, I find only a handful that I consistently use as a practicing nurse. These include:

- Impaired gas exchange
- Ineffective tissue perfusion
- Acute/chronic pain
- Fluid volume excess/deficit
- Impaired skin integrity
- Risk for infection
- Risk for falls
- Risk for impaired skin integrity
- Knowledge deficit
- Anxiety
- Spiritual distress

Practical nurse thinking does not lend itself to a three-part NANDA nursing diagnostic statement with "related to" and "as evidenced by" that laid the foundation of care planning in nursing school. This became obvious once I was a nurse in practice. Like David who brought down the giant Goliath with five small stones, I, too, have five small stones. Each stone represents an objective reason why this giant should be brought down and its current emphasis re-examined in nursing education to develop nurse thinking in students.

My Five Stones

1. NANDA (and step 2 of the nursing process as it is currently taught) does NOT reflect how a nurse thinks in practice.

2. NANDA does not identify the nursing priority when rescue is needed.

3. NANDA contributes to "failure to rescue" when there is a change in status.

4. NANDA is not on the NCLEX.

5. NANDA statements are NOT used in most electronic medical records nursing care plans.

Stone #1–NANDA does NOT reflect how a nurse thinks in practice

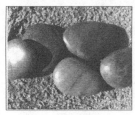 The nursing process has been the bedrock of nursing education for decades to operationalize the thinking of the professional nurse. The nursing process is one of the very first things taught in nursing education so students can begin to develop needed nurse thinking to safely care for patients. The nursing process as it is currently taught in nursing education and by fundamental textbooks (Berman & Snyder, 2012) consists of the following five steps:

1. Assessing
2. Diagnosing
3. Planning
4. Implementing
5. Evaluating

Once the systematic and continuous collection of clinical assessment data is done by the nurse in step 1, this data must be analyzed and clustered to determine the most relevant data and to formulate the best and correct nursing diagnosis. Step 2 of the nursing process requires the student to formulate the correct nursing diagnosis using one of the 216 NANDA statements and then complete it with a three-part nursing diagnostic statement that includes the following key components:

NANDA statement
• Related to…
• As manifested by…

There is only one problem with this traditional approach: this is NOT how a nurse in clinical practice thinks and establishes nursing care priorities, especially when there is a change of status. As you reflect on your experience as a nurse who practiced at the bedside, did you think and set care priorities using only NANDA statements and then formulate a three-part statement?

Students often ask, "Is NANDA used by a nurse in practice?" I honestly have to state, "No. The use of NANDA nursing diagnostic statements is not how I and nurses in real-world practice think." So how can I justify teaching this taxonomy? I started asking students to list the top three PROBLEMS after assessing a patient (not necessarily use a nursing diagnosis). I found that this led to a more meaningful problem list, and if not, led to a thoughtful discussion with the students.

The ongoing use of NANDA nursing diagnostic statements is an example that the practice-education gap is alive and well in nursing education. It makes nurse thinking much harder than it has to be and is a barrier that makes it difficult for to students to transition successfully to the bedside after they graduate.

To further illustrate my point, let me use an example of a critical change in patient status. Upon entering your patient's room, it is apparent that something is terribly wrong. You come closer and determine that your patient is not breathing and has no pulse. To determine what to do next and establish a correct clinical judgment would you step back and formulate the following NANDA statement before providing needed nursing interventions?

NANDA STATEMENT: Ineffective tissue perfusion-cardiac-neuro and renal
RELATED TO: Ventricular fibrillation, but oops…I cannot use the medical diagnosis but must state instead that this is a condition in which there is uncoordinated contraction of the cardiac muscle of the ventricles in the heart, making them quiver rather than contract properly.
MANIFESTED BY: Absence of pulse, absence of BP, absence of respirations, and ashen pale skin color

Though this correctly worded three-part NANDA statement would get an A on a written care plan, it FAILS to prepare a student to think like a nurse because it does not capture the simplicity and essence of clinical reasoning, which represents nurse thinking. Instead of this awkward and complicated three-part NANDA statement, nurses in practice use clinical reasoning that captures the "essence" of the current clinical scenario to recognize the most RELEVANT clinical data is and identify the nursing PRIORITY.

When a nurse clinically reasons in this same scenario, the essence of this scenario is simply: NO PULSE, NO RESPIRATIONS, and the nursing priority: Call a code and begin CPR! Life-saving interventions can then quickly begin.

Stone #2–NANDA does not identify the nursing priority when rescue is needed

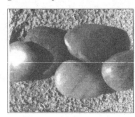 If the taxonomy of NANDA nursing diagnostic statements is the primary methodology to establish care priorities in your program, how is the student going to formulate a nursing judgment when there is not one NANDA statement that even comes close to describing the current problem? Though thinking in action and grasping the essence of the current clinical scenario is a component of clinical reasoning, the use of NANDA nursing diagnostic statements may be unable to capture the essence of change in a patient's status. The following is a common clinical scenario derived from a case study that I created that illustrates this dilemma.

Ann Smith is a 45-year-old woman who had an open hysterectomy earlier today. She is on a hydromorphone patient-controlled analgesia (PCA) at 0.1 mg bolus every ten minutes. She has been complaining of increased pain and has been using her PCA every ten to twelve minutes for the past two hours. You enter the room to bring her clear liquid dinner tray and she appears to be sleeping comfortably with a respiratory rate of 16. Her O2 sat is 98 percent. You attempt to wake her, but she does not arouse to verbal stimuli. She does arouse with vigorous physical shaking but after a few seconds falls back to sleep.

Recognizing that a problem is present, these are the NANDA statements that have a neurological emphasis and have relevance to this scenario:

- Altered sensory perception
- Alteration of operations of thought
- Impaired tissue perfusion...neurological
- Acute confusion

Do any of these NANDA statements accurately capture the essence and identify the current problem so the nurse can begin needed rescue? Not ONE! The inability of NANDA to identify the correct nursing priority and the seriousness of the current problem is also a contributing factor in failure to rescue (del Bueno, 2005).

But if your students have been taught to think like a nurse by situating clinical reasoning to the bedside, they would NOT rely on NANDA alone to identify the current nursing priority and make a clinical judgment. By using the nursing process, they would first cluster the relevant assessment data, simply state the nursing PRIORITY (narcotic over-sedation) that captures the essence of the current problem, develop a plan of care, appropriate nursing interventions and expected outcomes. In this scenario, the most important assessment data that needs to be clustered includes:

Assessment (RELEVANT data)
- Hydromorphone patient controlled analgesia (PCA) at 0.1 mg bolus every ten minutes

Increased pain and has been using her PCA every ten to twelve minutes for the past two hours
- Respiratory rate of 16
- O2 sat is 98 percent
- Attempt to wake her, but she does not arouse to verbal stimuli
- Does arouse with vigorous physical shaking but after a few seconds falls back to sleep

Nursing PRIORITY
- Narcotic over-sedation
- Plan

Administer naloxone IV stat

Implementation
- Dilute naloxone 0. 4mg (1 mL) with 9 mL of saline and titrate 0.04–0.08 mg (1–2 mL) every two minutes until the patient's level of consciousness returned to the desirable level
- Closely monitor neurologic status for any improvement to rescue this patient.

Stone #3–NANDA contributes to "failure to rescue" when there is a change in status

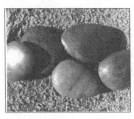

The inability of NANDA to capture the essence of a change in status translates to failure to rescue when a change in patient status occurs. del Bueno (2005) found that new nurses were unable to exercise correct clinical judgment at a basic level to "rescue" (identify the problem and then intervene) their patient in a simulated scenario due to inappropriate use of NANDA nursing diagnostic statements to make them "fit" when there was a change in status (del Bueno, 2005).

For example, when a patient had a condition change consistent with a stroke, the nurse used the NANDA statement "alteration in sensory perception" or "alteration in nutrition." In another patient having symptoms consistent with a myocardial infarction, the nurse used "activity intolerance related to pain." del Bueno (2005) summarizes her research findings with the following statement,

"Many inexperienced RNs also attempt to use a nursing diagnosis for the problem focus. Whatever the original intent for its use, the results are at best cumbersome and at worst risible." (p. 280)

Stone #4–NANDA is not on the NCLEX

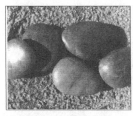

There is not one NANDA nursing diagnostic statement that students must identify on the NCLEX. The NCLEX is a clinical reasoning exam that emphasizes applied clinical reasoning for every question. Therefore, if you want to increase the NCLEX first-time passing rates of your program, strongly situate clinical reasoning in your program, NOT NANDA!

Stone #5- NANDA statements are NOT used in most electronic medical records nursing care plans.

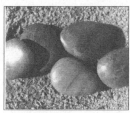

Electronic medical records (EMR) simplify care planning for the bedside nurse and are the dominant charting platform in acute care settings across the country. Where I practice, Epic is the most common EMR platform. In Epic, once the primary medical problem has been identified in the care

plan tab, the nurse can choose the problems that are relevant to the patient in their care.

But there is NO NANDA nursing diagnostic statement to identify the nursing priority for each type of illness that can be selected as the primary problem. Instead, Epic uses a problem-based approach to establish nursing priorities that are based on body systems throughout the care plan. This is also how other EMR platforms are also patterned. This body system approach to nursing priority setting is consistent regardless of the type of care plan chosen.

To illustrate this approach to care planning, on a general medical care plan in Epic, the following are the problems the nurse can select from:

- Care priority
- Hemodynamic stability
- Respiratory stability
- GU stability
- Nutrition
- GI stability
- Comfort/pain
- Activity
- Skin integrity/infection risk

Once the nurse chooses the relevant problems, the outcome is identified and a series of nursing interventions are automatically populated. In addition, every plan of care begins with the option for the nurse to choose a "Care Priority." The intervention for the nurse under care priority is defined by this statement: "Establish patient/family care priority for the day." It is open-ended so the nurse can simply and concisely state the current care priority. The essence of clinical reasoning is situated in Epic by asking the nurse to identify the nursing PRIORITY, NOT the diagnosis.

Thoughts from a Former Student

I recently asked a new nurse, who had just graduated from a local program, his perspective on NANDA while he was a nursing student. This is his response:

"Over the years NANDA and its nursing diagnoses have become a stumbling block rather than a tool as I have grown as a nurse. Nursing diagnoses to the nursing student are very much like reading glasses. Being new and overwhelmed with such copious amounts of information to learn, NANDA allows the student to focus in on something (hopefully) important. If my pa-

tient had shortness of breath, nursing diagnoses served as a helpful tool to find outcomes and interventions. "The problem with reading glasses is they make it awfully hard to really see where you are going. As I grew as a (student) nurse, I learned that these glasses I used to see had also blinded me. My patient was much more than a nursing diagnosis! Labs, imaging, PT, OT, procedures, medications, lifestyle, genetics, health and medical histories, and co-morbidities all contributed to the shortness of breath of my patient. NANDA often distracted me from important details. It was when I grew aware of the big picture and took my reading glasses off that I truly grew as a nurse." (L. Thorsgaard, personal communication, September 7, 2014)

Written Care Plans

Traditional care plans that emphasize the nursing process and a three part NANDA nursing diagnostic statement are best suited at the fundamental level. Build on this foundation with clinical reasoning applied to practice. The limitations of a written care plan are obvious. Students often copy interventions from their care plan text and do not take the time to personalize the plan of care to their patient. Their plans often contain interventions that are NOT even realistic for their patient!

Instead ask your students to look at what needs to be done for the patient that day, how often the tasks are done, and WHY they are done. Once they compare what is actually done for the patient by the staff, review the actual care plan, and individualize the plan of care for the patient, this will help students to think like a nurse and write a plan of care that more closely reflects real-world clinical practice.

Emphasis on "NCLEX Success"

I (Keith) received an email from Julie, a new nurse who is working nights in med/surg at a large metropolitan hospital. She was frustrated, overwhelmed, and struggling because she felt inadequately prepared for practice.

"I have been feeling completely overwhelmed the past two months off of orientation as I make the transition from student to staff RN. Every shift feels task oriented, as I struggle to find my groove with time management. I have a difficult time being able to critically think about the processes going on with my patients, and often feel rushed and flustered when I'm required to go

beyond my brain sheet list of to-dos. After finishing my shift (and having time to reflect on what I could have done better), I could kick myself when I realize I had the knowledge all along, I just wasn't able to apply it in the moment. I want to truly understand what is going on with my patients so that I am able to recognize if/when a patient is deteriorating and ensure I am providing the best and safest care possible."

Though graduate nurses struggle to transition to clinical practice because of clinical inexperience, students need to be taught and equipped to manage time, priority set, give bedside report, and delegate appropriately with multiple patients. Without possessing and practicing these essential skills in school, new nurses will continue to struggle to transition to clinical practice.

The opening scene of the movie *Saving Private Ryan* is harrowing and hard to watch. As the military unit approaches Omaha Beach in Normandy, France, during World War II on D-Day, June 6, 1944, with bullets whizzing by and some finding their intended target, the fresh recruits quickly realize that they are no longer in boot camp. War is a matter of life and death. But what if the emphasis of boot camp and basic training prepared a soldier to pass a written exit examination but not the battlefield?

This would be unacceptable. Soldiers must be prepared for the real-world realities of combat. But take a closer look at the most common assessment of nursing programs success or failure...the pass rates of the written NCLEX examination, with no other relevant assessment to gauge students' preparedness for real-world practice. Reflect and determine if your program emphasizes passing the NCLEX, or is it doing all that is needed to prepare students for the rigors of real-world practice?

Conference presentations at nurse educator conferences have variations of the theme "Do this or do that for NCLEX success." The NCLEX assesses that students meet basic levels of safety in practice. It does not guarantee that students are well prepared for the rigors and realities of real-world clinical practice with multiple patients. To transform nursing education, the emphasis on passing a written multiple-choice test needs to change. Like soldiers preparing for the battlefield, nursing education needs to do what is needed to intentionally and practically prepare students for real-world clinical practice.

If you implement the paradigm shifts advocated by *Educating Nurses* that includes an emphasis of clinical reasoning, you will prepare your students for both the NCLEX and clinical practice. Integrate clinical reasoning and provide opportunities for students to practice this nurse thinking skill. Then make it a priority to do all that you can to prepare students with practical principles and skills that will help them successfully transition to practice after graduation.

Here are some practical ways you can practically prepare students for real-world practice:

1. **Multiple patient assignments.** Do you provide advanced students with opportunities to manage more than one patient in the clinical setting? Though there may be limitations in the clinical setting to do so, try to consistently provide your advanced students two patient assignments. One approach to encourage multitasking with first year students is to begin the clinical day with one patient and later in the day add skills/assessment with another patient.

2. **Time management.** Most students can easily time manage one patient. If students have downtime, redeem this time with supplemental clinical reasoning tools, or better yet provide a second patient assignment to develop time management skills.

3. **Priority setting.** Setting priorities with one patient can be handled by most students. Like time management, this skill requires caring for multiple patients in the clinical setting. Can you see the pattern? Prepare students to priority set by giving a second patient whenever possible, especially at the advanced level.

4. **Professional communication.** Students don't typically talk directly to primary care providers to communicate a concern in clinical. Using the SBAR format must be consistently practiced in simulation and the clinical setting.

5. **Simulation whenever possible**. In addition to practicing professional communication, simulation is essential to safely develop the nurse thinking skill of clinical reasoning: Think in action, recognize relevant data, and establish correct care priorities that capture the essence of the current situation. Clinical experiences can vary widely in the clinical setting. This problem can be minimized when simulation standardizes nurse thinking and practical priority setting. Provide as many opportunities for simulation in your program. Using clinical reasoning case studies in the classroom also accomplishes this essential objective.

6. **Emphasize clinical reasoning.** This is an essential paradigm shift that is required to radically transform nursing education (Benner, et al., 2010). I have developed a simple step-by-step template that breaks down this essential thinking skill so that students can readily understand and apply it to practice.

Emphasis on "Student Success"

Students will struggle in the clinical setting. Most who struggle are able to successfully remediate and continue to grow and develop as novice nurses. But some were unable to put it all together in the clinical setting despite doing well in the classroom. Others struggled, but had little to no insight. Still others would blame the nursing instructor or nursing program instead of taking personal responsibility for their struggles. What do these last two student groups have in common? Regardless of their desire to complete the nursing program and graduate, they should not be assured of "student success" until they can demonstrate basic safety, clinical reasoning, and clinical competence.

Some programs emphasize "student success," which is an educational philosophy that every student who has enrolled in the program should succeed; despite concerns they are unable to safely transfer learning to the bedside. Nurse educators have a duty and responsibility to protect the public from students who consistently demonstrate an inability to be safe in practice. The failure to fail nursing students who are not able to demonstrate acceptable progression is also a contributing factor to the growing and unacceptable preparation-to-practice gap in academia (Docherty & Dieckmann, 2015).

When nurse educators have a choice between patient safety and student success, our guiding principle as educators must be patient advocates who protect public safety. Therefore, PATIENT/PUBLIC SAFETY must take precedence over STUDENT SUCCESS.

I am for student success! As a nurse educator, I give my all to promote the learning of my students. I willingly choose to do what is needed to guide and develop their learning to translate skills and knowledge to the bedside. I tell my students who fail that I have seen other students who struggled, who reflected and improved their skills.

They devoted additional time in the skills lab, and using the text, notes, and online resources, were able to succeed.

Nursing is a difficult major. Some students require more time to be successful. Failure at any level can be a new beginning that can lead to student success! By retaining a struggling student, this may not serve the needs of the student and their needed learning in the long run. It is often in the student's best interest to give them TIME to make a current weakness a strength. Therefore, allowing a student to drop or to fail, if done in a supportive manner, can strengthen long-term development as a nurse! I have observed struggling students who failed come back the following semester stronger and better prepared and hit it out of the park! Failure, when done in a supportive way, allowed them to reflect, strengthen their weaknesses, and be successful because they were allowed to fail and not allowed to be retained in the program at all costs.

"Make Learning Fun"

In order to cater to the needs of the current generation of students, there is an underlying assumption that learning needs to be fun, and that the use of games is needed to promote engagement and get them to participate. Games can help students memorize content and facilitate student participation, but the emphasis of CONTENT knowledge and memorization that games tend to emphasize is unable in and of itself going to develop clinical salience and clinical reasoning that students require for practice.

One nurse educator sent me her reflections regarding games in the classroom:

"I have used Jeopardy in the past, when this was promoted in a nursing education conference as a way to engage students in class. You leave some conference sessions thinking this is best teaching practice so I implemented this in my class. But I found that games promoted students' recall of content and not a deep understanding that they needed to solve a clinical problem. Games trivialize patient care and underestimate the seriousness of recognizing early clues in a patient's condition in order to rescue a patient from a potential complication. Games do not bring the ethical and moral aspect of nursing care into a classroom. Not all students can keep up with participating in a game and become frustrated. Not all students liked it and it was not an effective use of class time."

The reliance on and use of games in nursing education was also questioned by the co-authors of *Educating Nurses.*

"Although the students' attention is gained through games, the quality of their attentiveness may fall short of serious engagement with the practice of nursing. Whether the teacher intends it or not, games can reinforce the idea that guessing is acceptable and that memorization is the primary objective in nursing education...students may infer a subtle message that the intellectual projects and caregiving issues of nursing practice are not appealing enough to draw students' attention." (Benner, et al, 2010, p.74)

The educators who wrote the paradigm cases of learning in *Educating Nurses* did not use games. They engage their students by giving them intellectual and moral challenges of reasoning based on real patient scenarios. They actively involved students in developing clinical imagination, and exploring the ethical dilemmas that may be present in cases presented. They understand that every aspect of the education experience that trivializes patient care conveys a message and this may adversely impact their formation as a professional nurse (Benner, et al., 2010).

These observations also parallel with master teacher Parker Palmer who would also question the need to make learning fun and rely on games to engage. Though not a nurse educator, his philosophy of learning is timeless and relevant to nurse educators. His classic book, *The Courage to Teach: Exploring the Inner Landscape of a Teacher's Life* explains in depth the relevance and simplicity of a subject-centered classroom.

Palmer's thoughts on teaching stressed that for learning to take place, teachers need *"to get students inside the subject,"* and *"the subject inside the students,"* otherwise students do not see the importance of the subject (content) to their learning (Palmer, 1990). Lectures and the use of games do not allow this to happen; students may not be able to thread the connections between the "subject" and how this "subject" is SALIENT and RELEVANT to fit it into caring for a patient in nursing practice.

Overreliance on Technology

As our society embraces technology that has rendered the cassette tape, CDs, and the last generation of cell phones obsolete, this trend can also influence the way that nursing is taught. It is not enough to have a basic Sim-Man, but the highest fidelity of simulation manikins must be sought after, even if they approach six figures in cost. There is a latent assumption that the latest in technology including clickers, computer-based simulation, etc. equals an improved way to teach. Though technology engages even toddlers as they swipe and flip through tablets, does this translate to actual learning?

Though technology can facilitate learning, nurse educators must evaluate and determine if these expensive tools are NICE to have or NEED to have, based on their ability to develop nurse thinking and clinical practice skills. The decision to even consider using or adapting any technology needs to be based on the outcomes that need to be achieved, NOT because it is new and exciting. Educators must emphasize and continue to use innovative methods of teaching that engage students as active learners and partners in learning (Oermann, 2015).

Though technology can facilitate learning, Popil (2011) identified one pedagogy that is LOW tech but HIGH in learning value because it promotes critical thinking: a salient and relevant case study. I am NOT against the use of the latest technology that is available in nursing education, only the overreliance on it. The use of PowerPoint slides is a morality tale and an excellent example of how technology can make it easier to present content in the classroom, but does not guarantee transfer of knowledge and development of clinical reasoning. "Death by PowerPoint" is a powerful critique of the overreliance of this tool originally created for sales and business presentations.

Overreliance on PowerPoint Lectures

PowerPoint was never intended to be used as an educational tool. It was originally designed and marketed to salespeople for use in marketing presentations, beginning in 1987. PowerPoint slide design, how faculty typically use the slides, and the underlying technology actually create barriers that disconnect students from the learning process (Moellenberg & Aldridge, 2010). Educators struggle to engage students in the classroom. Could the ubiquitous use of PowerPoint be part of the problem?

Teaching by traditional lecture has been the norm for best teaching practice, as it was common for nurse educators to teach students in the manner in which they were taught (Emerson & Records, 2008; Lauver, et al., 2009).

For many years, lecture seemed to be an effective method to cover content needed to care for patients in clinical practice. Later, PowerPoint–enhanced lectures continued to emphasize a content-heavy curriculum (Benner, et al., 2010).

Technology has changed dramatically over the last ten years and how students are taught to care for patients in clinical practice has also changed dramatically. This includes bedside scanning of patients' identification bands and each medication before administration to ensure patient safety. Pyxis computerized systems are used to retrieve medications and intravenous bags. EMRs replaced "binders" that once contained printed copies and handwritten medical records and orders, all neatly sectioned by tabbed dividers.

As a result of a rapidly changing health care system, nurses are caring for patients who have acuity levels requiring highly skilled complex nursing care. Clinical reasoning, clinical judgment, critical thinking, and a spirit of inquiry are an expected and desired skill set of nurses today. Nurses need these skill sets so they can recognize early signs and symptoms indicating a decline, and reason through the patient's situation and condition, in order to rescue a patient and prevent a negative outcome (Benner, et al., 2010).

Why reflect on changes that have occurred over time in clinical practice? Because as nurses and nurse educators, if we are resistant to adapting how we teach and practice nursing in a clinical setting, we are holding on to past assumptions that are no longer relevant, despite evidence that we NEED to change.

It has been several years since Benner (Benner, et al., 2010) called for nurse educators to rethink how we conduct teaching in the classroom, clinical, and laboratory settings. It is time for you, as nurse educators, to reflect on your teaching practice, and honestly assess whether you are using classroom time to effectively develop, apply, and practice these essential and desired thinking skill-sets (Benner, et al., 2010). To meet the learning needs of students, and help them be prepared for professional practice, the status quo that relies heavily on PowerPoint lectures as the prime pedagogy needs to go and transition to meaningful active learning.

Are you ready to let go of your reliance on PowerPoint lectures? Are you going to be part of bringing NEEDED change to bring transformation to nursing education? Though it will require time and effort, as well as some speed bumps along the way, know that you will be using evidenced-based teaching practices for the betterment of your students and the patients under their care after they graduate. Use your expert nursing knowledge and experience to be creative and bring NEEDED change to your nursing classroom that does not rely so heavily on PowerPoint presentations.

Reflect

1. What golden calves are still standing in your program that need to be taken down or put out to pasture?

2. How will this impact student learning and/or department culture?

3. How will you champion this vision so other educators can join with you to strengthen student learning?

References

Benner, P., Sutphen, M., Leonard, V., & Day, L. (2010). *Educating nurses: A call for radical transformation.* San Francisco, CA: Jossey-Bass.

Berman, A., & Snyder, S. (2012). *Fundamentals of nursing* (9th ed.). Upper Saddle River, NJ: Prentice Hall.

del Bueno, D. (2005). A crisis in critical thinking. *Nursing Education Perspectives, 26(5), 278–282.*

Docherty, A., & Dieckmann, N. (2015). Is there evidence of failing to fail in our schools of nursing? *Nursing Education Perspectives, 36(4), 226-231.*

Emerson, R. J., & Records, K. (2008). Today's challenge, tomorrow's excellence: The practice of evidenced-based education. *Journal of nursing education, 47(8), 359-370.*

Lauver, L. S., West, M. M., Campbell, T. B., Herrold, J., & Wood, G. C. (2009). Toward evidence-based teaching: Evaluating the effectiveness of two teaching strategies in an associate degree nursing program. *Teaching and Learning in Nursing, 4(4), 133-138.*

Moellenberg, K.K., & Aldredge, M. (2010). Sliding away from powerpoint: The interactive lecture. *Nurse Educator, 35(6), 268-272.*

Oermann, M. (2015). Technology and teaching innovations in nursing education: Engaging the student. *Nurse Educator, 40(2), 55-56.*

Palmer, P. (2007). *The courage to teach: Exploring the inner landscape of a teacher's life.* San Francisco, CA: Jossey-Bass.

Popil, I. (2011). Promotion of critical thinking by using case studies as a teaching method. *Nurse Education Today, 31, 204-207.*

PART THREE

TRANSFORMING
THE CLASSROOM

13

Principles to Transform Classroom Learning

Keith Rischer, RN, MA, CEN, CCRN

"Students learn better...where educators make an attempt to integrate the classroom and the clinical."
—*Educating Nurses: A Call for Radical Transformation*, p. 12

The classroom is ground zero in the battle to transforming nursing education. This assessment was validated by the Carnegie Foundation's research detailed in *Educating Nurses*. Other leading voices in nursing education have been advocating for similar change for some time. Over ten years ago Tanner (2004) advocated a "pedagogy of engagement" that emphasizes guiding student learning by covering content in such a way that students are able to make connections with what is taught rather than playing the role of the content expert, so that authentic learning and thinking takes place.

Christine Tanner (2004) closed her editorial in the *Journal of Nursing Education* with the following thoughts that have relevance for every nurse educator today:

"Changing the way we teach is a journey, one of our own learning, reflection, and growth. When we begin to see ourselves as mentors and guides, rather than experts; when we become committed to hearing the students' interpretation of their experiences over our 'points to make;' and when we understand that to nurse well takes tending to the body, mind, and spirit, we commit to creating places for that growth to occur." (p. 4)

To prepare the way for transformation in your classroom and your program, and to create a classroom where faculty guide student learning and encourage thinking, the following principles derived from the literature as well as my own observations will lay a strong foundation for change. First there are general principles that must be incorporated, then specific steps to not only "flip" but transform your classroom!

Principles to Prepare the Way for Transformation

The following principles will prepare the way to successfully transform your classroom.

- Assess your strengths and weaknesses
- Have a high but realistic bar of student expectations
- Students come to class prepared
- Make learning active!
- Engage and involve students in learning
- Embrace adult learning principles
- Pursue passion!
- Don't "cover" the content
- Don't merely "flip" your classroom, TRANSFORM it!

Assess Your Strengths and Weaknesses

In order to change the way you teach, first honestly reflect on your current weaknesses and strengths as a classroom educator. The following questions will help you assess your current strengths and abilities and reflect on your current journey to determine what you are doing well, and how to strengthen your teaching abilities (Herrmann, 2016):

- Do you KNOW your content well enough to break

it down and present it so students can UNDER-STAND difficult concepts/topics?

- Do you have clinical experience in the subject matter you are teaching to provide personal insights and stories? If not, who can you go to bring this salience to your classroom?
- Do you create a classroom environment where students are encouraged to ask questions, clarify content, and consider alternatives?
- Do you present a positive role model for the profession and for the necessity to be a lifelong learner?
- Do you foster cooperation between students, encourage active learning, and communicate HIGH but realistic expectations?
- Do you respect the learning styles of diverse learners and include elements that are inclusive to meet the needs of auditory, visual, and kinesthetic learning styles?
- Do you have a consistent structure to your classroom that provides a consistent pattern that students are comfortable with and know what to expect in your classroom?
- Do you have the energy to teach with passion and enthusiasm?

Have a High but Realistic Bar of Student Expectations

At a faculty workshop for nurse educators, one statement jumped off the handout and into my educational philosophy:

"No student will RISE to LOW expectations."

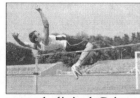

Only seven words, but it has since transformed the way I approach nursing education. The simplicity of this truth was illustrated when I taught advanced clinical. Prior clinical instructors had expected students to know the pharmacologic class of each medication they were to administer. I raised the bar by expecting them to know the mechanism of action in addition to the pharmacologic class. Once students knew my higher "bar" of medication knowledge, they quickly rose to this level of expectation and promoted their learning as a result.

Educators have a responsibility to do what is needed to prepare students for practice. One way we do this is by the level of the bar we set for safety and application of content to the bedside that is guided by the level of our students. Students will go no higher than what you expect of them. Set your bar too low and you will stunt their learning. Set your bar too high and they will be frustrated, stressed, and overwhelmed. Have a HIGH but REALISTIC bar of what students are capable of and hold them accountable to your "bar."

Some educators set the bar too low, even though it can and should be raised. One common example of an "acceptable" low bar is the expectation some educators have regarding student preparation for coming to classroom theory. Raise the bar in your classroom by EXPECTING your students to come to your classroom prepared and back it up with a pointed quiz from the readings or a posted case study that is a "ticket for admission" that has been worked through by your students. This will encourage buy-in and provide an incentive to transition to a paradigm of learning that will strengthen student learning.

Students Come to Class Prepared

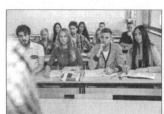

If a student came to clinical with no stethoscope and/or name badge because it was forgotten, most educators would have no problem sending this student home and would not allow this student in the clinical setting. Why? Because he/she was clearly UNPREPARED to enter this setting to learn and care for patients. But in nursing education classrooms, students typically come consistently unprepared. Students have not read the textbook and expect to be "spoon fed" content that must be known to pass the test. Take control of your class and change this low bar so students come to your classroom prepared as well as ready to engage as partners with active learning.

Class time needs to look like clinical to strengthen student learning and transform nursing education. The classroom should have the same level of PREPAREDNESS as the clinical setting because nursing is a PRACTICE-based profession. Educators must do what is needed to prepare students for professional practice. The educational culture can be changed, but it will require courageous faculty who are willing to risk the wrath of entitled students who overtly or covertly dictate how they should be taught.

This is a common struggle. Just as transforming classroom culture and teaching is a paradigm shift for nurse educators, it is also a paradigm shift for students. In order to be successful, students and faculty need to work collaboratively. Faculty must be prepared for student resistance and have the support of colleagues and departmental leadership to hold the line when educators do what is right by encouraging and expecting student engagement and partnership in their learning. Therefore, faculty must change the focus from covering the content so they pass the examination, to learning to learn (Morin, 2014).

To be SAFE in the clinical setting, students must deeply UNDERSTAND essential content from lectures and textbooks. This mastery does NOT come by just showing up for class but by being prepared as a partner in their learning. This partnership begins when the student reads the textbook BEFORE lecture. This often results in questions that can be clarified in class. Students who come to class prepared will facilitate the learning process. Memorizing content or writing out drug information verbatim out of the nursing drug manual on a med sheet in the clinical setting is not the same as UNDERSTANDING what has been taught. Once essential content is deeply understood, students must then be able to USE or APPLY this knowledge to practice. Students need to see themselves as an ACTIVE PARTNER in the educational process, not a PASSIVE ABSORBER!

Practical Steps to Change Classroom Culture

If you want to take the next step to raise the bar of student preparedness and change the culture of your classroom, here are three principles to get you started:

1. **Communicate expectations for classroom preparedness.**

   Just as you clearly communicate expectations for students to come to clinical prepared so they are not sent home, do the same in your classroom! Communicate that you EXPECT every student to have read from the textbook BEFORE the lecture. Then have an active learning tool that you have posted ahead of time (I used my case studies) and have them bring this to class, having worked through it as their "ticket" to class. As a new nurse educator, I quickly

learned that students will do just about anything for an extra point or two! Use this to your benefit by doing a short 3–5 question quiz at the beginning of class based on the textbook readings for 1–2 bonus points. Those who did not read will come better prepared next time!

2. **Bring ACTIVE learning to every lecture.**

   Students must be ACTIVE partners in learning, so bring ACTIVE learning to each lecture. Clinical reasoning case studies are an effective tool to teach any practice-based profession, including nursing. I have found that by dividing each lecture hour 50/50 with a hybrid flip—one half for lecture of NEED to know content, one half for ACTIVE learning/application. It was an effective model that transformed my classroom.

3. **Appeal to student desire to be the best.**

   Entitlement has become the new norm in our culture and society. Instead of working hard and reaping the fruit of what has been diligently sown, some students EXPECT a passing grade just because they showed up and paid for the credits. Call out this unprofessional behavior and make it clear that ACTIVE learning with required PREPARATION is needed to be the best nurse possible. Appeal to this higher motive to BE THE BEST nurse possible. Passive learning and spoon feeding may be enough to pass the test, but it will NOT prepare students to safely care for patients. Remind students that they are caring for people of infinite value and worth. The inability to transfer learning to the patient bedside can result in "failure to rescue" with a status change and lead to adverse outcomes, including patient death. Frame the argument this way and there is nothing your students can say to justify doing anything less than their very best!

Do NOT settle for the status quo, but do what is needed to bring needed change to your program by changing the culture in your classroom and expect students to come to class prepared. Make learning ACTIVE and give yourself permission to have fun by using relevant tools that will require your students to be engaged and participants in their learning. When I became the "guide on the side" instead of the "sage on the stage," I had a lot more fun teaching, and my students came to value and appreciate this higher bar of student preparation and participation as they transferred classroom learning to the bedside in clinical. This can be your experience as well! What do you have to lose by doing things differently? Take that first step and you will never look back!

Make Learning Active!

Being the "sage on the stage" and providing the majority of content through lecture is a barrier to student learning and can prevent students from integrating the professional apprenticeships of knowledge, skilled know-how, and ethical formation in your program (Benner, et al., 2010, p.82). In order to effectively integrate these apprenticeships, learning must be ACTIVE rather than passive engagement. How do you know if learning is active? It requires that students DO SOMETHING with the content that has been taught, versus listening to the teacher and taking notes (Oermann, 2004).

Though flipping the classroom and active learning are current buzzwords in nursing education, another perspective that can transform classroom learning is to make it INTERACTIVE. Make your classroom a safe place where students can share their thoughts and questions, and answer your questions. Your intent is to ENGAGE students with classroom content so they can think critically by applying what has been taught. This can be done when the educator embraces a paradigm that the classroom is going to be a conversation or discussion and that participation in this dialogue is NOT optional. It is imperative that faculty get away from the lectern at the front of the class and move around! Get close to students, especially those in the back, and let them be aware of your personable presence! Be creative with your content and include music, film clips, and anecdotal stories to illustrate key points (Moellenberg & Aldridge, 2010).

My first-year students commented that they will never forget my lecture on inflammation and immunity when I opened it up with the famous scene from the movie *Braveheart*. Mel Gibson starred as William Wallace, the defender of the Scots against the invasion of the English king, Edward Longshanks. As Wallace prepares the ragtag army of the Scots and yells, "Freedom!" I stop the video and ask, "What do William Wallace, this ragtag army of Scots and inflammation and immunity systems of the body have in common?" (They are both defenders against foreign invaders.)

Passive Learning

Passive learning is when students show up for classroom lecture, write down information from what they see and hear, and memorize this content. Though a large amount of information can be presented in a short amount of time, there is no way to determine if students UNDERSTAND what was presented. Because most students have been accustomed to passive learning in high school and college, they tend to prefer this pedagogy because they feel secure that memorizing content that has been "covered" will give them what they need to pass the test and be successful (Billings & Halstead, 2016).

The traditional classroom PowerPoint lecture that has been prevalent in nursing education is a passive learning strategy that has been shown to be ineffective for knowledge acquisition. In some studies, it has been shown that up to 80 percent of what was presented is forgotten 24 hours later! Though a typical classroom lecture lasts 50 to 60 minutes, students are most attentive for only the first 20 minutes. Then the slow fade of disengagement begins and they become easily distracted, heads begin to bob, and students start interacting with their cell phones. The role of students is also passive as they are expected to primarily absorb knowledge by taking notes, recording the lecture, and regurgitating content for the exam.

Active Learning

In comparison, when active learning strategies—case studies, small group discussions, or activities— are used in class, higher levels of student engagement are present in part because it is consistent with adult learning theory and how adults learn best. Active learning takes place when students ACTIVELY process what is being taught. Instead of being passive in learning, students are participants as they experience, apply, and construct knowledge (Herr, 2007).

The benefits of active learning include (Price & Nelson, 2011; Stevenson & Gordon, 2014):

- Increased attentiveness to learning
- Greater interest in learning
- Increased RETENTION of information
- DEEPER understanding of content taught
- Greater assimilation of learning
- Increased CRITICAL THINKING skills
- Increased PROBLEM-SOLVING skills
- Enhanced TEAMWORK skills

No Spoon Feeding!

Though an active learning classroom will promote learning, I have observed that students have a love/hate relationship with classroom lectures. Some will actively resist any attempt to create an active classroom learning environment! Many students prefer the security of having content spoon fed as it's covered in a traditional lecture and avoid having to read the textbook. Though nursing students are adult learners, some still communicate to faculty, "Tell me what I need to know" or "Will this be on the test?" Nurse educators need to demonstrate tough love and refuse to give in to this all-too-common demand. This desire to know only what is needed for the test is a reflection of ever-increasing amounts of content as well as stress in a high stakes field of study.

Engage and Involve Students in Learning

Students who are engaged in active learning will be more likely to be successful and APPLY concepts in the clinical setting (National Survey of Student Engagement, 2013). But based on feedback from educators, lack of student engagement is one of the areas that faculty continue to struggle with in the classroom. Students are responsible to become motivated and engage with the subject matter. They must be intrinsically motivated and desire to be the best possible nurse. It is the responsibility of the educator to use a variety of creative active learning strategies to facilitate and guide student engagement and participation (Billings & Halstead, 2016).

Since students are different and have varying learning styles, educators must employ a variety of strategies to engage students including videos (YouTube), case studies, or group activities and discussion. Case studies are a practical tool to apply classroom theory content to real-world practice. A strength of case studies is that they provide problem-solving practice and clinical reasoning in a safe environment. But case studies also require the students to be prepared. If not, students will learn less. This practical pedagogy will be discussed in detail in later chapters.

Embrace Adult Learning Principles

The following principles of adult learners (Peterson, n.d.) are derived from the work of Malcolm Knowles, a pioneer in the study of adult learning. These principles readily translate to nursing education and can help you become more effective as an educator.

1. **Adult learners want to know WHY something is important to know.** Adult students are searching for RELEVANCE in everything that is taught. Therefore, when the most important or relevant content is taught, adult educational best practice is supported.

2. **Adult learners want to learn with their dominant learning style.** Remember that most students are visual, auditory, or kinesthetic (hands-on) learners. Therefore, be sure to mix it up in your classroom and include active learning strategies that utilize all three! Make your slide presentation brief, but full of relevant visuals and then incorporate active learning for your kinesthetic learners.

3. **Adult learners want learning to be experiential.** To engage adult learners, active learning needs to be incorporated in the class. Educators struggle to engage students in the classroom. You could be part of the problem if you consistently use a content-heavy lecture format! Make learning active. This can take the form of case studies, group discussions, or small group activities. Remember to honor the life experiences that adult learners bring to your program and use them to encourage participation in your classroom.

4. **Adult learners want the process to be positive and encouraging.** I have observed that most students are extremely critical of their abilities and are in need of encouragement in a difficult field of study such as nursing. It may have been many years since some of your students have been in a classroom. In addition to teaching subject content, do not lose sight of the importance to inspire confidence and passion in each student.

Pursue Passion!

As I look back at nurse educators who had the greatest impact and made the greatest impression on me, they had one thing in common: a bright and burning passion for nursing, teaching, and learning. Passion is present when an educator has an intense, driving feeling of enthusiasm or excitement for what they do. In the context of nursing education, this passion is evident when an educator has a contagious enthusiasm for nursing and learning. This is the power of a passionate educator; they positively touch and impact those with whom they come in contact.

To be a transformational educator, curiosity, engagement, and passion for learning must be present in you. Educators must personify the very qualities they want their students to demonstrate. This ideal can be realized when the educator cares for and nurtures her or himself to be the best they can possibly be (Benner, 2013). As a result of living out this level of passion, the educator becomes truly alive. Eldredge (2004) also recognized the relationship between pursuing your passion and becoming alive. He writes,

"Don't ask yourself what the world needs. Ask yourself what makes you come alive, and do that. Because what the world needs are people who have come alive" (p. 200).

Do you possess this passion for nursing, teaching, and learning? Does teaching still make you come alive? Or did you once possess this fiery passion, but now have only a few glowing embers and wonder where the fire went? I have observed colleagues who were once alive, but are now just putting in their time, looking forward to retirement. Heinrich (2006) coined the term "joy stealing" that aptly describes the challenges of working in academia. The joy of teaching and learning that motivates many to pursue education can unfortunately be taken away by stress and ongoing demands that require immediate attention.

Don't "Cover" the Content

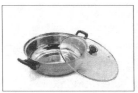 As a new nurse educator, I did what I saw modeled by more experienced nurse educators around me. This included the need to "cover the content" by summarizing a textbook chapter in PowerPoint slides with a content-heavy lecture. Patricia Benner has observed that when nurse educators "cover the content" by rushing through their stack of PowerPoint slides, they literally put a "cover" or lid on their content that prevents students from recognizing what is MOST and LEAST important.

Benner (1982) noted that novice nursing students see EVERYTHING that is covered in the textbook or lecture as EQUALLY important; they are unable to discriminate between what is most and least important because of their clinical inexperience. There is a better way. Students must be given the opportunity to PRACTICE nurse thinking and USE knowledge through relevant application in the classroom (Benner, et al., 2010).

Some faculty insist on covering the content because of the misguided notion that students must first learn classroom theory before they can apply it to practice. But in studies of teaching and learning a practice-based profession, students must first learn to transfer knowledge to the practice setting. Nursing students learn best when knowledge is put in CONTEXT (Benner, 1984). When faculty are focused on covering the content, they tend to pay too little attention to what students are actually learning. When content is isolated from context, students are left to figure out on their own how to make essential connections; because of their inexperience, they are unable to readily do so (Day, 2011).

Don't Merely "Flip" Your Classroom, TRANSFORM It!

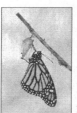 If there is one "hot topic" in nursing education, it is "flipping" your classroom. The flipped classroom is based on the premise that active learning is superior to passive learning. The essence of a flipped classroom is that the traditional passive lecture is prerecorded and available for students to review before coming to class (Hertz, 2012). This allows time for active learning strategies such as case studies, discussion, and small group projects to be done during class time. A fully flipped classroom requires a commitment from faculty to develop learning activities, pose clinical challenges, and guide student learning.

Students must commit to come to class prepared, having read the textbook and comprehended basic content so they are able to clarify concepts, connect them to clinical practice during class, and be an active participant (Billings & Halstead, 2016). If students and faculty are unable or unwilling to make these needed commitments, any attempt to implement meaningful active learning will be sabotaged and not get off the ground. One question that educators need to answer is, "Is flipping your classroom the same as transforming it?" From my perspective, it depends.

One of the current problems in nursing education is the vast amount of content that is presented and expected to be mastered by students. Over time, the curriculum becomes ADDITIVE (Tanner, 2004). Instead of revising lectures to reflect current practice, faculty simply add more (Benner, et al., 2010). This leads to superficial learning of a broad body of content, but prevents students from acquiring the DEEP learning of what is MOST important to practice. DEEP learning of what is most important must guide everything that is done in nursing education.

As a novice nurse, students see everything as relevant (Benner, 1984). This includes the content in a traditional lecture. If the same content-heavy lecture is merely repackaged as an electronic download to be reviewed before class, what has faculty done differently to emphasize the most important content that must be known deeply by students? Recognizing the need for relevance for novice nursing students, traditional lectures must be re-tooled to emphasize what is most important. If lectures are prerecorded, be sure they are as lean and brief as possible. Emphasize NEED to know content (Schlairet, Green, & Benton, 2014).

I have found that students value the security of having a condensed lecture in class that highlights the most important content or concepts to guide their learning. A win-—win for my students was when I did a hybrid "flip" by cutting my lecture in half, emphasizing the most important content, and then using the active learning pedagogy of a clinical reasoning case study that emphasized clinical application of what was just covered in class. This strategy will be discussed in more detail later in this chapter.

Steps to Classroom Transformation

The following six steps can be the start of your journey to transform your classroom.
  1. Key elements
  2. Start each lecture with a relevant story
  3. What content every lecture must address
  4. Decrease content overload (TMI)
  5. Contextualize your content
  6. Thinking is a skill that needs to be practiced

Step 1: Key Elements

Lecture remains relevant and needs to be done well to teach what is most important in the classroom. To replace the traditional content-heavy PowerPoint slide presentation and strengthen student learning and engagement in a classroom lecture, use Gagne's (1985) learning theory to structure a classroom lecture. Gagne identified specific events that are essential to student learning. By incorporating Gagne's nine events of instruction, you can

successfully restructure your lectures to be a more effective classroom educator (Miner, Mallow, Theeke, & Barnes, 2015).

1. **Get student ATTENTION**. Present an introductory activity that will hook and engage students. Consider using a relevant story or YouTube video.
2. **Inform students of class objectives.** Present and share objectives so students can see why they are relevant and apply to clinical practice.
3. **Recall PRIOR learning before presenting new content.** Review key aspects of relevant prior learning.
4. **Deliver the body of the lecture.** Keep main concepts in 10-15 minute segments. Use acronyms, stories and images consistently.
5. **Provide supplemental resources.** Record your lecture so students can download them as a podcast; create handouts and questions that represent expected learning.
6. **Provide PRACTICE.** Use case studies, simulation, or small group activities to use and APPLY learning.
7. **Provide immediate feedback.** Answer student questions immediately, have students raise hands to ensure understanding.
8. **Assess performance.** Use short pointed quizzes to ensure that students have understood new content BEFORE the examination.
9. **Enhance RETENTION to transfer of knowledge.** After an examination, break class into small groups to discuss specific test items and rationale.

Step 2: Start Each Lecture with a Relevant Story

Textbook content tends to be quickly forgotten, but the power of a relevant story that illustrates your information will impact your students years after they leave your classroom. Don't believe me? A story that was told more than two thousand years ago continues to have laws named after the lead character that emphasize the importance of coming to the aid of someone in need…the Good Samaritan!

Do you struggle to engage your students in the classroom? A relevant story will hook and engage students like nothing else! Make sure that every story told has a clear and practical point that you want students to take away. As a nurse educator, draw from your journey and experiences as a nurse in practice, and the patients you have cared for. Stories that illustrate timeless truths and essential concepts are desperately needed and must be told to the next generation of students. Another practical way to incorporate a good story into your content is to create case studies that use the power of a patient story to capture themes that promote student interest and engagement.

Step 3: What Content Every Lecture Must Address

After reading *Educating Nurses: A Call for Radical Transformation,* I realized that something had to give. I could not continue to cover the content and bring relevant active learning to my classroom. I cut my Power-Point presentation in half to make time for active learning. So, what did my NEED to know lectures cover to strengthen student learning? The following are eight essential components that I used in each presentation to emphasize NEED to know content that emphasized clinical reasoning. The following structure of my classroom presentations helped my students transfer learning to the bedside:

1. Pathophysiology review
2. Most important medications
3. Most important labs
4. Nursing priorities and plan of care
5. Worst possible and most likely complications
6. Nursing assessments to identify these complications
7. Interventions needed to rescue with a change of status
8. Patient education priorities

1. Pathophysiology review

Just because pathophysiology was covered as a prerequisite, there is no reason not to cover it again in class, but keep it brief and relevant. Make sure that students understand the complex physiology of some of the topics/concepts that are taught in your classroom. Memorizing content to pass a test is not the same as understanding and applying content.

For example, would your students understand the difference between right- vs. left-side vs. bi-ventricular heart failure and WHY patients typically develop SOB and orthopnea (left-sided) BEFORE fluid retention and pitting edema are present in the lower extremities (right-

sided)? This is an excellent example of the importance of applied pathophysiology to practice. When pathophysiology is deeply understood, the nurse's critical thinking dramatically improves as well.

2. Most important medications

Highlight and identify the most commonly used medications that treat the problem or concept you are teaching and why they are given. In addition to reviewing the medications, highlight the importance of understanding the mechanism of action. This is the most important content for any student to know and UNDERSTAND to safely administer a medication. It also reinforces the importance of applied pathophysiology to practice.

3. Most important labs

Identify the SPECIFIC labs in each panel with the disease process or concept you are presenting, and not the ENTIRE panel. For example, in a basic metabolic panel (BMP), the most important and RELEVANT labs include sodium, potassium, glucose, and creatinine. Ensure that students understand why these lab panels are relevant to every patient! When the physiology of fluids and electrolytes is readily understood, students will be able to recognize relevant clinical data, an essential component of clinical reasoning.

4. Nursing priorities and plan of care

Identifying nursing priorities is also an essential component of clinical reasoning. Though NANDA has been the taxonomy that has been used for over three decades to identify nursing priorities in academia, NANDA has limitations when it comes to practice. Students must be able to clearly state the nursing priority in their own words and not be held hostage to NANDA diagnostic statements! Though beginning or fundamental students should adhere more closely to this taxonomy, give your advanced students flexibility and freedom to simply state the priority as it fits for their patient. This is what nurses in practice do, so have your advanced students do the same!

5. Worst possible and most likely complications

Every patient can gradually or quickly change status and deteriorate with a complication. Sepsis is an excellent example of this slow fade that can be deadly if it is not recognized EARLY. Make it a priority to identify these complications in your lecture so students can transfer this learning to the clinical setting. For example, in heart failure, pulmonary edema would be a possible complication, especially if the patient was recently admitted. Deep vein thrombosis is also a potential problem for any patient who is immobile.

6. Nursing assessments to identify these complications

Once the most common complications are identified, what assessments does the nurse need to make to quickly identify this problem EARLY and not later? In the patient with heart failure, early signs of pulmonary edema would be tachypnea, lack of tolerance to activity, and increasing oxygen needs. Once the patient is in respiratory distress with decreasing O2 saturation, it is too late and could lead to an adverse outcome!

7. Interventions needed to rescue with status change

Once a problem has been identified EARLY, what will the nurse DO about it? This proactive thinking must be identified in the classroom so students can transfer this knowledge to the clinical setting with each patient in their care. This is a care plan within a care plan based on the need to rescue. Because failure to rescue is an ongoing problem in health care, it is essential that students are taught to develop a secondary plan of care based on the most likely or common complication. When the nurse is caught flat-footed by not anticipating or being prepared when a problem develops, this will ultimately affect the patient and can lead to adverse outcomes, including patient death.

8. Patient education priorities

The professional nurse is also an educator. Students tend to minimize or not make this a priority because they are students and feel incapable of teaching patients. By identifying patient education priorities and then teaching them, students can see how nursing partners with the patient to achieve beneficial outcomes.

Step 4: Decrease Content Overload (TMI)

Though educators may take for granted the ever-increasing size of nursing textbooks and the ever-increasing amount of content that students are expected to know, it

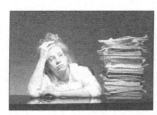

is the wise educator who recognizes that there is a limit to what students can handle and master. The growing amount of content that is present in nursing education is a barrier to student learning. del Bueno (2005) recognized that just because a student can recall and understand content or select the correct answer does not translate to being able to make correct clinical judgments. She also recognized the correlation between too much information in nursing education and the inability of new nurses to translate knowledge to the bedside. She weighs in by stating:

"The author believes that a highly probable cause (inability to translate knowledge to the bedside) is the emphasis on teaching more and more content in the nursing education curricula rather than a focus on use of or application of knowledge. A look at the size and plethora of nursing textbooks supports this conclusion." (p. 281)

Lessons from a Grey Whale

When I presented a clinical reasoning workshop in Orange County, California, I had the opportunity to catch a glimpse of migrating grey whales. The tour boat guide discussed how grey whales feed as they travel thousands of miles from Alaska to Mexico. To feed, a grey whale opens its mouth wide and filters thousands of gallons of water with its baleen teeth. It then partly shuts its mouth and keeps the small amount of krill and plankton that is left to eat to provide energy needed for its continuous migration.

This example from nature illustrates a foundational principle that transformational nurse educators must embrace and follow. FILTER the thousands of pages in the textbook as well as content in your PowerPoint presentations. Keep the most important content as the NEED to know to provide the needed sustenance for your students' professional growth! Apply the "faculty filter" to textbook readings for each lecture or unit as well. Are the entire chapter(s) really all NEED to know? I highly doubt it. Don't be afraid to identify the NEED to know pages in the textbook for students and even the most important slides in your PowerPoint presentation. Give students the option to read the remainder as NICE to know.

Even if you are a new nurse educator, you are also an experienced nurse who knows what aspects of nursing education are most important to practice. Be confident of what you do know. If you teach in a team, have this discussion and collaborate to decide what is NEED to know and NICE to know, using the lens of clinical practice. Do this and you will INCREASE the learning of your students and DECREASE student stress!

Cognitive Load Theory

Cognitive load theory (CLT) provides a framework that, when understood and applied, provides a rationale to be ruthless and filter content and decrease content saturation so student learning can be strengthened. CLT was developed in response to research that revealed that short-term memory can hold only a limited amount of information simultaneously. The ability of students to access recent content to use knowledge and clinically reason is limited. Long-term memory provides the scaffolding of knowledge and facilitates usage, but it is acquired over time and takes place over a lifetime (Bruning, Schraw, Norby, & Ronning, 2003). In other words, the MORE content students are expected to master, the LESS nurse thinking and learning takes place.

To DECREASE content overload and strengthen student learning in your classroom, implement these CLT principles by using the following strategies (Kaylor, 2014):

1. **Opening review activities.** Build on prior learning by asking true/false questions, ask a relevant question to open classroom discussion, or use a case study with clinical scenario to build on during class.
2. **Provide students with PowerPoint notes.** Use PowerPoint intentionally by using the "Notes Page" presentation view which reveals both the slide and the notes at the bottom of the slide. Write educator notes in concise bullet points so students know what is MOST important.
3. **Top 3-5 takeaways.** Help students break down major content/concept takeaways into 3-5 takeaways. Ask the question, "If you could learn only five things about…what would they be?" Do NOT write these down, but allow students to collaborate in small groups to determine and then share as a class.
4. **Determine what content is NEED to know vs. NICE to know.** Present NEED to know content with lecture and PowerPoint the first half of class, then use the last 30 minutes using active learning

strategies such as case studies to apply learning to practice. How do you decide what content is need and nice to know?

- NEED to know content. Answers the question, "What does a nurse need to know (about today's content) in order to safely provide care for a patient with…?"
- NICE to know content. Includes aspects of care that are important, but not essential. This content is also readily available in textbooks so students can read and review on their own.

Step 5: Contextualize Your Content

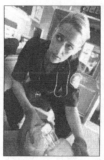

Once content has been filtered, and DEEPLY understood, it must now have a "hook" that CONTEXTUALIZES it to the bedside. Students must be able to recognize WHY this content is important to practice. This principle is not just for the classroom, but for EVERYTHING that is taught in nursing education.

Educating Nurses uses the term "clinical imagination" as a concept that needs to be consistently used in nursing education. Clinical imagination provides clinical contextualization to your content in such a rich way that students can imagine being in the clinical setting and able to practice what is needed to become proficient (Benner, et al., 2010). The classroom must be an active learning environment that situates clinical realities.

When I taught fundamentals, our program taught the typical skills of medication administration, sterile technique, and Foley catheterization but with no simple scenario to contextualize these skills to practice. I created short scenarios that contained the "hook" of contextualization so students could begin to use this knowledge, develop clinical salience, and see how these skills would be used in practice.

In the classroom, students can use knowledge and apply it to the bedside using clinical reasoning case studies that allow them to see its relevance to practice. Regardless of the active learning strategy you choose to use, make sure that the "hook" of contextualization is threaded through everything that is taught in your program so students can not only acquire knowledge but, more importantly, use it!

Step 6: Thinking Is a Skill that Needs to Be Practiced

To become proficient with any clinical skill, it must be practiced over and over again. When I taught fundamentals and the clinical skill of sterile technique/Foley catheterization, students immediately recognized the need to PRACTICE and most spent hours practicing sterile technique over and over until they were confident they were proficient and could pass the skills checkoff.

This obvious need for PRACTICE in nursing education was also recognized very early in the modern era of nursing by Isabel Hampton Robb, a nursing leader/educator who founded the American Nurses Association (ANA) and the American Journal of Nursing. She wrote in her textbook, Nursing Ethics (1900):

"Only by constant REPETITION can you become really familiar with the work; only by doing a thing well AGAIN and AGAIN can you obtain confidence, accuracy and precision. It is this constant, intelligent PRACTICE that constitutes the difference between the skilled trained professional woman and the amateur." (Emphasis mine-Hampton Robb, 1900, p. 69)

Though it is obvious that practice is essential and needed for clinical skills, Alfaro-LeFevre (2013) states that THINKING is also a skill that needs to be practiced for students to acquire the knowledge, skills, and experience required for practice. *Educating Nurses* also affirmed the importance of the classroom as a place to practice priority setting. In this context, students can safely make mistakes (Benner, et al., 2010). In one study that addressed nursing students' perceptions on developing clinical reasoning, they felt that the classroom was an excellent place to learn what was most important and ask why a course of action would be undertaken, but experiential learning in the clinical setting enhanced their development of clinical reasoning the most (Herron, Sudia, Kimble, & Davis, 2016).

Nursing education does not provide enough opportunities for students to consistently obtain this needed practice in clinical reasoning and thinking like a nurse. But if classrooms became opportunities to provide this needed practice, students could become more proficient to uncover signs of clinical deterioration and communicate recommendations. Providing opportunities to practice evaluation of clinical cues and communicating these

changes to the health care team will prepare students for complex clinical practice (Lancaster, Westphal, & Jambunathan, 2015).

The primary strategy that transformed my classroom was the creation of clinical reasoning case studies that incorporated a consistent template of clinical reasoning questions that can transfer learning to the clinical setting. By using a salient scenario that emphasizes clinical reasoning, students can practice "nurse thinking" in the safety of the classroom where no patient is harmed by the failure of the student to recognize the need to rescue. Dorothy del Bueno's (2005) research focused on the difficulties and inability of new nurses to think like a nurse by making incorrect clinical judgments agrees with the need to practice. "Like getting to Carnegie Hall, being an effective nurse requires practice, practice, practice" (p. 282). I wholeheartedly agree.

Reflect

1. What could you do differently to expect your students to come to class prepared?

2. How do you act as a "faculty filter" to decrease content and deepen the learning of what is most important?

3. If you "cover the content" with content-heavy lectures, what can you do differently to put your presentations on a diet and emphasize need to know content?

4. What active learning strategies could you use that provide practice of clinical reasoning?

5. What is one action step you can do to strengthen student learning in your classroom?

References

Alfaro-LeFevre, R. (2013). *Critical thinking, clinical reasoning, and clinical judgment: A practical approach.* (5th ed.). St. Louis, MO: Elsevier–Saunders.

Benner, P. (1984). *From novice to expert: Excellence and power in clinical nursing practice.* Upper Saddle River, NJ: Prentice Hall.

Benner, P. (2013). Teacher curiosity, passion, engagement and self-cultivation–Essential for transformative education. Retrieved from http://www.educating nurses.com/articles/teacher-curiosity-passion-engagement-and-self-cultivation-essential-for-trans formative-education/

Benner, P., Sutphen, M., Leonard, V., & Day, L. (2010). *Educating nurses: A call for radical transformation.* San Francisco, CA: Jossey-Bass.

Billings, D. M., & Halstead, J. A. (2016). *Teaching in nursing: A guide for faculty* (5th ed.). St. Louis, MO: Elsevier.

Bruning, R.H., Schraw, G.J., Norby, M.M., & Ronning, R.R. (2003). *Cognitive psychology and instruction* (4th ed.). Upper Saddle River, NJ: Pearson Education.

Day. L. (2011). Using unfolding case studies in a subject-centered classroom. *Journal of Nursing Education (50)*8, 447-452.

del Bueno, D. (2005). A crisis in critical thinking. *Nursing Education Perspectives, 26*(5), 278–282.

Eldredge, J. (2001). *Wild at heart: Discovering the secret of a man's soul.* Nashville, TN: Thomas Nelson.

Gagne, E.M. (1985). *The conditions of learning and theory of instruction.* New York: NY: Holt, Rhinehart and Winston.

Hampton Robb, E. (1900). *Nursing ethics.* Cleveland, OH: E.C. Koeckert.

Heinrich, K. T. (2006). Joy-stealing games. Retrieved from the Reflections on Nursing Leadership Web site: http://www.reflectionsonnursingleadership.org/pages/vol32_2_heinrich.aspx

Herr, T. (2007). Active vs. passive learning. Retrieved from http://www.csun.edu/science/ref/pedagogy/active-passive/active-passive-learning.html

Herrmann, J.W. (2016). *Creative teaching strategies for the nurse educator.* Philadelphia, PA: F.A. Davis.

Herron, E.K., Sudia, T., Kimble, L.P., & Davis, A.H. (2016). Prelicensure baccalaureate nursing students' perceptions of their development of clinical reasoning. *Journal of Nursing Education, 55*(6), 329-335.

Hertz, M. (2012). The Flipped Classroom: Pro and Con. Retrieved from http://www.edutopia.org/blog/flipped-classroom-pro-and-con-mary-beth-hertz

Kaylor, S.K. (2014). Preventing information overload: Cognitive overload theory as an instructional framework for teaching pharmacology. *Journal of Nursing Education, 53*(2). 108-111.

Lancaster, R.J., Westphal, J., & Jambunathan, J. (2015). Using SBAR to promote clinical judgment in undergraduate nursing students. *Journal of Nursing Education, 54*(3), S31-S34.

Miner, A., Mallow, J., Theeke, L., & Barnes, E. (2015). Using gagne's 9 events of instruction to enhance student performance and course evaluations in undergraduate nursing course. *Nurse Educator, 40*(3), 152-154.

Morin, K.H. (2014). Fostering student accountability for learning. *Journal of Nursing Education, 53*(10), 547-548.

National Survey of Student Engagement (NSSE). (2013). NSSE annual results 2013: A fresh look at student engagement. Retrieved from, http://nsse.iub.edu/html/annual_results.cfm

Oermann, M.H. (2004). Using active learning in lecture: Best of "both worlds." *International Journal of Nursing Education Scholarship, 1*(1), 1-9.

Peterson, D. (n.d.). 5 principles of teaching adults. Retrieved from http://adulted.about.com/od/teachers/a/teaching adults_2.htm

Price, K. M., & Nelson, K. L. (2011). *Planning effective instruction: Diversity responsive methods and management* (4th ed.). Belmont, CA: Wadsworth.

Schlairet, M., Green, R., & Benton, M.J. (2014). The flipped classroom: Strategies for an undergraduate nursing course. *Nurse Educator, 39*(6), 321-325.

Stevenson, E. L., & Gordon, H. A. (2014). Students as active learners and teaching partners in the clinical setting. *Nurse Educator, 39*(2), 52-53.

Tanner, C. A. (2004). The meaning of curriculum: Content to be covered or stories to be heard? *Journal of Nursing Education, 43*(1), 3–4.

14

The "Old School" Tool That Belongs in Every Classroom

Keith Rischer, RN, MA, CEN, CCRN

"Classroom teachers must step out from behind the screen full of slides and engage students in clinic-like learning experiences that ask them to learn to use knowledge and practice thinking in changing situations, always for the good of the patient."

—*Educating Nurses: A Call for Radical Transformation*, p. 14

One of the ongoing struggles that educators face in the classroom is a lack of engagement of students in the learning process who need to be actively engaged in the learning process. As adult learners, students are looking for RELEVANCE. Though there are many forms of active learning, case studies are one of the easiest and most consistent ways to bring relevant active learning to develop nurse thinking and breathe new life into the classroom (Popil, 2011). Case studies are an active learning strategy that have been shown to improve students' confidence levels by helping them develop clinical reasoning skills required for bedside practice (Evenson, 2013).

Case studies facilitate the development of nursing students' critical thinking skills. Problem-based learning uses salient scenarios that contextualize a problem that needs to be solved. Students need to rely on what they already know and identify what they need to know to resolve the problem (Niemer, Pfendt, Gers, 2010). A case study with a salient scenario and open-ended questions connects prior learning, and can even incorporate controversial psychosocial elements to elicit diverse opinions and increase student engagement (Duch, 2009).

Case studies used in the classroom are a low-fidelity simulation experience that provide opportunities for students to use clinical reasoning decision skills, apply theory to practice, and bridge the gap between classroom and practice (Billings & Halstead, 2016; Benner, et al,

2010; McNelis, et al., 2014). *Educating Nurses* illustrated the radical transformation needed in nursing education, with educators who used case studies to develop the skill of inquiry and connect knowledge learned in the classroom to the clinical setting (Benner, et al., 2010). *The Essentials of Baccalaureate Education* endorse and recommend the use of unfolding case studies as an active, collaborative, and integrative learning strategy (AACN, 2008).

A well-designed case study requires active involvement by students and incorporates problem-solving skills and decision making in a nonthreatening environment. A case study that develops clinical reasoning provokes student thinking and teaches them to think professionally using knowledge that they have been taught to resolve the clinical problem. Clinical scenarios must illustrate clinical realities that allow PRACTICE of clinical reasoning in the safety of the classroom.

Developing clinical imagination is a concept that educators must strive to achieve in the classroom. This includes creating opportunities for students to explore the multiple aspects of a clinical scenario that literally places or immerses the student in practice-based realities (Benner, et al., 2010). A well-designed case study can accomplish this transformational teaching paradigm.

To transform the classroom, content must be contextualized to the bedside of patient care. Content taught straight from the textbook that is abstract and decontextualized from practice makes it difficult for students to understand and realize the relevance of what is being taught (Benner, et al., 2010). After reading *Educating Nurses,* I began to contextualize my lecture content with brief scenarios and case studies I created from my practice experience. But I quickly discovered that not all case studies are created equal. When I reviewed the case studies that were supplied by the textbook publisher our department was using, I observed two weaknesses that limited their effectiveness because they did not integrate educational best practices:

1. They emphasized application of CONTENT, but did not place a similar emphasis on the THINKING of clinical reasoning that a nurse uses in practice.

2. Answers for case studies were MULTIPLE CHOICE. In practice, you either know what to do or NOT; you do not have the luxury of multiple choice. This structure is the equivalent of a multiple-choice test. It does NOT mirror real-world clinical practice.

Five Strengths of Case Studies

Though there are numerous strategies to bring active learning to the classroom, well designed case studies are an effective tool that will engage and strengthen student learning. Though they are LOW-tech, they have HIGH educational value! Case studies are one of the most adaptable teaching strategies that educators can use and develop. Case studies tie together essential aspects relevant to patient care including nursing priorities; pathophysiology, pharmacology, clinical reasoning, and can even develop empathy. An engaging case study also tells a story and engages students in the human experience that ties together textbook learning with human encounters (Harrison, 2012). Popil's review of the nursing literature on case studies revealed the following strengths of this practical pedagogy:

1. Facilitate active/experiential learning.

Because case studies present a scenario with open-ended reflective questions, student engagement and participation is required! Case studies utilized in the classroom make it possible for educators to be the "guide on the side" instead of the "sage on the stage" and allow students to create, construct, and present what they have learned to one another and to the class.

2. Identify problems.

A key component of clinical reasoning is the ability of the nurse to recognize RELEVANT clinical data. Once relevant clinical data is recognized, a potential problem or complication is also revealed. The failure to recognize relevant data is the root cause of failure to rescue. When a nurse fails to recognize a patient complication, it needlessly progresses and can result in an adverse outcome or patient death.

3. Safe environment to practice.

When simulation is used in the skills lab, it may be only a matter of time before an adverse outcome or even patient death occurs if the student makes an incorrect clinical judgment. Fortunately, this is not an actual patient and essential takeaways will strengthen student learning. In the same way, a well-developed case study functions as low fidelity simulation because it represents salient clinical realities and provides an opportunity to bring this clinical context to the classroom. Case studies used in the classroom also provide a safe place to PRACTICE the thinking and priority setting required in practice. This makes it possible for learning to transfer readily from the classroom to the clinical setting.

4. Experience clinical dilemmas.

Nursing has clinical dilemmas that, though infrequent, the nurse must anticipate and be prepared to respond to appropriately when they occur. How should the nurse respond when a physician or surgeon is uncivil or has alcohol on his breath? What if the nurse is concerned when aggressive medical treatment is insisted on by the family, but is NOT what the patient may have wanted or communicated? What should the nurse do? Case studies can contextualize these and other dilemmas so that students are well prepared to respond ethically and professionally when a dilemma happens after they graduate.

5. APPLY theory/USE knowledge.

To be well prepared for a practice-based profession, students must not only pass a multiple choice test called the NCLEX, but must be able to USE and APPLY knowledge at the bedside. Case studies with salient scenarios can provide students the opportunity to use what has been taught and apply it to strengthen student learning. Just as clinical educators use questions to assess student learning and knowledge, questions that emphasize clinical reasoning can be integrated into a case study to evaluate student learning in the classroom. This provides educators immediate evaluation and recognition of what was not "caught" so it can be taught and addressed before the test!

Case studies are effective teaching strategies that promote active learning and encourage the development of critical clinical thinking skills. Despite the overwhelming evidence regarding the effectiveness of case studies to prepare students for practice, case study pedagogy is not consistently implemented by educators. Popil ends her article by stating, *"I call out to educators today to use case studies more widely"* (Popil, 2011, p. 207). Though not the only pedagogy to bring active learning to the classroom, case studies are uniquely suited to be the foundation of methodology used by nurse educators who want to transform their classrooms. The greatest gift a teacher can bestow upon a student is not to require the regurgitation of textbook facts, but to ignite the spark of imagination that leads to personal, curiosity-based inquiry (Kaylor & Strickland, 2015). Case studies can accomplish this objective in nursing education.

Using Case Studies Effectively

I successfully integrated the transformational paradigm shifts advocated by *Educating Nurses* into the case studies I developed that were presented in my classroom. My case studies emphasized the THINKING that is required by the nurse using the clinical reasoning questions from the template of clinical reasoning questions I developed. Content was contextualized to the bedside with each patient scenario that brought clinical realities to class.

I have a structure that I use to create an effective clinical reasoning case study. I want to help you to do the same! Once you understand the essence of each step, you will be empowered to build your own clinical reasoning case studies based on the topics that you teach.

Components of Clinical Reasoning Case Studies

To develop case studies that have the power to transform your classroom, the following components or steps will bring clinical to class, contextualize content, and practice the nurse thinking skill of clinical reasoning and even the SBAR!

1. Develop an engaging scenario
2. Identify relevance and rationale of clinical data

- Presenting problem/social history
- Vital signs/nursing assessment
- Lab values

3. Template of clinical reasoning questions
   - Identify primary medical problem and pathophysiology
   - Identify nursing priority, related interventions, and expected outcomes
   - Identify priority body system to most thoroughly assess
   - Identify worst possible/most likely complication, assessments to identify, and interventions to implement if develops
4. Medical management. Rationale for treatment and expected outcomes
5. Priority setting of orders. Which orders are implemented FIRST and why?
6. Reflection questions on caring
7. Use reflection to THINK like a nurse
8. SBAR professional communication

Step 1: Develop an Engaging Scenario

Since case studies are another way of telling a story, consider using the narrative components of a well-written book. Intentionally incorporate the following into a case study that you create and develop (Harrison, 2012):

1. **Setting.** Where does it take place? Acute care, home care, clinic, or transitional care. Consider changing the setting as the case study unfolds. The setting will be determined by your objectives, focus, and emphasis of most common real-world scenarios you want to prepare students for.
2. **Plot and plot structure.** This is the action aspect and organization of the narrative scenario. Consider using multiple variables for advanced students including race, ethnicity, age, gender, socioeconomic status, substance abuse, and homelessness.
3. **Character.** Include distinct qualities that put a human face on your patient to increase student engagement.
4. **Elements of style.** Consider how much to disclose in the initial scenario so that there is more than one obvious solution to the case. Include essential data that needs to be recognized as well as trivial data, otherwise known as "distractors"' If it is good

enough for NCLEX test questions, prepare your students for this examination by doing the same in your case studies!

The foundation for a case study that will engage your students and capture their imaginations depends on the patient scenario. Avoid a short "just the facts" initial presentation, but use common themes that you have seen in practice as a nurse. Your goal is to create a salient case study that will mirror clinical realities so students are immersed in them. As a result, they will be well prepared to encounter these same situations in practice.

Make the subject or the patient central to the narrative. Faculty must role model the inquiry and curiosity that professional nurses utilize in practice. Once the goal of the class and content areas are identified by the educator for the case study, the narrative scenario is developed. To determine the direction you want the scenario to take students, ask what you want the case to do and who the patient will be. This includes the clinical setting and a patient who represents common themes seen in practice (Day, 2011).

Here is an example of a "just the facts" scenario that I created for a teenager entering the acute care setting with an eating disorder that does not "hook" or engage students with a salient scenario. My first draft was as follows:

Mandy White is an 18-year-old woman who has struggled with bulimia since the age of 14. She presents to the emergency department this evening with complaints of increasing weakness, lightheadedness, and a brief syncopal episode this evening. She has been inducing vomiting after meals for the past 3 weeks. She is 5'5" and weighs 83 pounds (BMI 13.8)

Though this scenario is concise and emphasizes the facts, it does not provide enough background information to promote student ENGAGEMENT and the relevance of psychosocial care priorities in the patient story. To promote engagement as well as provide a much-needed context for this scenario, I added relevant psychosocial clinical data of the themes I have observed practicing in the ED. By including this information the importance of the "art" of nursing and holistic care becomes evident. A salient scenario emphasizes not only the obvious physical needs, but also the underlying emotional and spiritual needs that need to be identified and addressed by the nurse.

This is my revised scenario:

Mandy White is an 18-year-old woman who has struggled with bulimia since the age of 14. She was sexually abused by her stepfather who was convicted and sent to prison. She lives with her mother and has recently been engaging in self injurious behavior (SIB) of cutting both forearms with broken glass and razors causing numerous scars.

She presents to the emergency department this evening with complaints of increasing weakness, lightheadedness, and a brief syncopal episode this evening. She has been inducing vomiting after meals for the past 3 weeks. She is 5'5" and weighs 83 pounds (BMI 13.8). Mandy is brought in by her mother. She does not want to be treated. You hear her say to her mother, "I am so tired of living, I wish I were dead!"

As you compare these two scenarios, the second scenario clearly promotes a higher level of engagement and addresses the importance of psychosocial care priorities in addition to the pressing physical priorities. Even though students have not met Mandy, her story engages them in such a way that Mandy matters to them. This is the same principle that we want to encourage with our students in the clinical setting. Every patient matters.

A significant weakness of textbook learning is that it is linear and can only present one concept at a time. It is also decontextualized from practice. In contrast, patients in practice present with multiple problems at the same time that must be prioritized and sorted out by the nurse. This is the strength of contextualizing any content to practice with a scenario that vividly illustrates the mastery of a wide body of information.

For example, in this scenario with Mandy, numerous problems/priorities that are interwoven include:
- Bulimia
- Dehydration
- Electrolyte abnormalities
- Depression
- Suicidal ideation/hopelessness

Each one of these content areas must be deeply understood by students so that the relationship of one problem to the other can be identified, the "fit" recognized, and the clinical puzzle can be put together. Deep understanding of pathophysiology and the applied sciences is essential to critical thinking and anticipating the nursing priorities because of Mandy's induced vomiting, which has resulted in dehydration and electrolyte abnormalities.

Students need to know the electrolytes that would most likely be depleted and the signs of the "hypo" of these electrolytes. This scenario illustrates how F&E content can be brought to the bedside using salient clinical reasoning case studies.

Step 2: Identify Relevance & Rationale of Clinical Data

Identifying relevant clinical data is the foundation of clinical reasoning and essential to providing safe patient care. This important nurse thinking skill can also be practiced when a patient care scenario situates the most common themes of abnormal clinical data seen in practice. In addition to recognizing the most important clinical data, students must also understand the clinical significance or WHY this data is relevant. When clinical data is recognized as relevant, and the rationale is concisely stated, the clinical and critical thinking of the student can be readily determined.

Just as in practice, the student must be able to "cherry-pick" and select relevant clinical data from the case study. Because the question is open-ended, the most important clinical data is recognized or it is not; there are no multiple-choice answers to select! This structure promotes student learning and provides immediate faculty evaluation by validating correct selection and identifying any areas of weakness.

The following sections from the case study scenario require the student to identify the most important (relevant) data and why:

- Presenting problem/social history
- Vital Signs
- Nursing assessment
- Lab values

Below is the initial presenting scenario from an actual case study on sepsis that I created and the corresponding faculty answer key. The case study requires students to identify the relevant data from the presenting history and why it is relevant.

Jean Kelly is an 82-year-old woman who has been feeling more fatigued the last 3 days and has had a fever the last 24 hours. She reports a painful, burning sensation when she urinates as well as frequency of urination the last week. Her daughter became concerned and brought her to the emergency department when she did not know what day it was. She is mentally alert with no history of confusion. While taking her bath today, she was weak and unable to get out of the tub and used her personal life alert button to call for medical assistance.

Step 3: Template of Clinical Reasoning Questions

The following questions capture the essence of clinical reasoning to PRACTICE and represent how students need to THINK to transfer learning to clinical practice.

1. What is the primary problem that your patient is most likely presenting?

2. What is the underlying cause/pathophysiology of this primary problem?

3. What nursing priority will guide your plan of care?

4. What interventions will you initiate based on this priority?

5. What body system(s) will you most thoroughly assess based on the primary/priority concern?

6. What is the worst possible/most likely complication to anticipate?

7. What nursing assessment(s) will you need to initiate to identify this complication EARLY if it develops?

8. What nursing interventions will you initiate if this complication develops?

9. What psychosocial needs will this patient and/or family likely have that will need to be addressed?

10.How can the nurse address these psychosocial needs?

Step 4: Medical Management: Rationale for Treatment and Expected Outcomes

In addition to understanding the nursing plan of care, students need to understand the essence of the primary care provider's plan of care and rationale for orders and interventions that are ordered. This essential skill can be practiced in a clinical reasoning case study by selecting the most common medications and treatments likely to be ordered for the problem-based scenario you have created.

Using the case study I created on sepsis, this is the medical management section with the answers included for faculty.

Step 5: Priority Setting of Orders: Which Orders Are Implemented FIRST and Why?

Because of a lack of clinical experience, novice students struggle to establish priorities (Benner, 1984). If

What data from the PRESENT PROBLEM are RELEVANT and must be interpreted as clinically significant by the nurse?	
RELEVANT Data from Present Problem:	**Clinical Significance:**
More fatigued for the last 3 days	*Though a general complaint, when clustered with the other symptoms of fever, this indicates that there is a likely PROBLEM present.*
Fever the last 24 hours	*Fever reflects the systemic inflammatory response initiated by the immune system and is there for a reason—to help the body fight off invading micro-organisms by increasing the production of neutrophil,; the first responders of the immune system—that are macrophages. The elevated temp also makes it less hospitable for bacteria to thrive and multiply.*
Painful, burning sensation when she urinates as well as frequency of urination the last week	*These symptoms are classic with a urinary tract infection (UTI). Suspecting a urinary infection, the nurse needs to know that if a patient meets the SIRs criteria, they should suspect sepsis.* *With an infection of any kind, sepsis is identified by having 2 or more of the following criteria of Systemic Inflammatory Response Syndrome (SIRS):* *• Temp > 100.4 or < 96.8* *• HR > 90* *• RR > 20* *• WBC > 12,000 or < 4000* *• Bands > 10%*
Did not know what day it was. She is mentally alert with no history of confusion.	*New onset of confusion is always a clinical RED FLAG in the elderly, and when CLUSTERED with other symptoms does not represent a neurologic problem, but is commonly seen with an infection such as a UTI.*
While taking her bath today, she was weak and unable to get out of the tub and used the help button to call for medical assistance.	*This confirms the weakness and fatigue she has had the past 3 days. It is severe weakness and a clinical RED FLAG if she is unable to get out of the bathtub and needed to call for assistance.*

students are given opportunities to PRACTICE priority setting, it can be strengthened. To situate priority setting in a case study, students take the same orders that were listed in step 4, place them in order from most important to least, and identify the rationale for the order they have chosen.

This exercise simulates what students will experience in clinical practice when multiple orders are written at the same time. Priority setting using the A, B, Cs or other practical strategies can be taught and contextualized to practice. This knowledge will also translate to the NCLEX because the client need category Management

Collaborative Care: Medical Management		
Care Provider Orders:	**Rationale:**	**Expected Outcome:**
Establish peripheral IV	*Need IV access to initiate IV fluid resuscitation.*	IV established
0.9% NS 1000 mL IV bolus	*Early fluid resuscitation is a standard of care in sepsis due to fluid volume deficit secondary to third spacing with inflammatory process as well as resultant vasodilation.*	Improvement in fluid volume deficit manifested by decrease in HR and elevation in SBP.
Acetaminophen 650 mg PO	*Though a fever can be beneficial in sepsis, most care providers will order to promote patient comfort.*	Lowering of fever
Ceftriaxone 1g IVPB…after blood/urine cultures obtained	*As a third generation, broad-spectrum cephalosporin, it binds to the bacterial cell wall membrane, causing cell death. Therapeutic Effects: Bactericidal action against susceptible bacteria. Spectrum: Like that of second-generation cephalosporins, but activity against staphylococci is less, while activity against gram-negative pathogens is greater.*	Will not see immediate response in resolving infection, but would expect to see improvement over the next 24 hours
Morphine 2 mg IV push every 2 hours PRN-pain	*Opioid narcotic. Bind to opiate receptors in the CNS. Alter the perception of and response to painful stimuli while producing generalized CNS depression*	Pain decreased

of Care emphasizes the ability of the graduate nurse to identify priorities and has the highest percentage of questions on the NCLEX.

Using the same case study I created on sepsis, this is the priority setting section with the answers included for faculty:

Step 6: Reflection Questions on Caring

To communicate the importance of caring to the nursing profession, and transfer this legacy to the next generation of nurses, caring needs to be incorporated in the curriculum. One simple way is to discuss the following two questions at the conclusion of the case study. These two questions provide an opportunity to develop caring, nurse empathy and engagement in the patient story by asking students:

1. What is the patient likely experiencing/feeling right now in this situation?
2. What can I do to engage myself with this patient's experience, and show that he/she matters to me as a person?

PRIORITY Setting: Which Orders Do You Implement First and Why?		
Care Provider Orders:	**Order of Priority:**	**Rationale:**
• Establish peripheral IV • 0.9% NS 1000 mL IV bolus • Acetaminophen 650 mg PO • Ceftriaxone 1g IVPB…after blood/urine cultures obtained • Morphine 2 mg IV push every 2 hours PRN-pain	1. Establish peripheral IV 2. 0.9% NS 1000 mL IV bolus 3. Ceftriaxone 1g IVPB…after blood/urine cultures obtained 4. Morphine 2 mg IV push every 2 hours PRN-pain 5. Acetaminophen 650 mg PO	1. C-Circulatory priority—required before IV fluids can be adminis tered 2. C-Circulatory priority—Low BP and obvious need for IV fluid re suscitation 3. Must treat and go after the source of the present problem! Is not tech-nically a C priority, so falls to #3. 4. Pain control is always a higher priority and needs to be addressed sooner vs. later, but is not an ABC priority.. 5. Fever is beneficial and will not harm the patient.

Step 7: Use Reflection to THINK Like a Nurse

Reflection-IN-action (Tanner, 2006) is the nurse's ability to accurately interpret the patient's response to an intervention in the moment as the events are unfolding to make a correct clinical judgment. Using Tanner's model of clinical judgment, these two reflection questions can identify key takeaways from the case study that can be transferred to the clinical setting.

1. What did I learn from this scenario?
2. How can I use what I have learned from this scenario to improve patient care in the future?

Step 8: SBAR Professional Communication

Just like any other skill in nursing education, SBAR is a skill that needs to be practiced. SBAR can be incorporated in any case study whenever communication needs to take place between the nurse and primary care provider, or a nurse-to-nurse report. Use the template that is included in the supplement to this book. Miscommunication between members of the health care team is the

root cause for the majority of sentinel events that result in patient death or serious injury (Joint Commission on Accreditation of Health Care Organizations, 2006). When students role played giving an SBAR, it was found to be more effective than classroom teaching alone (Kesten, 2010).

Unfortunately, this practice and structured learning and evaluation of students' handoff reporting does not take place in most nursing programs (O'Toole, Stevenson, & Good, 2013). To address this current deficiency in nursing education, one study recommended that faculty should incorporate innovative teaching strategies on handoff reporting throughout the curriculum so students have the knowledge and skills needed to be safe.

Instruction and contextualization of handoff communication should be done early in the curriculum. Using principles of situated learning, faculty can guide and strengthen SBAR communication. This, in turn, will reduce the number of adverse events linked with poor communication during clinical handoffs (Lee, Mast,

Humbert, Bagnardi, & Richards, 2016). Practicing SBAR with a salient case study will not only prepare students for practice, it may even save patient lives!

Steps to Transform Your Classroom

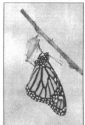 Once a clinical reasoning case study has been created or obtained, how do you structure your classroom to utilize this transformational tool? This is what I found effective as I implemented this pedagogy in my classroom and is based on the best practice recommendations from *Educating Nurses*. Use the following guidelines, be creative, and use the unique abilities you have been given as an educator to bring your classroom to life!

1. Take an Axe to Your PowerPoint Presentation and Cut It in HALF!

- Use the faculty filter of NEED to know vs. NICE to know discussed earlier. Use your lens of clinical practice to determine the content that is least and MOST important. Emphasize salient concepts to practice. Remember that students are adult learners and can read what is not covered in class! This will be the most difficult step for some because of the investment and development in your presentations.
- With a typical 50-minute time block of lecture, I lectured no more than 20 to 25 minutes.
- This gave me 20 to 25 minutes that I used to present the clinical reasoning case study that dovetailed with the content I just taught and provided the "hook" of application and contextualization to practice.

2. Create a PowerPoint Presentation of the Blank Student Version of the Case Study to Present for the Class

You can quickly create a PowerPoint presentation of a clinical reasoning case by following these simple steps:

- Make a PDF of the blank student version of the clinical reasoning case study that you have created or obtained.
- In the "Edit" menu at the top left of the PDF form, open the "Take a Snapshot" selection in the drop-down menu.
- A crosshairs icon becomes visible. It will go where your mouse directs it. Once you LEFT click your mouse, you can create a rectangle of any size that will automatically copy what is within this box.
- Go to your PowerPoint slide and RIGHT click your mouse. This will give you the option to paste directly to the slide. Be sure to choose the "Paste" option that is the icon of a document on the left side of the drop-down. This option provides greater clarity than if the "Picture" icon is chosen.
- Once the PDF has been copied to the slide, the size can be adjusted with the mouse to make it fit.
- Go sequentially through the clinical reasoning case study and copy and paste each section into your PowerPoint slides.

3. Student Responsibilities

Knowledge acquisition is a two-way street. It not only requires educators to use relevant active learning strategies in the classroom, but also requires students to be motivated and engaged in the learning process. To facilitate this partnership I had the following student expectations that were clearly communicated when I implemented my clinical reasoning case studies in the classroom.

- Students will come to class prepared by reading the assigned textbook readings BEFORE class.
- Students will be expected to work through the clinical reasoning case study that was posted one week before class, either individually or preferably in small groups.
- Students will be prepared to participate in classroom discussion.

One strategy I did not utilize but other educators have implemented successfully in their classroom was having students bring the filled-out case study as their "ticket" for admission to class. If you did not have your case study you were not allowed to enter the classroom because you were not prepared. Another way to use this approach is to give points for completing this assignment before class. Points could be either bonus, or built into the classroom theory grade.

4. Faculty Role

Nursing students are stressed. Stress levels will rise even higher when change is introduced. Communicate the following to students:

- Class is a "safe" place to make mistakes. No harm will come as we practice nurse thinking, but we will learn from one another if any errors in judgment take place.

- Instead of being the "sage on the stage," I will be the "guide on the side" who facilitates discussion, redirects as needed, and emphasizes salient points as students respond to the open-ended questions throughout the case study.

- I will stand alongside you to guide your learning. This will be done through the discussion of textbook content, and I will use my clinical experience to highlight and emphasize what is most and least important in my classroom and why.

5. Another Approach

Educators across the country have successfully incorporated this active learning strategy in their classrooms. One educator submitted an alternate approach to encourage student participation for a smaller classroom of 30 to 40 students.

- Divide the class into ten small groups of three to four students. Make this random so other students who do not normally mix together do so.

- Assign one to two questions from the clinical reasoning case study to each group.

- Give ten to fifteen minutes for students to collaborate, using textbooks or other resources to answer their assigned questions.

- Each group presents its answers to the questions they were assigned to the class and discussed the rationale for the answers they chose.

With this approach, student engagement will be heightened because they will need to be prepared before coming to class. They may also be responsible to present to the entire class! Use peer pressure in a positive way to push and encourage some students to become full partners in the learning process.

How to Construct Knowledge in the Classroom

Construction of knowledge is the highest level of Bloom's cognitive taxonomy but also a difficult objective to attain! You can use a clinical reasoning case study to create knowledge by flipping the paradigm of a case study and how it is traditionally used. Instead of having a case study that has the scenario and clinical data already created, have students CREATE the case study

after the topic/concept has been presented in class using a skeleton structure that you create or use what I developed (included as a supplement to this book). This teaching strategy is also known as a "reverse case study" because students develop the scenario using analysis and evaluation of course content to create the specific details of the case study (Atkinson, 2014).

Once you have presented the content (either by textbook reading, classroom lecture, or online delivery) do the following:

1. Give students a blank template of the case study that has a place for the opening scenario, nursing assessment, vital signs, lab values, and clinical reasoning questions.

2. Have students USE the knowledge that has been presented and use it to write a typical scenario of the problem that is being covered in class. What would be the expected abnormal findings in vital signs, assessment, and labs with this problem? What physician orders would be expected to manage this problem as well as the rationale?

3. Once the case study has been created by students, they need to INTERPRET the clinical data and answer the clinical reasoning questions that follow.

4. Have students share their case study in class and present their scenario with clinical data. Have the rest of the class answer the clinical reasoning questions. The educator is the "guide on the side" as learning is facilitated in your classroom!

Pursue Needed Change Together

Change is difficult. Though I knew that my clinical reasoning case studies represented educational best practice, I experienced resistance from some faculty. I have consulted with educators across the country and many have shared this same struggle. In order to bring lasting change to your content and program, the most important priority, and also the most difficult, is to get your entire teaching team pursuing transformational change together!

When I read *Educating Nurses* over winter break in early 2011, I began to rework my content and created active learning case studies that required students to come to class prepared. Since I implemented the changes of my content over break, I was the only one on our teaching team implementing these paradigm changes. The other faculty did not have an opportunity to read *Educating Nurses* and get on the same page so that we could be consistent in how we taught and work through these transformational changes together. Though my team lead was supportive when I informed her of what I was planning and had already created, other faculty were less enthusiastic and did not have the time or desire to make any changes to their traditional content lectures.

Since I was the only one doing things differently in my classroom, this did not provide a structure for long-term success to bring needed transformation to the program. Though I proceeded with my original plan and integrated the clinical reasoning case studies I developed, its impact would have been far greater had this paradigm shift been done as a team with each educator implementing the same transformational changes together.

Student Response

Since traditional content-heavy PowerPoint presentations gave students the security of what they needed to know to be pass the test, some resisted this pedagogy change. Some students will still prefer the passive path of being spoon fed and told what is needed to pass the test. If you begin to implement these transformational changes in your classroom, expect some push back and resistance from students, but do not let it deter you from doing what is needed to promote student learning and develop clinical reasoning in your classroom.

As I continued to implement active learning that emphasized clinical reasoning week after week, students began to appreciate and value this new way of teaching. It was helping them to think more like a nurse and transfer their knowledge to the clinical setting. I persisted with this pedagogy through the remainder of the semester.

At the end of the semester, I conducted an anonymous written survey to obtain feedback how students felt about the changes I had introduced and I received 60 responses. I was shocked to see that NOT ONE student said to go back to the traditional content-heavy lecture. Many wanted other faculty to teach in this same manner. One student's response was typical of many that I received:

"It was very helpful. I didn't feel like I was memorizing for the test. I felt like I was able to APPLY the information. It helped put KNOWLEDGE into PRACTICE and made it clear why it was RELEVANT" (Emphasis mine).

Nurse educators who have used these clinical reasoning case studies have shared that they also encountered student resistance at first, but also student buy-in as the benefits to their own learning became evident over time.

Strengths of Clinical Reasoning Case Studies

The following are seven reasons why clinical reasoning case studies have a place in your classroom, to not only teach students to think like a nurse, but also realize the needed transformation in nursing education!

1. Implementation of educational best practice from *Educating Nurses:*
   - Contextualizes content
   - Integrates classroom and clinical learning
   - Emphasizes clinical reasoning
2. Practices thinking like a nurse
3. Emphasizes knowledge usage and application of content
4. Rehearses for most common changes of patient status
5. Active learning strategy
6. NCLEX principles reinforced
7. Mirrors clinical realities

Implementation of Educational Best Practice from Educating Nurses

These clinical reasoning case studies bring clinical to class and integrate the three essential paradigm shifts from *Educating Nurses* that are needed to transform nursing education.

- Contextualize content to the bedside of patient care so students can see why it is relevant.
- Integrate classroom and clinical learning. These components of nursing education are no longer in two separate orbits but are now integrated.
- Emphasize clinical reasoning, which captures the essence of how a nurse thinks in practice.

Because these case studies incorporate all three of these paradigm shifts they really are a literal "tool of transformation"!

Practice Thinking Like a Nurse

Clinical experiences are never standardized for all students. They are random, and the quality of learning is influenced by the patients your students will care for. At the end of a clinical rotation, some students had opportunities to strengthen and develop clinical learning because of their challenging patients, while other students cared for patients who were not as complex. But when a clinical reasoning case study is used in the classroom, EVERY student gets the same opportunity to develop and practice the thinking that will directly translate to the bedside regardless of the quality of clinical experiences they may have had.

Emphasize Knowledge Usage and Application of Content

Content is taught; it must be placed into clinical context and applied to the bedside for students to recognize its relevance. Though nursing education has traditionally emphasized knowledge acquisition, the emphasis of my clinical reasoning case studies is on USING knowledge as well as APPLYING this knowledge for the good of the patient.

Rehearse for Most Common Changes of Patient Status

It is not likely that a student will care for a patient in the clinical setting who will have a change in status that will require the nurse to "rescue." But this needed practice can take place with a clinical reasoning case study. Addressing "failure to rescue" can be taught in your program through the use of these case studies that will help students identify common complications and care planning priorities needed when the patient's status begins to change.

Active Learning Strategy

The classroom must move from passive spoon feeding to an ACTIVE learning environment where students are required to participate and partner in their learning. These case studies require students to become active participants in the learning process.

NCLEX Principles Reinforced

The NCLEX is essentially an examination that assesses the ability of every graduate nurse to clinically reason. By integrating clinical reasoning throughout your program, in the classroom as well as clinical settings, you will prepare students for the NCLEX— and professional practice.

Mirror Clinical Realities

Once in practice, students do not have the luxury of multiple choices to determine the nursing priority or the most important clinical data. You either know it or you do not. If a student is unable to determine relevance of clinical data or recognize the need to "rescue," they will be unsafe in clinical practice. This approach most closely mirrors real-world clinical practice and identifies any weaknesses that can be addressed so they can be made a strength!

Barriers to Transformation

Though the need for transformation persists in nursing education, there continue to be barriers that limit or oppose radical transformation. To see change realized, these barriers need to be confronted and addressed head-on. The most common barriers that I encountered and other educators have shared include:

1. Department culture that resists change
2. Faculty who oppose change
3. Lack of self-confidence/fear of failure
4. Not enough time

1. Department Culture that Resists Change

Some faculty continue to resist needed change. I have not been in academia long enough to fully understand the dynamics of this problem, but it remains an issue, or Patricia Benner and the co-authors of *Educating Nurses* would not have chosen the subtitle A Call for Radical Transformation! The gravity of this title and the conclusions of the Carnegie Foundation's educational research make the state of nursing education painfully clear. Radical change is needed and must be implemented. Educators need to determine if they are going to remain part of the problem or be the solution.

Though you may be ready to change the world—or at least your program—reflect and determine the current culture of your department.

- Are innovative and educational best practices embraced so student learning is strengthened?
- Do numerous faculty resist needed change and target educators who challenge the status quo?
- Does nursing leadership in your department support, encourage, and expect educational best practice that requires change?
- Is nursing leadership part of the problem or part of the solution?

These reflections are essential to determine if creative active learning will be supported by colleagues or if you will be the "lone ranger" who is recognized by colleagues and students as a problem and not valued for the innovative teaching you bring. In one study, institutional administrative support and academic freedom to implement new strategies were essential to create an environment and culture that embraced transformational innovation in the program (Schlairet, Green, & Benton, 2014).

2. Faculty who oppose change

When I consult with educators, one of their current struggles is overcoming faculty resistance to change. This is unacceptable and difficult to overcome. This is where strong and visionary leadership is needed in nursing education. Academic freedom that allows faculty to teach the way they want needs to take a backseat to educational best practice, which is what the paradigm changes in *Educating Nurses* represent. Nursing leadership must hold faculty to this new standard.

Those who oppose or are indifferent to the transformational changes advocated in *Educating Nurses* need to recognize that it is hypocrisy to insist that students write papers on evidence-based best nursing practice if educators are unwilling to embrace evidence-based educational best practice themselves. You cannot have it both ways. We must practice what we preach. Therefore, nurse educators must embrace transformational change because it is founded on educational best practice.

3. Lack of self-confidence/fear of failure

Though educators are inherently creative, to actually implement creative strategies that you or other educators have created includes an element of risk and putting yourself out there. This increases vulnerability and with it, the fear of failure. Who wants to increase their stress level with additional fears, especially when you are a newer nurse educator? Playing it safe and doing what your colleagues have done for years can appear to be safer, but in the end it will leave you and your program stuck. This contributes to barrier number one, resistance to change.

If you are a newer educator, your first priority is to get comfortable with the content that you are teaching (Herrmann, 2016). Once your knowledge and expertise of the content is strengthened, your confidence will increase and you will become more comfortable using creative strategies in your program. If you tend to be a turtle who is more comfortable in your "shell," now is the time to do what is needed and stick your neck out. Be part of the needed change in nursing education!

4. Not enough time

Time is a precious commodity for any nurse educator. The challenge of doing anything differently is that it requires a significant investment of TIME that is already in short supply. That is one of the reasons I wrote this book and created the numerous clinical reasoning case studies and tools that educators can access and put to use in their program. I want to facilitate and make it as easy as possible to bring down this barrier to transformational change.

Reflect

1. How do you provide opportunities to practice the critical thinking that is required for the clinical setting in the classroom?

2. How consistently do you integrate case studies or other types of active learning in your classroom?

3. What barriers prevent or hinder your ability to bring needed change to your classroom?

4. What can you do to overcome these barriers?

5. What steps do you need to take to integrate case studies consistently in your classroom?

References

American Association of Colleges of Nursing. (2008). The essentials of baccalaureate education for professional nursing practice. Retrieved from http://www.aacn.nche.edu/education-resources/essential-series

Atkinson, T.N. (2014). The "reverse case study:" Enhancing creativity in case-based instruction in leadership studies. *The Journal of Leadership Education, 13*(3), 118-128.

Benner, P., Sutphen, M., Leonard, V., & Day, L. (2010). *Educating nurses: A call for radical transformation.* San Francisco, CA: Jossey-Bass.

Billings, D. M., & Halstead, J. A. (2016). *Teaching in nursing: A guide for faculty* (5th ed.). St. Louis, MO: Elsevier.

Day, L. (2011). Using unfolding case studies in a subject-centered classroom. *Journal of Nursing Education, 50*(8). 447-452.

Duch, B. (2009). Problems: A key factor in PBL. Retrieved from: http://www.udel.edu/pbl/cte/spr96-phys.html

Evenson, M.E. (2013). Preparing for fieldwork: Students' perceptions of their readiness to provide evidence-based practice. *Work, 44*, 297-306.

Harrison, E. (2012). How to develop well-written case studies: The essential elements. *Nurse Educator, 37*(2), 67-70.

Herrmann, J.W. (2016). *Creative teaching strategies for the nurse educator.* Philadelphia, PA: F.A. Davis.

Joint Commission on Accreditation of Healthcare Organizations. (2006b). Root causes of sentinel events 1995-2004. Retrieved from http://www.jointcommission.org/NR/rdonlyres/67297896-4E16-4BB7-BF0F-5DA4A87B02F2/0/se_stats_trends_year.pdf

Kaylor, S.K., & Strickland, H.P. (2015). Unfolding case studies as a formative teaching methodology for novice nursing students. *Journal of Nursing Education, 54*(2), 106-110.

Kesten, K.S. (2011). Role-play using SBAR technique to improve observed communication skills in senior nursing students. (2011). *Journal of Nursing Education, 50*(2), 79-87.

Lee, J., Mast, M., Humbert, J., Bagnardi, M., & Richards, S. (2016). Teaching handoff communication to nursing students: A teaching intervention and lessons learned. *Nurse Educator, 41*(4), 189-193.

McNelis, A. M., Ironside, P. M., Ebright, P. R., Dreifuerst, K. T., Zvoner, S. E., & Conner, S. (2014). Learning in practice: A multisite, multimethod investigation of clinical education. *Journal of Nursing Regulation, 4*(40), 30-35.

Niemer, L., Pfendt, K., & Gers, M. (2010). Problem-based learning in nursing education: A process for scenario development. *Nurse Educator, 35*(2), 69-73.

O'Toole, J.K., Stevenson, A.T., & Good, B.P. (2013). Initiative for innovation in pediatric education-pediatric research in inpatient settings accelerating safe sign-outs study group. Closing the gap: a needs assessment of medical students and handoff training. *Journal of Pediatrics, 162*(5), 887-888.

Popil, I. (2011). Promotion of critical thinking by using case studies as teaching method. *Nurse Education Today, 31*(2), 204-207.

Schlairet, M., Green, R., & Benton, M.J. (2014). The flipped classroom: Strategies for an undergraduate nursing course. *Nurse Educator, 39*(6), 321-325.

15

Tools to Transform the Classroom

Keith Rischer, RN, MA, CEN, CCRN

"Nursing students need to learn for a practice, and every class should contribute to their clinical imagination."

—*Educating Nurses: A Call for Radical Transformation*, p. 79

I developed the following tools to support and strengthen the educational practice of those educators who are willing to step out and do things differently!

Tool #1:
Transform My Lecture Template

This template addresses each of the eight components of an effective classroom lecture so educators can quickly simplify their presentations and put them on a diet! The goal is to lose 40–50 percent of its original weight. Take your current lecture and format it into this document to ensure that you are addressing the need to know content that students must know to transfer learning to the bedside. By integrating and implementing these eight components in every classroom lecture, you can be confident that you are covering what is most important so that your students will be able to clinically reason and be well prepared for clinical practice!

Tool #2:
Clinical Reasoning Case Studies

I initially developed three levels of synthesis care studies that are titled "Fundamental," "Rapid," and "Unfolding Reasoning." Each case study level has the same scenario but progressive levels of difficulty and complexity based on the level of the student. For example, "Fundamental Reasoning" can be used in practical programs or funda-

mentals/first semester; "Rapid Reasoning" is best suited for basic med/surg; while "Unfolding Reasoning" is the most complex, with a change of status that will push your advanced students to put the entire clinical puzzle together before graduation!

Though these case studies were effective tools, the longer length made it difficult to integrate into the classroom. I recognized the need to design smaller, "bite-sized" case studies that are much shorter and can be used at any level of the program. I created three complementary case studies with the same scenario, "Clinical Reasoning 1-2-3". They are two to three pages in length. These case studies can be reviewed in 15–20 minutes in the class or post-conference setting and are ideal for practical and first-year RN students. Clinical Reasoning 1-2-3 heart failure case study is included in the appendix of this book.

Clinical Reasoning 1-2-3

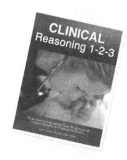

These three smaller case studies or "steps" have the same scenario, but emphasize a different aspect of how a nurse thinks in the clinical setting. Each case study stands alone, but student learning will be strengthened when all three case studies are used, because they have a relationship to one another.

Case Study Step #1:
Recognize RELEVANCE and PRIORITIES

This case study emphasizes the essence of clinical reasoning and the following four principles of clinical reasoning:

1. Identify and interpret RELEVANT clinical data
2. TREND relevant clinical data to determine current status (stable vs. unstable)
3. Grasp the "essence" of the current clinical situation
4. Determine nursing PRIORITY and plan of care

Case Study STEP #2:
Recognize Clinical RELATIONSHIPS

This case study builds on the essence of clinical reasoning by emphasizing the skill of pattern recognition or recognizing clinical relationships. This concept was addressed earlier in the book.

The six essential clinical relationships are:

1. RELATIONSHIP of the past medical history and current medications
2. RELATIONSHIP between RELEVANT present problem data and the primary medical problem
3. RELATIONSHIP between RELEVANT clinical data and the primary problem
4. RELATIONSHIP between the primary medical problem and nursing priority
5. RELATIONSHIP between the primary care provider's orders and primary problem
6. RELATIONSHIP between diseases in PMH that may have contributed to the development of the current problem

Case Study STEP #3:
Care Like a Nurse by Providing Holistic Care

This case study emphasizes the importance of holistic care and the relevance of the "art" of nursing by addressing psychosocial priorities.

The holistic care priorities are:

1. Integrate caring, empathy, engagement, and presence while providing care
2. Care for the entire person (physical-emotional-spiritual)

3. Identify educational and psychosocial needs
4. Determine psychosocial PRIORITY and plan of care

Synthesis Case Studies
FUNDAMENTAL Reasoning (Practical/Fundamental students)

- Identify relevant clinical data in the opening scenario, nursing assessment, vital signs, and lab values.
- Additional emphasis on the applied sciences of pharmacology and F&E to strengthen the "walls" and develop critical thinking
- Learning activity that situates home medications (make these medications the most common or most important of your content or clinical rotation) and requires the student to identify the pharmacologic classification, mechanism of action in their own words, and the most important nursing assessments/considerations.
- "Lab Planning" creates a plan of care with a priority lab, and based on interpretation of all lab panels, determines if the nursing priority has changed.
- Dosage calculation exercise that can situate an oral or parenteral medication that requires a correct calculation by the nurse
- Identify basic clinical relationships of data to put the clinical puzzle together.
- Instead of incorporating the full template of clinical reasoning questions, the focus is on identifying the nursing priority, and care planning using nursing process.

RAPID Reasoning (Basic med/surg)

- Identify relevant clinical data in the opening scenario, nursing assessment, vital signs, and lab values.
- Twelve clinical reasoning questions that provide a template for "nurse thinking"
- Rationale and expected outcomes for medical management
- Priority setting exercise to determine which orders from management of care should be done first with rationale
- Dosage calculation exercise that can situate an oral or parenteral medication that requires a correct calculation by the nurse

- SBAR report at the end of the case study to the nurse who will be assuming care

UNFOLDING Reasoning (Advanced med/surg)

- All aspects of RAPID Reasoning including the template of clinical reasoning questions
- Identify relationship of illnesses in past medical history (PMH) that influenced present problem and the order that they most likely occurred.
- Cardiac telemetry interpretation (if appropriate to scenario) and clinical significance
- Dosage calculation exercise that can situate an oral or parenteral medication that requires a correct calculation by the nurse
- "Lab Planning" creates a plan of care with a priority lab, and based on interpretation of all lab panels, determines if the nursing priority has changed.
- Evaluation of status. Has it improved or is there a need for rescue?
- SBAR report is introduced and allows students to practice this important skill by providing a SBAR at the end of the case study to the nurse who will assume care or to the primary care physician if there has been a change of status.
- Supplement of QSEN competencies and National Patient Safety Goals. This content is reworded as questions that can be used in a case study that you create. Choose the questions to incorporate.
- This level is ideally suited for simulation because it incorporates a change of status that must be recognized. The evaluation component can show improvement that also must be recognized by the nurse.

For more information on clinical reasoning case studies go to: KeithRN.com/clinical-reasoning-case-studies

References

Oermann, M. (1997). Evaluating critical thinking in clinical practice. *Nurse Educator, 22*(5), 25-28.

16

How One Educator Successfully Transformed Her Classroom

Patricia Pence, EdD, MSN, RN

"Unless we are making progress in our nursing every year, every month, every week, take my word for it we are going back."

—Florence Nightingale

My TRANSFORMATION to best teaching practice is shared with you, not as the only "fix-it" solution to any and all problems ailing nursing education, or to force you to teach your classes my way, but to describe what I learned during my journey struggling to TRANS-FORM my teaching practice. Whether you are a new or experienced teacher in nursing, I want to EMPOWER you to reflect on your own teaching practice and begin a conversation with me on how to make active learning a part of your own nursing classroom. We can collectively bring NEEDED CHANGE to improve the quality of nursing education, so that we can better prepare our students to be successful graduates in our nursing program and, most importantly, to practice safely, accurately, and compassionately in professional practice (Benner, et al., 2010).

Have you ever stepped back and asked yourself, "Why do I teach the way you do?" There are many internal motivations for all that we do in life that are subconscious and beneath the waterline of our awareness. Could it be that your own past learning experiences as a nursing student influenced or shaped your teaching practice as a nurse educator? If you are a newer nurse educator, have you observed and are you doing what you see other educators do in the classroom, not knowing that there could be a better way?

My Beginning

Traditional lecture has historically been and continues to be the primary pedagogy regarded by teachers in nursing as an efficient method to cover nursing content (Caputi, 2010; Lauver, West, Campbell, Herrold, & Wood, 2009; Young & Diekelmann, 2002). In the late 1970s, walking through the halls in our community college, you would catch a glimpse of a large lecture classroom with the teacher standing in front of the class at the podium, lecturing nonstop using an abstract taxonomy format that categorized the definitions of diseases, the pathology, signs and symptoms, diagnostic tests, and nursing care of patients, or other nursing concepts, for two or three hours depending on the nursing course. Using abstract taxonomies has since been shown to NOT help nursing students imagine how to use and apply the information in actual patient care (Benner, et al., 2010).

I was one of those nursing students sitting in that class who was part of a captive audience, where learning consisted of DUAL student responsibilities: hearing the teacher speak and being responsible for quickly writing notes. There was little interaction between teacher-to-students or students-to-students during class. As students, we hoped we "got it all" between the translation of hearing FACTS spoken by the teacher and writing it all down in our notes; let alone to be able to UNDERSTAND our notes later when reviewing for our test. From a student perspective, hearing an abundance of FACTS during lecture did NOT lead to a MEANINGFUL and DEEP understanding of the course content; it led to MEMORIZATION of FACTS and sometimes confusion. There was no opportunity to clarify our understanding of the course content before the test, and most importantly, no chance to clarify our learning before performing hands-on care of our patients in the clinical setting.

Active Learning

During my bachelor and master's degree nursing education, I experienced a gradual transition of learning expectations that required students to be responsible for their own learning, be prepared for class, work in small groups or teams, be an active participant in class, and conduct presentations related to the course content. This was an unexpected class requirement that I was not prepared for. Students could not be DEPENDENT on the teacher for all of their learning and sit PASSIVELY in class writing notes. In each nursing course, we were guided by our teachers to think critically about the course content, relate the content to providing EVIDENCED-BASED patient care, evaluate current policies, recommend changes in policy development, and research the current status of the health care system. Each class was an open DIALOGUE between the teacher and students.

I was extremely shy and nervous in front of others. When I learned that I would have to present and lead a discussion before my peers and teachers in every class, I panicked. The announcement for this expectation was a SHOCK, which presented an area of personal growth that I had to master. Each time I had to talk before my peers and teachers, I felt every sign and symptom of stage fright imaginable—flushed face, sweaty palms, pounding heart, shaky knees, and trembling voice, which was so awful that I could barely get my words out at times. At this time I did not realize that I was experiencing what Malcolm Knowles, a pioneer in adult learning theory, referred to as *"culture shock,"* when students are confronted with a new teaching model and are not prepared for this transition (Knowles, Holton, & Swanson, 2005). In the midst of my culture shock experience, despite my uncomfortable and uneasy feelings and thoughts I had during this transition, I began to gain an understanding of how teaching and learning could be DIFFER-

ENT. ACTIVELY participating during each class led to a more MEANINGFUL and DEEPER understanding of the course content, compared to my previous learning in lecture classes.

The waterline of awareness to good teaching practice was almost perceptible; an awareness that was about to surface some time later after I became a teacher.

Novice Educator

When I became a novice educator, I did not have any formal coursework or preparation on teaching nursing students. I entered my teaching role with a nursing background as a LPN, and later RN for 23 years. My professional work experience was medical-surgical nursing, home health, and long-term care. I was a director of nursing in long-term care facilities for eight-and-one half years and led staff education meetings. I later returned to staff nursing while pursuing my master's degree in nursing, and continued to work as a nurse as needed while teaching until I enrolled in a doctoral program. I present to you my perspective on why we need radical change in nursing education through my personal and professional lens as a nursing student, staff nurse, nurse leader, and nurse educator.

To prepare for my first nursing course as the "lecture" teacher, I adopted the course materials and teaching style of my previous teachers. Lecture remained the primary pedagogy for this nursing program where I had started my nursing education 24 years ago. Lecture seemed to offer some advantages:

- It provided the teacher with maximum control.
- It kept all students focused on the same point.
- It ensured efficient use of time.
- Teachers could cover a large amount of material in a short amount of time.
- The teaching method was familiar among teachers and students.
- A high student-to-teacher ratio was cost effective.
- It presented a common base of KNOWLEDGE to all students (Caputi, 2010, p. 687).

Over time, the health care system had rapidly become more complex and high-tech, resulting in increasing standards and difficulty for graduates to pass the NCLEX examination. There were higher expectations of the teacher to teach more content to keep up with the changes occurring in health care and the NCLEX. Predictive testing for students, such as Health Education Systems Incorporated (HESI) examinations administered after each semester, was added to the curriculum (HESI exam guide, 2016). Students then faced more significant consequences if they did not meet the established benchmarks for passing the examinations, such as remediation.

Gradually, the already content-heavy curriculum became even more ADDITIVE, in response to the assumption among teachers that content must be "covered" in class so that learning will take place. Ironside (2004) wrote that there has been a common *assumption* among nursing teachers that "if important content is *'covered,' thinking* necessarily follows" (Ironside, 2004, p. 5). Nursing teachers also assume that thinking should transfer knowledge of abstract facts to answering higher cognitive-level test questions and application to caring for acutely ill patients in our clinical settings (Benner, et al., 2010).

Our classrooms were and are still arranged in an orderly manner that requires students to sit in desks facing the teacher who stands at the front of class, delivers a direct nonstop lecture, now heavily relying on a PowerPoint slide-by-slide method. The students expect to be told *"everything that is on the test."* And the teachers expect nursing students to "apply" important content from their textbooks and lecture to practice during clinical. First-year students are expected to *"remember"* and *"apply"* this important content in second-year nursing courses.

For some time I accepted traditional teaching practice as *this is the way teachers teach in academia.* I held on to this assumption about teaching practice until, as a nursing instructor of a few years, I was asked to participate on a college committee charged with developing a college-wide "blueprint" to guide teaching and learning for our faculty. The committee was assigned to read *The Courage to Teach: Exploring the Inner Landscape of a Teacher's Life* by Parker Palmer (1990) as a springboard for discussion. In his book, Palmer, a national author, expert, and speaker on best teaching practice, wrote that "by non-stop lecturing, where our efforts to 'cover the field' often do exactly that—they bury topics in a *blizzard* of information, obscuring them from students view" (Palmer, 1990, p. 10–16).

Lessons from a Blizzard

I live in central Illinois where we have had a number of historic blizzards! The last blizzard (the Super Bowl

Blizzard) was from January 31 to February 2, 2015, that dropped a hefty 19.3 inches of snow in the Chicagoland area (wgtn.com). I have driven home from college in extremely hazardous conditions, heading south into a storm, praying to God to keep me safe on the road. When you drive into a windy, blowing blizzard that creates a *"whiteout"* with winds more than 35 mph, there is zero visibility. The highway lanes may be reduced to one snow-packed lane with huge snowdrifts. In whiteout conditions, *you do not know whether you are driving on the road or heading in the right direction!*

Palmer stated that delivering a nonstop lecture is the *"least desirable"* way to teach. During a lecture class, students become overwhelmed by the blizzard of information and may misinterpret the information during translation to their notes. The students' *visibility is blurred by the whirling whiteout of words.* They do not know what is NEED to know versus NICE to know from the blizzard of FACTS and words given by the teacher. Lecture does not allow time for students to process and use the information so that they can learn and have a MEANINGFUL and DEEPER understanding of the content. *Students leave class not knowing if they are heading in the right direction!*

Palmer recommended the following as an alternative to using lecture alone:

- Have students read and review information from their textbooks BEFORE class. Resist student demands to be spoon-fed content!
- Use this additional time to USE the information to promote critical thinking or application of what has been taught.
- In nursing classrooms, practice CLINICAL REASONING by developing a sense of SALIENCE, CLINICAL IMAGINATION, and ETHICAL FORMATION. (Benner, et al, 2010)

SUBJECT-Centered Classroom vs. CONTENT-Centered

Palmer's thoughts on teaching stressed that for learning *to take place, teachers need "to get students inside the subject,"* and *"the subject inside the students,"* otherwise students do not see the importance of the subject (content) to their learning (Palmer, 1990). Most lectures do not allow this to happen. Students may not be able to thread the connections between the "subject" and how this "subject" is SALIENT and RELEVANT to contextualize it into caring for a patient in nursing practice.

Palmer's philosophy about what is and is not good teaching led me to consider making small changes in my nursing courses. I thought of ways to bring active learning into my classroom by developing brief activities to complete after my lecture was done. Most often this was done *if there was time.* I still felt compelled to hold on to the tradition of lecture. This was the norm for teaching in our nursing program, and there were expectations among faculty that students had to be provided with detailed information by the teacher during face-to-face class time. *Is not a larger part of learning that leads to a deeper understanding of the material held back and deeply submerged by delivering a heavy-content lecture?*

Questioning My Practice

My continued desire for personal and professional growth as a nurse educator led to pursuing further education, not in nursing, but in education and curriculum. Would this change my teaching practice? One of my colleagues told me, as I considered enrolling in a doctoral program, *"A doctorate will change the way you think about teaching."* At the time, I did not realize how true my colleague's statement was and led to a much NEEDED RADICAL TRANSFORMATION of my nursing classes.

As a doctoral student, you are an adult learner who is responsible for your own learning. You seek out the resources needed to complete coursework and a research study, you are expected to critically think about evidenced-based research and latest teaching pedagogy, and collaborate with other learners as a team to solve problems. The instructor serves as a facilitator who guides you in learning the course content. The teaching model used by teachers in my doctoral classes was a stark contradiction to how I was teaching my nursing students.

I began questioning my teaching practice after reflecting on my experience over the years as an adult learner and a novice teacher. A dichotomous teaching practice existed between lecture in community college courses and active learning in higher level university courses. If active learning is being used as a teaching practice at the university level, why is the lecture model used in nursing classrooms today in our community college nursing program, and other schools of nursing, in

which our graduates need to be better prepared for safe, EVIDENCED-BASED contemporary nursing practice? If we require our nursing students to research EVIDENCED-BASED nursing practice in our curriculum, why are we not teaching according to the best EVIDENCED-BASED teaching practice, such as what is proposed by Dr. Patricia Benner and her colleagues in *Educating Nurses?*

Embracing Educational Best Practice

Dr. Patricia Benner's educational research described in *Educating Nurses* was published in 2010. Her research found a significant gap existed between the quality of nursing education and professional nursing practice. Her findings were based on two national surveys and observations of the quality of teaching practice in the classroom, clinical, and lab that clearly indicated a critical NEEDED CHANGE toward RADICAL TRANSFORMATION away from lecture. Why is there a culture of resistance to change the status quo in nursing education? Why do teachers in nursing education resist changing the way we teach such as traditional lecture, when evidenced-based research calls for radical transformation toward more innovative and effective ways to teach nursing students to think like a nurse?

Change is difficult. I have to admit there was a time that I was not ready for change. I am sure that there are many of you who, like me, get caught up and overwhelmed by the day-to-day routine of teaching, out-of-class prep, and post-class and clinical work. This leaves little to no time to reflect on good teaching practice, to assess the status of your teaching practice, and diagnose what could be improved. Many nurse educators find little time or opportunities for reflection (Benner, et al., 2010). However, there comes a time when change is CRITICALLY NEEDED and RISK TAKING is necessary so that we do what is best for our students and the patients that they care for in our clinical sites.

Emerson and Records (2008) wrote, *"It may be time to sacrifice some of our sacred cows in educational practice"* (p. 363). Just as nurses have held on to old outdated ways of nursing practice, as *"this is the way we have always done it,"* teachers in nursing have preferred to teach students in the same traditional model as they had been taught (Caputi, 2010; Emerson & Records, 2008). Teachers in nursing must *"accept that change is the only con-*

stant" (Emerson & Records, 2008, p. 369). To face the educational challenges in Dr. Patricia Benner's CALL to RADICAL TRANSFORMATION, teachers must be *"willing to step out of old comfort zones to engage in designing imaginative and innovative ways to educate nurses in the future"* (Rich & Nugent, 2010, p. 228).

Struggles in the Classroom

I reflected whether learning how to critically think and reason as a nurse was a reality in my classroom?

My observations of the classroom climate in my nursing courses while lecturing:

- Students were unprepared for class and tests
- Disruptive student behaviors occurred in class
- Students challenged teaching: "Mrs. Pence didn't say it so she didn't teach it."
- Expectation: the teacher was responsible for all learning and test grades
- Students were not able to transfer content and skills to the clinical setting or second-year course tests
- Assumption: "So it must not have been taught during the first year."

In our nursing program, we had created a classroom climate and expectation where students were PASSIVE learners. Students expected the teacher to tell them everything they needed to learn for clinical practice and needed to know for their tests. The sole responsibility for learning fell on the teacher. *Is this really the best teaching practice?*

We've probably all experienced a lecture where students come to class and do everything but listen to the teacher. I have observed unprepared students strategically sitting by the wall or in the back of the classroom so they can sleep after working the night before (hoping that you do not notice), interrupting my lecture to ask me to repeat what I said, or bringing a buffet of food to eat in class. Some students felt compelled to have side discussions while I was talking. Some students accessed their personal mobile devices for email or texting during my lecture. During this time, we had an attendance policy that required students to be in class. However, there was no policy that outlined what was acceptable or unacceptable classroom behavior. Consequently, students "met" the attendance requirement by being a warm physical body in my class while not consciously making any effort to listen to my lecture or take notes. Oftentimes in class I would say, "You need to write this down!"

Another concerning observation was that some students reviewed 20 minutes before an exam. Hearing that some of my students had not prepared for their exams was extremely disappointing and frustrating. It became clear to me that as the lecturer I was bearing the responsibility for their learning and grades and putting more time and effort into the class than some of my students! Would their failure to pass my exams reflect on my credibility and skills as a teacher? If students did fail, would other teachers question my ability to teach that course?

High-stakes testing (our course tests and the HESI tests) continued to be the prime assessment of student learning in our nursing program. There are no opportunities to assess student learning prior to these tests when you lecture nonstop. The only way to tell whether they "got it" or "did not get it" was by their grades, albeit a superficial impression of their understanding or lack of understanding of the course content.

I believe that when students listen to teachers talking at them during a lecture, it creates silos of each individual student's understanding or misunderstanding about the abundance of facts spoken by the teacher. Talking at students is somewhat similar to the television studio business term "talking heads," which is defined as the head and shoulders shot of a person who is "talking all content, but no action" (Talking Head, 2016). Teachers become "talking heads" during a nonstop lecture class when they stand behind a podium or instructor's desk (head and shoulder view) and try to cover all the content. Teachers make the *assumption* that conveying an abundance of facts will translate to learning for nursing practice.

Another common *assumption* in teaching, is that by lecturing, "all students are learning at the same pace," a pace that is actually dependent on the teacher's pace of talking (Caputi, 2010, p. 690). If students are not able to keep up with the teacher's pace of talking through a long list of PowerPoint slides, they leave class and later take a test without having an opportunity to clarify any misunderstandings or clear their confusion about the course content. How many of you have experienced this as well, as a student or an attendee at a conference, when the teacher or speaker just keeps talking? Adult learners need time to process chunks of information before moving on to another topic; otherwise we have TMI that will cause our students to SHUT DOWN!

One student's quote from *Educating Nurses* research clearly illustrated the errors with this common assumption of teaching by lecture: "*A very prescribed, static environment that moves at a certain pace and there's no room to stop if a quarter of the class isn't following. It's not an interactive environment*" (Benner, et al., 2010, p. 72). If we continue to lecture, how will we know whether our students really understand the course content after leaving class? Will their thinking be headed in the right direction? In a high-stakes testing nursing program, does teaching by lecture really prepare our students for practice?

I also continued to observe situations in clinical practice where students were not prepared and not able to thread the connections between theory and content to practice and problem solve during patient care. How many times have you said to a student during a clinical day, "We talked about this yesterday in class"? According to the findings in *Educating Nurses,* there *are* significant differences in the problem-solving skills of associate-degree nurses compared to baccalaureate-degree nurses. Reading knowledge-based abstract information in textbooks decontextualizes learning, making it difficult for students to imagine how to apply clinical reasoning and gain a sense of salience to problem solve a patient's condition that likely changes during clinical practice. Classroom strategies that make it a priority to contextualize content will help bridge this current gap (Benner, et al, 2010).

For example, students may read a list of nursing interventions to provide for a patient who has a medical problem, such as chronic lung disease. By reading or hearing about facts in the care of patients with diseases, will the student be able to recognize what is the most important and RELEVANT clinical data to respond to when a change in the patient's respiratory status, such as a drop in oxygen saturation and increased dyspnea, to prevent a potential adverse outcome? How could I better prepare my students to connect learning from the classroom to the clinical site?

I was becoming disillusioned with teaching and often asked myself, "Why do I continue to lecture?" The disrespectful and unprofessional behaviors in the classroom and students not taking responsibility for their own learning had taken a toll on my desire to continue teaching. I was beginning to experience what Palmer calls lose heart in teaching (Palmer, 1990).

Transitioning to Active Learning

I had become a skilled lecturer. Although student feedback on my lecture skills was positive, this seemed to be a passive method to teach what was essential for safe competent nursing care. I imagined a nursing classroom where teacher and students both shared in learning. In October of 2012, after hearing a conference session on using active learning in the classroom, I realized I could no longer teach the same way I had for the past 12 years. During this session, the speaker described how she recorded her lectures as podcasts to be posted prior to class and had in-class assignments for students to complete in an iPad classroom. There was another way to teach nursing students!

Active learning has the following advantages compared to traditional lecture:

- Promotes enthusiasm for learning.
- Develops higher-order thinking.
- Increases engagement and participation.
- Creates an inclusive learning environment.
- Supports learning among a diverse group of students.
- All students are engaged and participate. (Caputi, 2010, p. 691)

Baby First Steps

I began researching how to pilot and implement active learning in my first-year second-semester medical-surgical nursing course that was scheduled in about five months. At the time, there was not much literature to guide this transition to a new teaching model (Hessler, 2017). I planned my course based on the speaker's examples at the conference, any literature I could find at that time, and any online textbook resources for teachers.

My usual lecture content was prerecorded as podcasts and made available as a link in my Blackboard course. Podcasts allowed my students to play, rewind, and play it again to hear my lecture at their convenience and own pace as preparation for my class (Delaney, Pennington, & Blankenship, 2010). Readings from their textbook were also required as class preparation. I posted an announcement about these requirements before the class began.

On the first day of class I explained to students how an active learning model would be a benefit to their learning and that I was there to help lead them through this transition. Students were given handouts on assignments to complete in class. So you would think that students would value this new approach that would increase their participation, right? Wrong.

Student Resistance

My first few weeks of introducing active learning in class did not go smoothly even though I had spent months planning. I was introducing a new model for learning that they had not experienced in their previous courses, which resulted in "culture shock" for my students. It seems that students also have some assumptions regarding how they should be taught. *"I don't learn that way"* was some students' rationale for wanting to go back to lecture instead of trying active learning. Some students' perception was, *"So I have to teach myself?"*

Instead of lecture, small group case scenarios with questions taken from their textbooks were given out as assignments. Initially, these assignments seemed to be the way to promote active learning. Some students complied with the request to form small groups, while others demonstrated their resistance. One student sitting in the back of class blurted out, *"This is stupid,"* while her friends sitting nearby laughed. Another student said, *"This isn't what I paid for."*

One of my students sat staring at me, while sitting in the back of the classroom, leaning back in her chair, arms crossed over her chest, and feet propped up on another chair, making it visibly clear that she had no intention to participate. Despite any encouragement to try a different way of learning, students sat passively in resistance during the assignments.

Many students in other classrooms prefer lecture and to sit passively in class and resist active learning, which is not an uncommon phenomenon among college students (Palmer, 1998). Some students made their case before my dean, "Can't she go back to lectures?" Their plea for a return to lecture showed their resistance to change, and possibly their own fears of not understanding the course content and failing the exams.

Another initial attempt at using active learning was to have students complete an online case study assignment in a computer classroom. At that time the technology was not always working in our classrooms, causing computer case study programs to freeze, among other technology problems, which caused frustration among some students. After a few class sessions, I realized that

I had only scratched the surface of what active learning could be during our in-class study time. I tried getting students to use their textbooks for case studies, such as a pathophysiology textbook that presented a brief scenario with questions. In retrospect, those questions might do well for independent learning as they read the book, but students were only asked to locate and recall knowledge from their readings. These assignments were not helping my students imagine how to connect my course content within the context of a nurse using clinical reasoning and critical thinking when caring for a patient who has a changing condition.

My confidence to pursue trying a new teaching model was challenged. Going to class everyday was another stressful encounter of dealing with conflict and resistance from some of my students. I knew I had to persist through these struggles and overcome my fear of failure as a teacher; a fear that might drive me backward into lecturing again. Palmer (1998) stated that fear could be both pathological and healthy. Fear may lead teachers to hold on to lecture or help teachers SURVIVE, learn, and grow. Fear is healthy when teachers are *"taking the risks that good teaching requires"* (Palmer, 1998, p. 39).

I continued to work hard to improve my teaching practice. As Florence Nightingale wrote over one hundred years ago, *"Unless we are making progress in our nursing every year, every month, every week, take my word for it we are going back"* (Nightingale, 1914, p. 1). Any movement backward to traditional lecture would have given in to my own and my students' fears and given into a teaching practice proven to not adequately prepare students for professional nursing practice. I had to face these fears in order to transform to best teaching practice. Palmer (1990) explained, *"Good teaching requires courage."* The courage to overcome our fears instead of letting them be a *"driving force behind the kind of teaching that makes students into spectators, that pedagogy that tries to protect both teacher and subject"* (Palmer, 1990).

Start with Case Studies

During the second week of class, one student suggested KeithRN's clinical reasoning case studies. Her friend's instructor in another nursing program had used Keith's clinical reasoning case studies and said those students

"LOVED THEM." My student's suggestion led to contacting Keith to learn more about how to implement his clinical reasoning case studies into my course. Keith was extremely encouraging and supportive of this "newbie" to active learning.

In the next class I asked students to complete one of his case studies in small groups, and then we discussed their findings as a whole-class activity. Students were actively engaged and applied content to care for *"our patient for the day."* Instead of standing in front of class lecturing, I was able to circulate among the small groups to offer assistance and learn what my students were thinking *before the exam.* These were things that normally would not occur in my lecture class.

Although this was early in my teaching efforts at using an active learning model, I could see that the classroom was beginning to be TRANSFORMED into a "CLINICAL SITE." Students were less focused on resisting active learning. I was beginning to feel more satisfied in my teaching practice because the burden of who was responsible for learning was slowly being transferred to my students. Students were now beginning to learn how to take responsibility for their own learning and develop better study habits.

Keith's clinical reasoning case studies set the stage for active learning and promoted clinical reasoning, critical thinking, and engagement in class. His clinical reasoning case studies served as a formative assessment; a way to assess my students' understanding or misunderstanding prior to our tests. As our class discussion involved higher-level questions and content, I adapted my test questions to be at an application or higher Blooms' taxonomy level. My students were THINKING about the content I planned each day! Keith's clinical reasoning case studies continue to be a "staple" item in my toolkit of active learning strategies. *The students and I were slowly adapting to a new model of teaching!*

Published Article

My first two years of piloting active learning was published in the April 2016 issue of *Teaching and Learning in Nursing*. My article describes my initial pilot on *flipping* a class by recording lectures and using active learning strategies in my classroom. But my classroom has evolved to more than just a *flipped* class with active learning. Per Keith's recommendations, I read Dr. Patricia Benner's book, *Educating Nurses: A Call for Radical Transformation."* This book has become indispensable in guiding my teaching practice. The three exemplars of teachers illustrate other strategies to bring CLINICAL IMAGINATION into the classroom and integrate the classroom with clinical practice, "always for the good of the patient" (Benner, et al., 2010, p.14). I continually strive to bring the essence of these research findings into my nursing classroom. I also teach with the intention to lead my class in a way that is for the "good of my students."

Let me share a few of the recommendations for quality teaching in nursing education proposed by Dr. Patricia Benner and her colleagues that I bring into my nursing classroom.

- Every classroom is integrated with clinical practice.
- Every class contributes to clinical imagination.
- Teaching is patient-centered.
- Scaffolding teaching around patient care promotes reasoning about real patient situations.
- Cultivates habits of thinking for clinical judgment and skilled know-how.
- Develops situated knowledge, skills, and ethical comportment and formation.
- Effective classroom pedagogies are: Active learning, spirit of inquiry, unfolding case studies, narrative structures, simulations, and patient interviews.

Gaining Momentum

I have since transformed a first-semester fundamentals course into an active learning class. Because first-semester students were now introduced to active learning earlier in the nursing program, I thought of ways to help them take "baby steps" to become comfortable with active learning. This is the student's second fundamentals class that is very skills intensive. Sterile technique is taught and practiced in lab to administer injections, provide intravenous therapy, catheterization, or sterile dressing changes. Proper care of a patient who requires nasogastric tube and feedings, enemas, and oxygen therapy are taught.

On the first day of class I have students "buddy up" for a case study that illustrates ethical and legal implications in a scenario where a student makes an error while catheterizing a confused resident who lives in a long-term care facility, all while the instructor and assisting students may or may not have noticed the error. The student is faced with making a moral and ethical decision on the next course of action. I developed this activity to help stimulate a discussion to show students that they will now be learning procedures that require clinical judgment to protect their patients and prevent adverse outcomes, such as an infection. Our discussions help students to think beyond just the steps in a skill, but to develop their moral imagination about treating the patient as a person and acting as a patient advocate (Benner, et al., 2010). Students learn from day one that they will be expected to have a dialogue with other students and me during each class and that we will be thinking about safe and quality care for *"our patients for the day."*

Next Steps

I have gained the confidence to think of other ways to bring meaningful and relevant real-life learning activities into my nursing classroom, such as stimulating class discussion of nursing care and priorities after showing educational YouTube videos. For example, I begin a new unit in my medical-surgical nursing course by showing YouTube videos of physicians performing procedures on real-life patients, which I will share with you and explain in my active learning chapter. Students have to draw from their previous learning and new information to answer:

- How will you prepare for this patient?
- What are the risks and potential complications?
- What will you be looking for then?

Other questions aptly used by Dr. Lisa Day, one of the Educating Nurses exemplars, help to guide my classroom activities and discussion.

- What are your concerns about this patient?
- What is the cause of the concern?
- What information do you need?
- What are you going to do about it?
- What is (the patient) experiencing? (Benner, et al., 2010, p.133)

Students now come to my first class knowing "this is how I teach." They come to class better prepared and ready "to apply" what they learned and help each other. You might see students demonstrate how to solve medication calculations, or explain how they would help a family member with one of the diseases or problems we are learning about.

Students know that if they have a question, I will ask, "Where can you find that answer?" So, they open their textbook, or look in their notes from my podcasts, or search on their phone for the answer to report back to me and the rest of the class. By doing this, I help students "access just-in-time" information and increase their awareness that nurses are lifelong learners (Benner, et al., 2010, p. 221). We all learn from each other. Learning is student-centered and patient-centered.

My Classroom Today

My classroom does not look and feel the same. You will not see me standing in front of my class with students facing me sitting in desks all lined in rows waiting for me to convey my words of wisdom to write down in their notes. My classroom time is dedicated for students to use their knowledge to perceive, think, and imagine caring for patients. My PowerPoints are all pictures and diagrams that serve as a visual aid and backdrop for illustrating changes you would see in anatomy or appearance of a patient who has a disease.

Students now move their desks into small groups. Mobile devices are routinely accessed to find information for "our patients." I hear my students, even my quiet ones, working together to care for our "virtual patients." My classroom is a *clinic-like learning community* where students imagine caring for patients, collaborate, and work as teams, like working on the hospital or nursing home unit. I serve as a facilitator, guide, and coach for my students' learning.

Unprofessional and disrespectful behaviors, such as what occurred in the past, no longer occur in my classroom. We have adopted a professional behavior policy, which helps lessen disruptive behaviors and supports teachers who address this problem. I recommend that you have your own discussion with your nursing faculty about developing a professional behavior policy. However, I think that by keeping students actively engaged during the entire class time with MEANINGFUL and RELEVANT learning activities, you will find that your students are focused on learning instead. Sometimes they are so engaged they do not realize class has ended!

Final Thoughts

Teaching using active learning has completely changed the learning climate in my nursing classroom. I would never go back to lecturing for two to three hours. Instead of being a *Talking Head* talking AT my students, I am talking WITH my students. I am learning with my students every day in every class how to *THINK LIKE A NURSE* and care for our patients. My classroom is focused on a clinical situation, in which we all are solving a clinical puzzle (Benner, et al., 2010).

TRANSFORMING your teaching practice is not going to be easy. It is a gradual, evolving, and unfolding process. Initially what you think is an application level activity, may be at a remember-and-understand level. Avoid letting your active learning strategies become *"as stale as the traditional classroom-lecture format"* (Edie, 2013). At first, you may only sense the direction of where you will be heading, regarding good teaching practice, but realize that you are taking a risk for NEEDED CHANGE to RADICAL TRANSFORMATION.

Plan time to REFLECT on your own learning and self-growth in your teaching practice. We expect our nursing students to reflect on their learning during clinical and lab experience for personal and professional improvement: *What did you accomplish? What went well? What did not go so well, and what would you do better next time?* Why not reflect on what is working well and what needs to change in your classes as the teacher? R*eflecting on our teaching practice "allows us to uncover our underlying assumptions about the education process in which we participate"* (Emerson & Records, 2008, p. 368).

I consciously make notes when I am leading a class. Noting what did not go so well or making a reminder for future revisions eases my way as I tweak it for the next time. Hessler (2017) recommends revising your active learning course soon after it is over.

Although my journey to transform my teaching practice has not always been easy, it has been worthwhile and rewarding. My classroom has changed from a PASSIVE to an ACTIVE learning environment. I experienced tremendous personal and professional growth as a nurse educator by following through with a vision and taking risks to transform my teaching practice. The responsibility for learning is now transferred back to my students and the classroom climate is focused on learning to better prepare my students for professional nursing practice. In-stead of holding on to the sacred tradition of lecture, why not embrace a new assumption in teaching practice

that expects students to take ownership and "direct their own learning" and transform your classroom for active learn-ing (Benner, et al., 2010, p.106)?

I now come to class with excitement and anticipation of having a dialogue with my students about *"our patients for the day."* As one of my students commented, "We are ready to apply our learning." I have once again regained my heart for teaching! Because my journey to bring needed change and transformation is based on educational best practice, I am confident that my story can become your story.

Are you willing to take that all-important first step?

Reflect

To reflect on your teaching practice, ask yourself these questions:

1. What assumptions do you have about classroom learning that need to be reconsidered?

2. What is your greatest fear that prevents you from bringing needed change to your classroom?

3. Is this fear founded or unfounded?

4. What is working well in your classroom?

5. What would you change about your teaching practice as a nurse educator?

6. How would you envision your transformed nursing classroom?

7. Once you have taken time to reflect, take a closer look at your nursing classroom by asking these questions adapted from those suggested by Dr. Patricia Benner:

8. What kinds of responses are expected from your students during your class?

9. Does you class provide opportunities for clinical imagination?

10. What level of information is presented and represented by the exchange of questions and answers between you and your students?

11. What is the extent of integration between classroom and clinical education in your classroom?

12. What support and resources will you need to make the transition to transforming your classroom to active learning?

References

Benner, P., Sutphen, M., Leonard, V., & Day, L. (2010). *Educating nurses: A call for radical transformation.* San Francisco, CA: Jossey-Bass.

Caputi, L. (2010). *Teaching in the classroom. In Teaching Nursing: The art and science* (2nd ed.), Glen Ellyn, IL: College of DuPage Press.

Delaney, E., Pennington, N., & Blankenship, M. B. (2010). The role of podcast lectures in associate degree nursing programs. *Teaching and Learning in Nursing, 5*(2), 54-57.

Edie, A. H. (2013). My flipping journey. *Reflections on nursing leadership, 39*(4).

Emerson, R. J., & Records, K. (2008). Today's challenge, tomorrow's excellence: The practice of evidenced-based education. *Journal of nursing education, 47*(8), 359-370.

Hesi exam guide (2016). Retrieved at http://www.hesi-exam.com

Hessler, K. (2017). *Flipping the nursing classroom: Where active learning meets technology.* Burlington, MA: Jones & Bartlett Learning.

Ironside, P. M. (2004). "Covering content" and teaching thinking: Deconstructing the additive curriculum. *Journal of Nursing Education, 43*(1), 5-12.

Knowles, M., Holton, E. F., III, & Swanson, R. A. (2005). *The adult learner: The definitive classic in adult education and human resources development,* 6th ed. San Diego, CA: Elsevier, Inc.

Lauver, L. S., West, M. M., Campbell, T. B., Herrold, J., & Wood, G. C. (2009). Toward evidenced-based teaching: Evaluating the effectiveness of two teaching strategies in an associate degree nursing program. *Teaching and Learning in Nursing, 4*(4), 133-138.

Nightingale, F. (1914). *Florence Nightingale to her nurses.* London: Macmillan and Co.

Palmer, P. J. (1990). Good teaching: A matter of living the mystery. *Change magazine, 22,* 10-16. Retrieved at https:// www.CourageRenewal.org

Palmer, P. (1998). *The courage to teach: Exploring the inner landscape of a teacher's life.* San Francisco, CA: Jossey-Bass.

Process coaching center (2001-2016). The unconscious mind & the iceberg metaphor. Retrieved at https://www.processcoaching.com

Rich, K. L., & Nugent, K. E. (2010). A United States perspective on the challenges in nursing education. *Nurse Education Today, 30,* 228-232.

Sacred cow (2016). Merriam-Webster Dictionary. Retrieved at http://www.merriam-webster.com/dictionary/sacred%20cow

Self-reflection (2016). Merriam-Webster Dictionary. Retrieved at http://www.merriamwebster.com/dictionary/self–reflection

Talking Head (2016). Merriam-Webster Dictionary. Retrieved at https://www.merriam-webster.com/dictionary/talking%20head

Young, P., & Diekelmann, N. (2002). Learning to lecture: Exploring the skills, strategies, and practices of new teachers in nursing education. *Journal of nursing education, 41*(9), 405-412.

17

Additional Strategies to Successfully Transform the Classroom

Patricia Pence, EdD, MSN, RN

"Nursing students need opportunities to safely practice reading situations, imaginatively see possibilities, and draw on knowledge in particular situations"
—Educating Nurses: A Call for Radical Transformation, p. 36

Before I attended a conference session on active learning in 2012, I realized that my teaching practice had come to a standstill. Relying totally on lecture prevented me from moving toward a meaningful and creative teaching practice. The conference speaker's presentation provided innovative ideas that bridged the gap between lecture and active learning. Her inspiration motivated me to set aside my hesitation and fears so that I could move forward to transform my teaching practice and the quality of learning for my students.

When I began my journey to transform my classroom from passive to active learning, I did not know whether this change was going to be a success or a failure. Even though I had not completely planned how to actualize this change, I had a clear VISION of a nursing classroom where students took ownership and responsibility for their learning and the classroom was focused on patient care. As I reflected on the last three years of transforming two first-year nursing courses, five steps came to mind that evolved during this transition to an active learning environment. In sharing these steps, my hope is that you will learn from my experience and avoid the mistakes that I made. My goal is to provide you with additional strategies to help you succeed in transforming your nursing classroom.

These five steps are:

- ASSESS the need for change
- PLAN to bring clinical to class
- IMPLEMENT active learning strategies
- Obtain student FEEDBACK
- EVALUATE and revise

Step One: ASSESS the Need for Change

There are many nurse educators who advocate for the traditional lecture model of teaching (Lauver, West, Campbell, Herrold & Wood, 2009). I also was comfortable with teaching in this manner and I am not totally against lecturing. Even after using active learning strategies, I still plan "short bursts" of lecture to introduce or expand on a topic, supplement the students' discussion, or clarify a misunderstanding— just not for an entire class. I have students in my class for two to three hours depending on the nursing course. I need to break up the monotony of lecture for my own sanity and maintain my students' attention to learn nursing concepts being taught.

As I learned about adult learning theory and the best teaching practices, I realized there were more diverse ways to teach nursing concepts than simply to lecture. I spent a great deal of time reflecting on and assessing my teaching practice. Using the first step in the nursing process (assessment), assess teaching and learning that occurs in your classroom.

- *Are you satisfied with the quality of teaching and learning in your nursing classroom?*

- *Do students take ownership for their own learning?*
- *Is there interaction between students-to-students, and teacher-to-students?*
- *Do students use their critical thinking, clinical reasoning, and clinical judgment skills in the classroom?*
- *Does your nursing classroom stimulate clinical imagination?*

When I think back to my traditional lecture classes, I would have answered NO to all of the above assessment questions. My assessment clearly identified a need for RADICAL change. Do you identify with any of the above questions in your nursing classroom? Let me offer my suggestions and ideas to guide you to bring about RADICAL change to your own nursing classroom.

In my classes, I stress the importance of students establishing baselines in their assessments of patients. I encourage you to adapt these additional strategies as a "baseline" to develop your own strategies that will work best for you and your students. As you become more comfortable with this new model of teaching, you will develop your own active learning strategies.

Step Two: PLAN to Bring Clinical to Class

As I made the initial decision to transition to an active learning classroom, I envisioned a gradual, evolving change that would be adapted, revised, and evaluated in one specific nursing course—my eight-week first-year medical-surgical course. I chose to change the entire course, so that my students would experience a consistent teaching and learning method throughout the nursing course. This was a huge undertaking at that time. You might consider discussing your plan with another instructor and enlisting their help and support during your transition to active learning (Bergmann & Sams, 2014; Hessler, 2017).

You might feel more comfortable with a gradual transition and change one *"class"* or *"classes"* within a nursing course to begin. That is up to you. As I explain my strategies for active learning, I will refer to a *"nursing course."* You can certainly apply these ideas to one class or classes and gradually make the change when you feel more comfortable and confident with this model of teaching.

The following suggestions will help guide this important second step.

1. Decide what nursing course you want to transform.

- Which nursing course are you most comfortable teaching?
- Would this nursing course be easily transformed to an active learning model?

To answer this first question, think of a nursing course that you are most confident teaching, while anticipating that *there will be* additional questions that will arise from students during your in-class time (Hessler, 2017). Active learning opens up opportunities for students to explore new ways of thinking and often leads to new questions related to your course content that you had not thought of before.

For example, I had been teaching a first-year medical-surgical course for about 12 years prior to transforming this class to active learning. This was the most likely course for me to transform, as I had worked a number of years as a RN on a medical-surgical and skilled nursing unit and continued as a clinical instructor in both areas of nursing.

Because students were applying med-surg content during class, we could work on gaining a deeper understanding of patient care for these diseases, which often prompted new questions to answer. Although I tell my students that *I still have to look things up,* which is a great example of lifelong learning, this was the best course for me to be able to answer new questions from my students. It would have been a more difficult process if I were building a new nursing course or one in which I did not have much work experience as a practicing nurse.

A nursing class that requires many higher-ordered *"skills"* is easily transformed to an active learning model (Hessler, 2017). Think of the term *"skills"* in a broader context, more than having your students perform *hands-on* tasks. *Skills* can apply to activities that ask students to use their critical thinking, clinical judgment, and clinical reasoning skills (Benner, et al., 2010; Hessler, 2017). In my medical-surgical course, you will see students spend time in class with both hands-on practice and other learning activities that promote critical thinking, clinical judgment, and clinical reasoning.

2. Review Course and Unit Learning Objectives for the Class

Hessler (2017) suggests everything *"should flow from the existing learning objectives"* (p. 102). What are the overall key points of NEED to know content from the learning objectives that you want emphasized in your course? I intentionally plan learning activities for students and write my own notes to ensure these key points are stressed during class.

What content do you want available to your students to prepare outside of class? The out-of-class time should include activities that help students meet the lower-order learning objectives in your nursing course. The out-of-class prep time is used to *"cover"* content at Bloom's REMEMBER and UNDERSTAND level of learning and to gain knowledge about course concepts.

Students can complete text or article readings as preparation for the "remember" level objectives. My students also listen to a recorded lecture for each class. You decide on what required preparation is best for your students. Keep in mind that the goal for out-of-class preparation is to help prepare students to APPLY the content during your in-class time. Focusing on higher-order objectives during class will allow you as the nurse educator to guide *"students into a deeper understanding and comprehension of the material"* (Hessler, 2017, p. 89).

3. Allow Enough Time for Planning to Transform

Dr. Karen Hessler, a nurse educator and nurse practitioner from Denver, Colorado, recommends *"planning at least one semester or three calendar months prior to the time"* you will be implementing the active learning course (Hessler, 2017, p. 88). I took about five months (including Christmas break) to prepare a plan for my first active learning course that began in March 2013.

To begin planning active learning strategies in your nursing classroom, the following suggestions will help guide you:

1. Determine the MOST IMPORTANT content to "cover" during face-to-face time with your students (Bergmann & Sams, 2012; Hessler, 2017).

My learning activities are focused on key concepts that I want to spend class time helping my students to understand and apply before their test. These activities serve as a formative assessment to get a better idea if students have any misunderstandings or misconceptions about the course content before the test. In a traditional lecture class, you would not have an opportunity to assess your students' learning prior to administering a test.

I also plan the essential content for my students to know as a practicing nurse, so that I can best help them *"develop a sense of salience, clinical reasoning, and clinical imagination necessary to become effective and ethical nurses"* (Benner, et al., 2010. p.15). I list the most salient concepts that I want my students to apply in class, after they have prepared for my class by listening to my recorded podcast lectures, reading their texts, and writing notes in a printed outline that I provide. I intentionally plan my in-class learning activities to help my students APPLY and ANALYZE these concepts based on the readings and my recorded lectures.

2. Create "compelling clinical situations" where students are nurses along with the teacher to solve clinical puzzles in class (Benner, et al., 2010, p.141).

Lecturing a taxonomy or abstract categorical list of diseases focused on a *medical model* does little to help students learn the true essence and clinical realities of the *"nursing aspect"* of what occurs at the bedside during patient care. Since I have transformed to active learning, I focus my in-class activities on nursing priorities necessary to care for patients safely and competently.

3. Refer to the educator version of the National Council Licensing Examination (NCLEX) test blueprint and the Quality and Safety Education for Nurses (QSEN) initiatives for the competencies necessary for nursing practice.

These competencies are embedded in my learning activities (Beischel & Davis, 2014). I highly recommend reviewing the ncsbn.org and qsen.org websites to guide your active learning strategies, which will better prepare students for the NCLEX examination as well as professional nursing practice.

4. Filter the content for NEED to know.

In my teaching experience, first-year nursing students are

overwhelmed with the vast amount of reading, usually required from several nursing textbooks per nursing course. Students are *expected* to read through all this information and know what is most important to learn to be successful in the course and to be able to apply in clinical nursing practice. Filter the content of your textbook by identifying specific pages that are the NEED to know, while the remainder of the chapter is NICE to know. What I have learned is that novice students might not have any health care experience to base their learning on. ALL information appears to be important to these students.

As a nurse educator for 17 years, I have learned to view my teaching practice thru the lens of a first-year novice student, who is learning this information for the *first time.* Therefore, I try to emphasize through our learning activities what they NEED to know as a nurse to provide safe and quality nursing care. Any NICE to know information is suggested for those students who desire to further research a topic. For example, some online resources are suggested for more practice with a topic.

Set Expectations for Active Learning

Your students will be adapting to a new model of teaching and learning. To set the stage for active learning, I recommend adding statements in your course outline or syllabus regarding expectations for active learning. Outline your expectations for class preparation and active participation during class. The first time I transformed a class to active learning, I arranged with another instructor to meet with the students during the previous nursing course so that I could introduce the change in teaching method and tell students what they could anticipate for class preparation and active participation.

On the first day of class, I began with an interactive activity that eased students into an active learning model. For my fall semester fundamentals course (the students' first experience with active learning), students partner with another student to read about a real-life clinical dilemma that presents an error requiring students to reflect on and respond to the potential ethical and legal implications. This is a prime example of an active learning strategy that promotes students' formation to think and act ethically as a nurse (Benner, et al., 2010).

Determine Active Learning Strategies

The following are the wide variety of approaches I used in my classroom for active learning. This will keep both you and your students from getting into a rut. Be creative and have fun!

1. Clinical Reasoning Case Studies

After one of my nursing students suggested to try Keith's clinical reasoning case studies, I went to Keith's website and ordered all the case studies that related to the rest of my medical-surgical nursing course. Needless to say, my students also loved them! They remain a staple in my toolbox for my active learning strategies. We have since used his clinical resources for most important labs and medications, and have adopted his textbook, *Think Like a Nurse,* for our first-year nursing students.

Keith's clinical reasoning case studies transformed teaching and learning for my nursing classes. My nursing students were now engaged in a discussion about our *"patients for the day"* and were beginning to critically think, clinically reason through the case scenario, and imagine caring for these patients *in class.* That initial step in changing my teaching practice was the impetus that shaped my active learning approach for teaching my nursing classes to be *"all about our patients for the day."* I *listened* to my students and *adapted* to how they wanted to learn. This small, but very important step, opened the doors to create other relevant active learning strategies and an authentic teaching practice.

Keith's textbook and clinical reasoning case studies have met the approval of well-known national leading nursing education experts including Dr. Patricia Benner. His clinical reasoning case studies have been referenced and reviewed by other nurse educators and are ready to implement into your nursing classroom with a student version and fully developed answer key for faculty.

2. Research available instructor online resources

As a nurse educator, new to active learning, I initially did not feel confident in my teaching practice to develop my own active learning strategies. I first spent time researching available online textbook student and instructor resources. I gleaned the instructor online resources, such as TEACH for Nurses Evolve instructor online resources from Elsevier, for short case scenarios and other ideas on active learning strategies that I would be most comfortable using in class

The TEACH for Nurses instructor online resources are available with each textbook. If you are new to teaching, I suggest contacting your textbook representative if you are not familiar with what instructor online resources are available for you.

In addition to a test bank and PowerPoint slide for each chapter, you will find a lesson plan with these suggested activities:

- Mosby's Nursing Video Skills program and review questions
- Discussion topic questions
- Ideas for small group activities
- Case scenarios with five NCLEX-style questions

For my nursing courses, I selected TEACH for Nurses active learning strategies from each textbook. The selected short case scenarios, NCLEX-style questions, and other types of activities, such as ordering steps in a task, were typed up as a handout given to students to complete in small groups. For my fundamentals class, I have shown the Mosby's skills video on preoperative and postoperative care so students could observe a nurse perform a pre-and post-op interview and assessment. We critiqued the video and completed the review questions as a whole-class activity. In my medical-surgical nursing course, I showed the skills video on blood transfusions to begin a discussion on this topic. You can engage students by asking them to create a short video with their cell phones on various skills or topics. Although these activities were not as in-depth as Keith's clinical reasoning case studies, they helped me during the transition to an active learning class before I learned about his resources.

3. Use animations, video clips, pictures, and graphics

In my experience, many first-year nursing students are not aware of the online student resources available to them with each textbook. I often use student resources in class to help them realize that additional resources are available to support their learning. One common online student resource available with textbooks today is animations and video clips.

Even though the medical-surgical textbook would begin a chapter with a review of the anatomy and physiology for each body system, rather than lecturing a review of what is already in the textbook, I will start class with

signing into the Evolve online student resource program (evolve.elsevier.com) from the computer and play any animations or video clips that related to the in-class content.

For example, to begin my respiratory and cardiac units in my medical-surgical nursing course, students listened to animations of heart and lung sounds, viewed a narrated animation of blood flow through the body, conduction system of the heart, and changes in the lungs that occur with asthma. Using animations or video clips stimulates visual and auditory senses and connects previously learned content from anatomy and physiology (A&P) class to our current nursing class. Students now have to apply A&P to patient care. A discussion follows about how abnormal changes in the patient's A&P would alter the function of the patient's body systems, result in a disease process manifesting in signs and symptoms, the need for nursing care, and a nurse's careful watch for potential complications.

Another way I address pathophysiology and bring the science underlying nursing care into a classroom is through pictures or graphic items shown in my Power-Point that compare and contrast normal and abnormal organs (Flood & Robinia, 2014). This strategy is based on my past students' curiosity about visualizing how disease processes alter normal body structure and functions in their patients. My PowerPoint is a visual tool composed of pictures illustrating our patients for the day, as well as a graphic illustration of key concepts or disease processes. One of the effective teaching strategies recommended in *Educating Nurses* was using PowerPoint presentations with pictures and graphic illustrations (Benner, et al., 2010).

Audio clips, video clips, and graphic items are currently a few examples of alternative formats used to develop test-item questions for the NCLEX exam. Students have practice with these types of alternative formats during my classes. My students can expect test questions with alternative formats in my exams. I will explain how to create test questions using alternative formats later in this book.

4. Connecting new content to prior learning

In my class, you might hear me say, "Remember when we talked about… Now let's think about this in relation to our patients with…."

Because I have taught fundamentals and basic medical-surgical nursing course, I can plan activities that connect previous learning to new content as we progress through both courses. The class discussion guides students to make connections between their previous learning with new learning to care for patients. For example, students gain a basic understanding of and learn how to interpret simple arterial blood gas (ABG) results in their fundamentals course, and later in their medical-surgical nursing course apply this learning to abnormal ABG results for our patients who have respiratory, cardiac, gastrointestinal problems, diabetes, and renal failure.

Lisa Pestolesi, one of the exemplars described in *Educating Nurses,* aptly uses this active learning strategy. She teaches by *"building on what students have already learned in other classes and introduces new knowledge that she expects students to integrate"* (Benner, et al., 2010, p. 109). Pestolesi teaches in a simple to complex manner, connecting "old and new" information to create coherence throughout the course (Benner, et al., 2010, p. 110). Lisa Day, another exemplar, skillfully applies questioning and dialogue to draw from her students' earlier learning to their current learning (Benner, et al., 2010).

5. Relate content to real-life examples from clinical practice

Recently I transformed my first-year fundamentals nursing course, the students' second course in our nursing program, into an active learning class. The first course in our nursing program is taught by lecture. An early approach I used related the students' textbook content to real-life examples that occurred in my clinical practice with students.

For their first unit on Infection Prevention and Control, students were divided into small groups and given a printed handout outlining various activities for that class session. Students used my list of real-life patient examples illustrating a break in the body's natural defense mechanism to compare to the table content in their textbook, and then used the boxed section on prevention measures to determine appropriate patient teaching. Students created their own case scenario that illustrated a person experiencing the four stages in the course of an infection that is listed in another section of their textbook. When they discussed medical and surgical asepsis, students identified whether my list of real-life examples were medical or surgical asepsis. Students went to the

cdc.gov website to review evidenced-based care of patients with an emerging infection, which at that time was Ebola. The care plan in that chapter was reviewed for any significant data, such as the patient's white blood cell count and neutrophil count, any risk factors exhibited by this patient, any potential complications, and the nursing priorities related to the patient's infection.

By leading students through the content in their textbook for the first unit, students learn how to study, think about the infection prevention and control content, and relate the content to real-life nursing practice. Students realize that class time will best be used to develop *clinical imagination* and the ability to *think like a nurse.* Students become more comfortable with collaborating and working together with each other in small "teams," which is how they will need to perform for safe nursing practice. Actively using key information from their textbook for patient-based learning activities brings life to their textbook readings and integrates theory (content) to real-life clinical nursing practice.

Clinical imagination defined:

Students "imagine being with a patient" and "rehearse how they might act in a clinical setting," "deciding what needs to be done next and why."
Students are invited to "form a vision for practice, and to focus... on developing the most appropriate responses to patient situations"
(Benner, et al., 2010, pp.102, 160).

6. Bring "real-life" patients and health care providers into the classroom

One of the active learning strategies that I have found effective when I begin a unit in my medical-surgical nursing course is showing a YouTube educational health care video illustrating a patient undergoing a procedure or diagnostic test. There are many more credible educational YouTube videos available now than when I first began using active learning strategies. It is best to find videos that are not too lengthy in time. (Or fast-forward through the NICE to know content.)

Most units in my medical-surgical nursing course begin after an exam, when my students have not had time to prepare for the next unit's content. I provide students a handout with questions to answer in small groups after viewing the video. Showing these videos places students in a virtual health care setting in which they can imagine being with and caring for this patient as we begin a new unit.

Medical Procedures and Diagnostic Tests

Not all students have an opportunity to observe medical procedures and diagnostic tests in other departments. With the rapidly changing health care system, I cannot always count on patients scheduled for procedures or tests during my clinical day. But my exams include questions on the nursing care of patients who undergo medical procedures and diagnostic tests. To help my students, I will often show YouTube videos in class to provide this "observational clinical experience."

For example, when beginning my gastrointestinal unit, I show a YouTube video by Dr. Oller, an emergency room physician, who performs a paracentesis on a patient with cirrhosis that resulted from an adverse response to a medication (Oller, 2012, August 19). Students learn that this is another example of why a patient might have cirrhosis. Students see that this patient is jaundiced and has ascites, observe how the physician preps and drapes the patient, hear the physician explain the procedure, and see eight liters of pale yellow ascitic fluid removed during the procedure. Students then break into small groups to discuss questions, such as *"What is your role and priorities as the nurse for this patient?" "What is the worst thing that could happen to this patient?" "How will you monitor this patient to prevent this from happening?"* This video is available at https://youtu.be/6d-L6Hni6A4?t=4s

Some examples of other YouTube videos that I have shown are patients and health care providers in a bronchoscopy and other endoscopies, a thoracentesis, pulmonary function tests, angioplasty with stent placement, lithotripsy, and skin biopsies. I find that students can relate the textbook content to medical procedures and diagnostic tests much better after viewing YouTube videos in class and following up with discussion about the nursing care of patients undergoing these procedures and tests.

Patients and Nurses

Another strategy I use is showing a YouTube video where a nurse or a patient explains a procedure, such as a hemodialysis or peritoneal dialysis treatment. Students hear from real-life patients how they manage their daily life around dialysis treatments or hear a nurse explain what their role is during the procedure. Students work in small groups to compare and contrast the nursing care, priorities, and potential complications for hemodialysis and peritoneal dialysis patients.

Other topics that I have used YouTube videos in class are of young adults exploring issues with public's perception of a person who has an ostomy and a toddler who explains his ostomy care. For "covering" a colonoscopy procedure, I have used a YouTube segment showing well-known television anchors, Katie Couric and Harry Smith, describe a live colonoscopy procedure performed on Smith for the morning CBS Early show. You can find the news segment at https://youtu.be/zLAPQdlXgdU

YouTube and Web Links

My first-year medical-surgical course that I teach includes pediatric care. YouTube videos and web links can incorporate technology to stimulate an engaged discussion with students in class about class content. In a rural area, we do not very often see pediatric patients or patients with some of the rare teen or adult problems seen in our hospital clinical sites.

These videos "simulate" being with the child or teen, as well as any other patients, at the bedside in place of a clinical experience. You could apply this active learning strategy for any nursing course. Use videos during class or post them before class to stimulate discussion. This is an excellent strategy to bridge clinical with theory in a large lecture class. What topics in your nursing class would you supplement with YouTube videos?

Here are ten questions to ask:

1. What did you notice in the video?
2. What other questions would you ask your patients?
3. What treatments or medications are needed?
4. What is the purpose of using these treatments or medications?
5. What teaching will you provide these patients?
6. Why is this patient teaching so important?
7. What complications will you be on the watch for?
8. What will be the cues or signs to alert you of an early complication?
9. What orders will you anticipate?
10. How will you evaluate the outcome of patient care that you provide?

Patients and Family Members

YouTube videos can also promote effective learning and

an understanding of the concept of caring, which is foundational to nursing practice and is an essential integrated nursing competency included in the NCLEX exam. Students hear from the patient and/or family member about what they are experiencing during a time of illness or chronic disease.

Instead of lecturing about cystic fibrosis in my class, students can gain a much *deeper* and *meaningful* understanding of this disease process by hearing firsthand from a patient and family member's lived experience, such as that of a young single mother's struggle to maintain a positive outlook on life while managing the care for her three-year-old daughter who has cystic fibrosis (Jennings, 2016, March 9). Students can observe the child crying during her daily respiratory treatments, the number of medications taken every day, how her mother needs to adjust her child's nutritional needs, and other aspects of her child's daily life. What better teaching strategy can you use to ignite compassion and caring in the hearts of your students than hearing from a real patient's and family member's experience?

Educating Nurses research found that the practice of caring was absent in formal lecture classes (Benner, et al., 2010). To foster caring practices essential for compassionate nursing practice, nurse educators must teach students during class *"to be with a patient and bear witness to the patient's plight"* (Benner, et al., 2010, pp. 194–95). We cannot expect that students fully develop the competency of caring during the little clinical time they have prior to graduation. In my nursing program, students have clinical one day per week. Therefore, nurse educators should integrate teaching students about caring and compassion during each class.

YouTube videos stimulate my students' visual and auditory senses to help them imagine caring for patients undergoing these procedures or those living with an illness or disease. I find that using YouTube videos as an active learning strategy provides a more *authentic* learning experience for my students than if I were to spend class time lecturing on the procedures and diagnostic tests, diseases, and nursing care, as I had done previously. I have compiled a list of my favorite YouTube videos of these procedures for you at the end of this chapter.

7. Adapt your simulation program for an in-class learning activity

After simulations were added to our nursing program, I began using our simulation resources to create in-class learning activities. Due to the obvious limitations of being in a classroom with approximately 40 students, I adapted simulation scenarios to what is possible for an in-class learning activity. For example, when discussing the perioperative unit in the fundamentals course, I provided a handout on the background and assessment information for several simulation patients of different gender, age, and medical history who were undergoing different surgeries.

We *"walked"* through the pre-op phase of the simulation as the *"interview nurse"* by analyzing and comparing patients' pre-op history for risk factors, medication history, possible interview questions, and what pre-op patient teaching is needed, and determined whether they have any concerns about these patients. Later we were the *"medical-surgical nurse"* as these patients "returned to our unit" with post-op orders that included labs and medications to review, nursing priorities to establish, and interventions to prevent potential post-op complications. By the end of the simulation activity, I found that this was a much more realistic and meaningful approach to *"cover"* the perioperative content, than when I lectured.

Benner (Benner, et al., 2010) called for nurse educators to bring clinical imagination into the nursing classroom so students can imagine being with the patient and have an opportunity to rehearse and decide on what needs to be done next as the nurse. Engaging students in simulated case studies helps students consider how they would act in a clinical situation. Simulated case studies are an excellent active learning strategy that helps students integrate knowledge, develop skilled know-how, and ethical comportment (Benner, et al., 2010).

8. Connect textbook content to real-life health care issues in your community

At times, I suspect my nursing students might wonder whether the nursing content that I "cover" really matters to them as a student and as a future practicing nurse. To answer that question, I searched for course-related health care issues in my community that gained attention from our local news station.

Last spring when the topic of lead poisoning came

up in my medical-surgical nursing course, a local television station had broadcast a news segment describing how a school building in a school district in Peoria, Illinois, was contaminated with lead, causing the administrators to close the school building. School administrators, teachers, students, and staff were redirected to other temporary buildings. The reporter interviewed several parents who were concerned about the potential effects on their children. In the video you also see a RN, who is the disaster coordinator and a nurse at one of our hospital clinical sites, performing a blood test on children to screen for lead exposure.

I used this news segment to lead a whole-class discussion about lead poisoning, addressing the parents' concerns, the potential effects on a child's development and health, and information to include when educating the parents. This active learning strategy was an excellent way to add relevance to the topic of lead poisoning and demonstrate leadership exemplified by one of our local nurses during a time of crisis. The video can be seen at http://www.centralillinoisproud.com/news/local-news/parents-worry-about-kids-lead-exposure. I encourage you to think of any "hot topics" related to your course content that might be illustrated in your local news media.

9. Connect classroom with real-life nursing care from clinical practicum

Here are a few strategies that I use to "situate learning" so that it helps students imagine being the nurse caring for patients on a medical unit.

Protocols and Procedures

I often use my clinical practicum site's hospital protocols and procedures, such as for a heparin drip and venous thrombosis embolism (VTE) prophylaxis screening, to create an active learning strategy in my medical-surgical nursing course. For example, in the respiratory and cardiac unit we discuss different scenarios that might lead to the risk for pulmonary emboli or VTE. We used a heparin drip protocol from our clinical site to evaluate a patient's lab results in the scenario. Students respond to the situation and determine their next course of action based on the hospital protocol and lab result. We also reviewed the screening protocol for VTE prophylaxis and review how to administer lovenox and heparin subcutaneously, and discuss required patient teaching.

Another protocol I used was for hypoglycemia. We compared the nursing care for different patients with Type 1 and Type 2 diabetes and walked through a scenario using the hospital protocol for management of a hypoglycemic reaction to determine the next nursing action based on the patients' conditions. Consider enlisting the help from your clinical site staff for their common protocols and procedures that could be used to bring real-life nursing practice in your class.

Clinical Patients as a Case Study

A second active learning strategy that is in alignment with *Educating Nurses* research is connecting learning with real-life nursing care (Benner, et al., 2010). I have enhanced classroom learning by using real-life exemplars from our clinical experiences (Flood & Robinia, 2014). We compared real-life patients from our clinical sites who have the same medical diagnosis.

For example, we compared assessment and laboratory data and the nursing care for three patients we cared for with heart failure who were in different stages of the disease process, from just newly diagnosed to end-stage heart failure. I projected the real-life cases in my PowerPoint slides (while maintaining HIPPA guidelines) and led a discussion on the gradual changes that occur in heart failure. My clinical students could share their personal experience in caring for these patients.

10. Use nursing equipment to address the learning needs of hands-on learners

In my teaching experience, I have observed that nursing students need repetition with nursing skills and to have their nursing skills *"leveled up"* as they progress through the nursing program. Nurse educators assume students gain full knowledge about the intricacies of complex nursing skills by reading a procedure in a textbook, and practicing the skill once in a lab. Therefore, nurse educators expect students to perform this skill competently in clinical practice (Benner, et al., 2010).

For example, in our second nursing course, students have hands-on practice in lab with drawing up medications from a vial and the steps to administer an injection. By the time they have their fourth eight-week class (my medical-surgical nursing course), the reality is that some students might not have had an opportunity to give an insulin injection in their clinical practicum, either by drawing up from a vial or using a pen. Not all students have experienced the repetition needed to skillfully perform hands-on tasks.

When I discuss insulin therapy in the endocrine unit of my medical-surgical course, I bring insulin supplies from the skills lab to my class. I divide my students into small groups and ask them to explain how to prepare insulin, put into order the steps to safely prepare and administer insulin by vial and pen, and discuss patient teaching strategies. Instead of another demonstration and lecture on this nursing skill, students need to critically think and clinically reason through the proper steps on their own with my guidance. Benner (Benner, et al., 2010) found in the national surveys that nursing students want to have the repetition with hands-on skills in the nursing classroom. Consider how you might bring nursing equipment into your classroom so that you will reinforce learning and how to correctly and accurately perform hands-on skills related to your course content.

11. Thinking about differences in "hypo" and "hyper" diseases

In the past when I lectured for my endocrine unit, students did not do well on the test. To address this problem, I developed a handout that included tables with questions based on *Educating Nurses* that asks students to compare the main diseases, with the resulting pathophysiology, medications, treatments, nursing care, patient teaching, and potential complications for patients with Type 1 and Type 2 diabetes, Cushing's and Addison's Disease, and hypothyroidism and hyperthyroidism. Some of the questions I included based on Educating Nurses (Benner, et al., 2010) were:

- *What will you see in your patient?*
- *How will you care for this patient?*
- *What complications will you look for?*

Using a table may seem very simplistic, but it is just one of the strategies that I have used in this unit that has been very effective. To help you understand how this table is used, let me explain my lesson plan for "covering" the endocrine unit. During this unit, students attend a two-hour lab where two guest speakers and another instructor explain diabetic diet, types of insulins, and oral antidiabetic medications. I have a one-hour class after

the previous test where I introduce basic concepts about diabetes using various strategies, such as YouTube videos of young patients with diabetes explaining their daily life struggles with this disease, and bringing insulin supplies into class for an activity. The next class is two hours and 50 minutes. I use Keith's clinical reasoning case study on Diabetic Ketoacidosis as one of our patients for the day. We compare "patients" illustrated in my PowerPoint for diabetes Type 1 and 2, and the other endocrine diseases. Students then break into small groups and create this table as a review and study tool. We regroup to discuss their findings before the end of class. Assessment questions on a handout are given for students to complete independently and turn in to me prior to the end of class.

Students have performed better on my tests when they determined for themselves the important content to include in their table.

12. Develop your nursing students' skill of inquiry

Dr. Benner's research found that the skill of inquiry has been a weakness in nursing education (Benner, et al., 2010). Nursing students need to ask clinical questions and follow up to answer these questions by using available literature and resources. They need to practice the skill of inquiry in the classroom to prepare for lifelong learning required in a complex and changing professional nursing practice (Benner, et al., 2010).

During my medical-surgical nursing course, students often ask new questions during our class, Caring for Our Patients. As a result, rather than answering the question, you might hear me redirect a student to search for the answer and report back to everyone in class. Cell phones and other mobile devices are commonly used for online Internet searches to access "just in-time information" to answer questions regarding care for our patients (Benner, et al., 2010, p. 221; Hessler, 2017). I intentionally guide students to discover new evidenced-based information during active learning activities throughout my course.

For my integumentary unit, I developed a handout listing directions for students to walk through decision making and patient teaching as a clinic nurse, office nurse, and a school nurse for patients with various skin problems. Students searched for information on website links listed in their handout with each scenario. Colored pictures of patients with these skin problems are given as a handout for each group. Students matched the colored pictures to the related scenario.

13. Prioritization, Delegation, and Assignments

Dr. Patricia Benner's (2010) research found novice students have difficulty setting priorities during a clinical practicum. Many novice students have not gained a sense of *salience,* so all tasks, requests, and concerns are urgent (Benner, et al., 2010). The ability to prioritize, delegate, and make assignments correctly has been an area of weakness noted in students in our nursing program. Consequently, I try to include an active learning strategy on prioritization in both lecture courses I teach.

One resource that I use to help nursing students prioritize, delegate, and make assignments appropriately is the *Prioritization, Delegation, and Assignment* online program by LaCharity, Kumagai, and Bartz (2014). To address this area of weakness, I downloaded and printed the "Unfolding Case Studies for Class Discussion" instructor PowerPoints from the *Prioritization, Delegation, and Assignment* online Evolve program to use as a handout in class. These case studies are not available to students; they purchase the printed book with other case studies.

To create my handout, I changed the white background to add color and added pictures of "patients" or nurses or graphic diagrams, such as a diagram related to the renal system. Students completed these as a small group activity as a review of the unit's content.

For my fundamentals course, I used the "Urinary Incontinence and Perioperative Care" PowerPoint presentations. In my medical-surgical nursing course I use "Acute Kidney Injury," "Complications of Chronic Kidney Disease," "Chronic Pancreatitis," "Hyperthyroidism," "Pediatric Asthma," and "Tuberculosis" PowerPoints. Other topics available are "Depression" and "Ectopic Pregnancy."

During a "debriefing" session, students provided a rationale for their group's answer. What I like about these case studies is that they place brief patient scenarios in the context of making priorities, assignments, and delegating tasks to other health care providers. Teaching students how to think about these tasks can easily be overlooked when planning active learning in a CONTENT-HEAVY curriculum. Oftentimes, students learn that what they have observed occurring during

their work experience may differ from the standards expected in nursing education literature or the NCLEX examination.

> **Sense of salience:** *"When a practitioner can discern what is more or less important in a clinical situation."* (Benner, et al., 2010, p. 25)

14. Summarize key concepts from learning

Memory Notebook of Nursing, developed by Zerwekh, Claborn, and Miller (2012), are a group of graphics, pictures, and mnemonics that are a favorite of my students, especially those students who are visual learners. I have included many of the *Memory* graphics in my fundamentals and medical-surgical nursing course to illustrate concepts. For example, at the end of the discussion on renal failure, we use the pictorials to compare the nursing care of patients with acute kidney injury and chronic renal failure. We will look for similarities and differences in the pictorial compared to our previous class discussion.

Once students are familiar with the style of graphics, I might ask them to create their own graphic on large Post-It Notes paper as a small group activity. *Memory Notebook of Nursing* are available in print and CD format at www.nursinged.com. The CD format allows you to download the graphics, save to your computer, and insert the graphics as a PDF document in your own PowerPoint.

Top Three

At the end of a class, students can summarize learning by writing down three "take-home points" on 3" x 5" index cards (Hessler, 2017, p. 226). I developed a similar strategy for students to summarize "take-home points" on six blood disorders. Students were asked to think of the top three key points that would help them differentiate these blood disorders from one another.

Instead of 3" x 5" index cards, I gave students a handout with images of six blood drops, one for each blood disorder that we discussed earlier during other activities. Students were instructed to write down the top three key points that would help them remember the differences among these blood disorders for questions on my exam. Although this "Blood Drop" handout is very basic, it helped my students summarize their learning for that content. They requested more visuals, such as this handout.

15. Formative assessments prior to testing

Based on a college-wide goal requiring all lecture instructors to report on assessment of student learning, I recently developed application level questions as a formative assessment activity for students to complete independently at the end of a unit. These questions are written at a higher application/analysis level and pose a scenario that includes the patient's subjective and objective data often in a table format, simulating a medical record. Students review the information and make a decision for their next course of action.

I collect and review their responses for the formative assessment and clarify any misconceptions or misunderstandings prior to their exam. My response is posted in my Blackboard online course prior to the exam. In the past when lecturing, I would not have any idea of the students' understanding prior to my tests. You may choose to use this type of question as a small group activity in class.

Step Three:
Implement Active Learning Strategies

When I piloted active learning strategies four years ago, there was not much research to guide me in successful implementation of this new model of teaching. I am sharing what I learned through trial and error so that you will avoid the problems I experienced and have a much smoother transition into active learning than I had. Along my journey, I experienced four basic, but vital phases that helped me implement my strategies.

Phase 1: Create a template listing the times for what will occur during each class session

When I first began planning my active learning strategies, I had not planned how much time to allow for each activity or knew how long it would take students to complete the activities. Once I had gotten through the first two units, I learned to create a template that listed the objectives for each day, instructions for students for small group activities, and estimated the amount of time each activity would take.

I would suggest allowing the first 10–15 minutes to take attendance, answer any questions from the text or article readings (or recorded lectures if you choose to do this), and introduce the plan for class (Bergmann & Sams, 2012). If you plan to show YouTube videos, list the amount of time to show the video and complete any

questions for a small group activity. Include time for breaks. Allow 5 to 10 minutes at the end of class to answer any questions before students leave and state any reminders of what to prepare for the next class. I found that allowing time for questions and reminders is another strategy to help your students adjust to a new model of teaching (Hessler, 2017).

Let's take a look at a sample template for the first 50 minutes of a class period in a medical-surgical course. This is on the next page.

Phase 2: Type a student and an instructor version of any handouts

I typed a handout for students and one for myself with my own notes and key points to address during each class. Last fall this strategy helped a new instructor teach a fundamentals course for the other half of first-year students. She had not taught the class before. Having typed lesson plans and handouts for each class helped ease her into teaching a new course and become comfortable with a new model of teaching. I encouraged her to add her own personal or professional stories or examples during class and to provide me with any feedback on each activity. It is also a useful tool for me to ensure that we all stay focused on what is NEED to know content.

Phase 3: Plan extra active learning activities

It is wise to plan extra activities in case your class or small groups finish early (Hessler, 2017). The reason you should do this is that each group learns at their own pace. In a lecture class, it is assumed that all students learn at the same pace (Benner, et al., 2010). Once you start bringing active learning into your classroom, you will find that one class or group might complete an activity earlier than another. I learned that some groups of students took much longer while others would get done quickly and then sit waiting or would get bored and start checking their emails or other social media on their cell phones. Coming up with on-the-spot activities was rather stressful for me. This approach did not help students smoothly transition to an additional activity. Having a plan for high-quality additional activities will help in the event you have groups or a class that finishes earlier.

Phase 4: Take notes on each class

I learned to take notes during each class or soon after re-

Sample template for a lesson in the Respiratory Unit:			
Lesson Plan	**Respiratory Unit** **Time: approximately 50 minutes**		
Opening	Q&A/ attendance	10 minutes	Instructor Notes: https://youtu.be/v30vHFz1ZAY https://youtu.be/noDxydboLrA Handouts for discussion questions application assesment questions Key points
Interactive activity	Review of A&P and assessment	5 minutes	
YouTube video	Bronchoscopy Thoracentesis	5:30 minutes 8:56 minutes	
Active Learning	Small group questions	10 minutes	
Debriefing	Entire class	5 minutes	
Application-level question	Individual activity	5 minutes	
Break		10 minutes	

garding how the class went. Taking notes will help you in the final steps of evaluation and revision. Here are ten questions that helped me reflect on the learning activities and plan revisions for my course for the next time:

- Did you and your students find the learning activities helpful?
- Did the learning activities provide a meaningful experience?
- Did the learning activities meet the learning objectives?
- Were there any revisions needed?
- Did you or your students notice any errors or typos in the handouts?
- Any changes in the format for handouts to make them more appealing and easier to read?
- Were there any other higher-level questions that could be added to the activity?
- Would there be a better active learning strategy to convey this nursing concept?
- Did you or your students have any innovative ideas for active learning to use for the next class?

- How much time did it take for students to complete each activity?

Step Four: Obtain Student Feedback

It takes much time and energy to adjust as a nurse educator and for a student to be comfortable when transitioning from passive lectures to active learning. To smooth this sometimes-bumpy transition it is imperative to obtain frequent feedback from your students on their perception about the transition and related learning activities. Do not allow their feedback to be the final word on the effectiveness of your teaching. Adapt your active learning strategies to their learning needs to show your students that you care about their learning and success in your class. Some active learning strategies that worked for my students one semester did not work well for my next group. Addressing your students' learning needs and preferences during the transition will help build a partnership with your students that are essential for the transition to active learning (Bristol, 2014; Hessler, 2017).

Not All "Rainbows and Butterflies"

I have faced many challenges in my life and career, so facing another challenge to transform to active learning was not new to me. I dived right into this new challenge to transform my classroom without fully realizing the struggles ahead. As mentioned earlier, my experience implementing an active learning model was "not all rainbows and butterflies"!

I struggled each day facing students who were angry, resentful, and resistant to the change that I was bringing to my nursing classes. One of the main concerns voiced by my students was requiring out-of-class time to prepare for class when they have work and family responsibilities. This is a common concern of students at the beginning of an active learning class (Towle & Breda, 2014).

In a traditional class, preparing for class is also expected, whether students choose to prepare or not. It takes time for students to realize and shift their thinking about who is responsible for their learning. Is the teacher responsible for teaching and learning, or are students responsible for what they learn or refuse to learn (Bergmann & Sams, 2012)?

Along my journey, I came to realize that no matter what type of teaching method used, traditional lecture or active learning; there would always be certain pitfalls to expect. I hope by sharing about the struggles that I experienced during my journey, you can avoid these pitfalls and have a much smoother transition. Even though I anticipated there would be some difficulties, it took a great deal of persistence and courage to overcome the barriers created by passive learning.

Here are three pitfalls that you should anticipate:

1. Not all students will be on board with a new way of learning.

During my initial attempts at transforming two first-year nursing courses, there was resistance by some students who did not want to spend time preparing before class or want to participate during class. Most college students are familiar and comfortable with lecture and being "spoon-fed" information from their teachers, expecting to be told whatever is necessary to be successful on the exam. Don't let this stop you from transforming your class. You will not be able to please all students, even if you lectured.

Using various active learning strategies will better address the different learning styles of your students, than if you continue with a strictly lecture style. Take extra time to explain how the learning activities will help address different learning styles of the students. This approach also helps students realize that each student in the class is unique and has specific learning styles that you are trying to address during class.

2. Active learning does not guarantee all your students will pass the test.

Based on their previous learning experience, some students perceived that if they could "repeat" what the teacher said (as heard in a lecture class) they had "learned" the material and should be able to pass the test. The traditional lecture model had created a passive learning environment, where students learned material at the Bloom's recall cognitive level just to pass the test. I needed to change my students' perception that learning to be a nurse requires more than just recalling or regurgitating content for the exam.

When reviewing test results with my students, I sometimes heard that if they failed or did poorly on the examination, they would state, "This is not the way I learn" as an excuse. But when I compared their test scores in another class taught by traditional lecture, I learned that these students also struggled with learning by lecture. It was not the new model of teaching that was the problem. These students were used to being "spoon-fed" content and perceived that lecture was the most effective method for teaching. Overall test results in my first active learning course improved compared to when I taught that class by lecture.

3. Not all students prefer lecture by Power Point.

In my teaching experience, even before changing to active learning, I learned that not all students wanted to listen to a PowerPoint presentation read by myself or other teachers, when they can read the PowerPoint themselves. Sometimes I would hear a student comment about teachers "reading the PowerPoint slides." Lecture by PowerPoint is not based on how adults want to learn, nor does it address the different learning preferences of students.

Student Feedback

During my first class taught by active learning in 2013,

student anxiety about the change lessened by midcourse. Students eventually became more focused on preparing for class and less resistant to active learning. By the end of the eight-week medical-surgical course, most students indicated positive feedback on the course evaluation. Students perceived the active learning strategies helped them to learn the course content. As expected, some students still preferred lecture and passive learning, which is common among nursing students (Oermann, 2015).

In the second year of teaching the course, I made revisions based on previous students' feedback. In the second-year course evaluation, the main comment was that there were too many case studies. That year we started using two new textbooks for the course. I had included previous case scenarios and added others from the new textbooks, as well as Keith's clinical reasoning case studies. In hindsight, the students were right. Doing case studies for almost three hours in a class can be monotonous. Therefore, that led to developing other active learning strategies that were explained in this chapter.

By spring of 2016, I had tweaked and revised the class four times. The strategies and examples seen in this chapter are the result of four years of teaching with active learning in my nursing classroom.

Step Five: EVALUATE and Revise

Implementing active learning strategies is an evolving process that entails planning, self-reflection, evaluation, revision, and refinement each time you teach the class (Bergmann & Sams, 2012; Hessler, 2017). Take time to reflect on how the class went for you and your students. Review your notes on the ten questions listed in the implementation section. Initially, you will find that some activities may not be as effective in engaging all students. You may decide to omit the activity or choose to revise it. Even when I found that an activity went well, I look for improvement, such as adding higher-order level questions (Hessler, 2017).

Student feedback at the end of a course is another method to evaluate the active learning class. The first time I taught using active learning, I posted an online survey in my Blackboard course regarding students' perception of their preparation for class and the course tests (Pence, 2016). Open-ended questions allowed students to type any other comments. The college course evalua-

tion was also used to provide data on the effectiveness of the course.

Be prepared for negative responses from some students, especially the first few times that you teach with active learning strategies. Reviewing negative or "neutral" responses from my students' evaluation has always been rather hard to swallow. Take their responses with a grain of salt. Students do not always realize all the time and effort that you put into a class to provide the best teaching and learning experience. Be assured that you are using evidenced-based teaching practices to improve the quality of nursing education. You will not be able to please all students even in a traditional lecture class. Resist the temptation to return to lecture.

Do use any constructive comments from your students' evaluation for improvement. Once you have completed your overall evaluation, make any needed revisions. It is best to revise shortly after the class is finished, while the necessary revisions are fresh in your mind (Hessler, 2017). This will ensure that your nursing course will be ready to teach for the next time.

When reflecting on your teaching practice, take time to acknowledge your efforts at bringing needed change into your nursing classroom. Give yourself credit for taking steps to transform your nursing classroom. Take a break and celebrate your accomplishments!

"Level Up" Active Learning Strategies

When I interviewed for my teaching position and presented my teaching topic, a faculty member commented, "Students don't know that yet." That insightful remark has "stuck" with me throughout my teaching career.

My examples of active learning strategies illustrate what my typical "lecture time" is like in class with my first-year nursing students. To help you understand the *"curricular context"* in which I have based my active learning strategies, I will provide needed context with our ADN nursing program. Because the curriculum in our nursing program had been based on a simple-to-complex philosophy, and I am teaching first-year nursing students who might have not been in an active learning class, and who are at a lower level of understanding and curricular expectations than our second-year students, I strategically plan my active learning strategies, so that they are *"leveled up"* as we progress through my courses, and nursing program. Our nursing program also includes practical nursing students in the same registered nursing courses during their first year. These practical nursing students take two additional nursing courses the following summer semester to complete their certificate in practical nursing.

My active learning strategies are *"leveled up"* from the first week to the last week of a course, and from first semester to second semester. For example, when I begin teaching my fundamentals of nursing course, my activities introduce students to the active learning model, such as how to "care for patients" with an infection. My style of questioning and clinical detail is simpler than what you would see in my class at the end of this course, when we are "caring for patients" with oxygenation needs, who are showing signs of shock, or exhibiting changes in their arterial blood gas levels. During the next semester, as we progress from week one to eight in my medical-surgical nursing course, you will see the expectations for my students' attainment of knowledge, clinical reasoning, clinical judgment, and inquiry *"leveled up,"* as they "care for patients" who have medical problems related to one or more of the six body systems in the course.

"Leveling up" is an approach that can be continued throughout all levels of nursing education. As nursing students progress to second-year nursing, an instructor could "level up" the cognitive level of questioning in class for critical thinking, clinical reasoning, and a spirit of inquiry. For example, Keith's "Fundamental Reasoning" case study that I use in the first year of nursing would be an excellent active learning strategy to "level up" in the second year medical-surgical nursing course, such as a patient experiencing a myocardial infarction (MI) with a higher-level complexity case study, "Rapid Reasoning." In first-year courses, I need to lead students through the care of a patient with an MI, and acquire a basic level of understanding about common EKG rhythms (what is the cardiac rhythm, possible causes, signs, and symptoms, and most important treatment/medications). At second-year, students could interpret a given EKG rhythm, as the patient is cared for in the immediate stage of an MI, and continue care for the patient in an unfolding scenario as the patient's condition changes and progresses to being discharged. Keith's "Unfolding Reasoning" series of case studies have this higher level of complexity needed for advanced students.

Nursing instructors who teach at the bachelor's de-gree level, could expand on the student's level of understanding, by including concepts of leadership, management, supervision, and facility policy development involving the nursing care of patients on a unit who have had an MI. A master's degree nursing student who is in a clinical nurse specialist or nurse practitioner course track would participate in an unfolding case study to learn to "manage the care and treatment" for this patient, in an unpredictable, changing, and complex health care clinical situation.

In Closing

My classroom emphasizes small groups of students learning how to provide nursing care for patients. Providing more opportunities for students to work as teams in the nursing classroom is critical for the future of the nursing workforce. *Educating Nurses* (Benner, et al., 2010) research and the National Council of State Boards of Nursing recommend nurse educators strengthen nursing education in communication, teamwork, and critical thinking (2016). These essential objectives can be practiced safely in the classroom.

Is this worth your time and effort? Absolutely! My pearls of active learning strategies are just some of the ways to integrate the classroom with clinical practice. You have your own unique nursing practice and nurse educator background to draw upon so be creative in your nursing classrooms. I know that you will create different ways to integrate clinical practice into your nursing classroom. As a result you will be part of the needed change and be leaders of transformation in nursing education!

Strategies from this chapter are taken from an article on my pilot study published in *Teaching and Learning in Nursing Journal* (2016) and a presentation at the *Organization of Associate Degree Nursing* conference on November 6, 2016.

Reflect

Now that you have learned some ways to transform a nursing class into a higher quality level of teaching and learning, take some time to reflect on how you can be a part of this needed change and take the initial steps to transformation.

1. Why do you hesitate making a change to active learning?

2. What fears hold you back from becoming the creative teacher that you want to be?

3. What concerns do you have about implementing active learning strategies?

4. Select one nursing class to transform to active learning. Use the assessment questions listed at the beginning of this chapter. How would you answer these questions?

5. What strategies would you feel most comfortable using as an active learning strategy?

6. How would you plan to use this strategy or strategies in your nursing class?

Resources
Respiratory Unit
Diagnostic tests and treatment
- Bronchoscopy http://youtu.be/v30vHFz1ZAY
- Thoracentesishttp://www.youtube.com/watch?v=ugIWa1Kl7ps
- Pulmonary function test
  http://www.youtube.com/watch?v=1rjN2_hDXEY
- CT scans http://youtu.be/mMOBgHkivtI
  http://www.youtube.com/watch?v=KZZ_kf3ByYw
- Peak flow meter-asthma
  https://youtu.be/6MK3xSkxFAg
- Sweat chloride test-cystic fibrosis
  http://www.youtube.com/watch?v=8UCWoz6gUp8

Assessment and Respiratory Problems
- Lung sounds
  https://www.youtube.com/embed/O8OC7EiqBKQ
- Nasal flaring
  http://www.youtube.com/watch?v=LJVfErMKRi8
- Croup
  http://www.youtube.com/watch?v=Qbn1Zw5CTbA

- Child with asthma
  http://www.youtube.com/watch?v=GUkh1EGXvaE
- COPD/Asthma
  http://www.youtube.com/watch?v=sCgah1rO2ik
  http://www.youtube.com/watch?v=UKl_Pv-Q3hk
- Pneumonia
  http://www.youtube.com/watch?v=nBqF7lOcUiU
- RSV
  https://www.youtube.com/embed/WLBnyk-C6iw
  https://youtu.be/lIE_UElOk3c?t=2m2s

Cardiovascular/Hematology Unit
Cardiovascular diagnostic tests, medical problems, and treatment
- Echocardiogram
  https://youtu.be/0eKdhHF-JLg
- Stress test
  https://youtu.be/PXay0q1kJVw
- Cardiac catheterization and stent
  https://youtu.be/JeH4zPzQgRc
- Telemetry lead application
  https://youtu.be/2aBI9FQQu44
- Unna boot
  https://youtu.be/esO_29qgGZaU
- Peripheral Arterial Disease
  http://heart.memorialhermann.org/peripheral-artery-disease/

Hematology diagnostic test and medical problems
- Bone marrow aspiration and biopsy
  https://youtu.be/NkdsLHBCreI
- Hemophilia
  https://youtu.be/ZMjI7f6EeSA
  https://youtu.be/RNc0yV69-cE
- Leukemia
  https://youtu.be/VfcomGt24Uo
- Sickle cell anemia
  https://youtu.be/bEYqP8iZ8TE
- Sickle cell crisis, complications, self-care
  https://youtu.be/2CsgXHdWqVs
  https://youtu.be/Y3eWxtKUE90
  https://youtu.be/4lNPRp2MMuY

Gastrointestinal Unit
Gastrointestinal diagnostic tests, procedures, and medical problems

- ABD ultrasound
  https://youtu.be/eM1qLM7VJw8
- Barium swallow (UGI)
  https://youtu.be/5QhBvXsJ53E
- Barium enema
  https://youtu.be/AwGt8TKOrnI
- EGD
  https://youtu.be/gDtAl4pGamw
- Colonoscopy
  https://youtu.be/zLAPQdlXgdU
  https://youtu.be/b5j-NCvOpjs
- Pyloric stenosis
  https://youtu.be/2v5U6M7cfyM
- Liver biopsy
  https://youtu.be/ug3n7bvq2Wg
- Paracentesis
  https://youtu.be/6d-L6Hni6A4
- ERCP
  https://youtu.be/IRdA2krJ6LQ
- Cholangiogram
  https://youtu.be/cjJKdNm-cLQ
- Ostomy patients
  https://youtu.be/eBry_MsqcVs
  https://youtu.be/mEZ3hxK4WEM

Renal Unit
Renal diagnostic tests
- Cystoscopy
  https://youtu.be/d9Vx3Lgz4sw
- Lithotripsy
  https://youtu.be/fR_CjlVXhzw
- Kidney biopsy
  http://bit.ly/2qIHCht
- Renal angiogram
  https://youtu.be/1iXlxX—t80
- Hemodialysis and peritoneal dialysis
  https://youtu.be/fKlY2SKi_dk
- Hemodialysis patient
  https://youtu.be/E8Uj-C1-HyU
- Peritoneal dialysis patient
  https://youtu.be/B5HGpLLE9Ko

Endocrine Unit
Endocrine diagnostic tests, procedures, and medical problems
- Diabetes review

  https://youtu.be/X9ivR4y03DE
- Living with diabetes
  http://www.youtube.com/watch?v=TIgsDlu3cxo&feature=relmfu
- Effects of diabetes
  http://diabetes.emedtv.com/diabetes-video/diabetes-and-its-effects-on-the-eyes-video.html
- Living with retinopathy
  http://www.youtube.com/watch?v=AU0krf1Bgec
- Hypothyroidism
  https://youtu.be/rNJI1MdGELQ
- Hyperthyroidism
  https://youtu.be/mad4hZqXJgE?t=2s
- Addison's Disease https://youtu.be/Zcyr8fV7deg
- Cushing's syndrome
  https://youtu.be/RfzCIDYNwVs?t=2s

Integumentary Unit
Integumentary diagnostic tests and medical problems
- Skin punch biopsy
  https://youtu.be/tH98alFT8JA
- Shave biopsy
  https://youtu.be/R0yvX-ty9VM
- Excisional biopsy
  https://youtu.be/Z_R2uMp6XN8?t=2s
- Psoriasis
  https://youtu.be/dQ_4EkmV1tM
- Scabies
  http://www.cdc.gov/parasites/scabies/index.html
- Acne
  http://www.webmd.com/skin-problems-and-treatments/acne/default.htm
- Eczema
  http://www.mayoclinic.org/diseases-conditions/eczema/basics/definition/con-20032073
- Burns
  https://youtu.be/UQu8qpwhtKM?t=1m24s
  https://youtu.be/Wf5Bn_9cv_c
- Impetigo
  http://www.nlm.nih.gov/medlineplus/ency/article/000878.htm
- Pediculosis
  http://www.cdc.gov/parasites/lice/
- Shingles
  http://www.cdc.gov/shingles/index.html

- Herpes
  http://www.healthline.com/health/std/herpes-sim-plex#Outlook
- Fungal skin problems
  http://www.nlm.nih.gov/medlineplus/ency/article/000878.htm

Other educational YouTube videos can be found at: https://www.**youtube**.com/**education**

References

Beischel, K., & Davis, D. (2014). A time for change: QSENizing the curriculum. *Nurse Educator, 39*(2), 65-71.

Benner, P., Sutphen, M., Leonard, V., & Day, L. (2010). *Educating nurses: A call for radical transformation.* Stanford, CA: Jossey-Bass.

Bergmann, J., & Sams, A. (2012). *Flip your classroom: Reach every student in every class every day.* Eugene, OR: International Society for Technology in Education.

Bergmann, J., & Sams, A. (2014). *Flipped learning: Gateway to student engagement.* Eugene, OR: International Society for Technology in Education.

Bristol, T. J. (2014). Flipping the classroom. *Teaching and Learning in Nursing, 9,* 43-46.

Flood, L.S., & Robinia, K. (2014). Bridging the gap: Strategies to integrate classroom and clinical learning. *Nurse Education in Practice, 14,* 329-332.

Hessler, K. (2017). *Flipping the nursing classroom: Where active learning meets technology.* Burlington, MA: Jones & Bartlett Learning.

Jennings, J. (2016, March 9). *Living with cystic fibrosis* [Video file]. Retrieved from https://youtu.be/hiyT68ClDko

LaCharity, L.A., Kumagai, C. K., & Bartz, B. (2014). *Prioritization, delegation, and assignment: Practice exercises for the NCLEX examination* (3rd ed.). St. Louis, MO: Mosby.

Lauver, L. S., West, M. M., Campbell, T. B. Herrold, J., & Wood, G. C. (2009). Toward evidenced-based teaching: Evaluating the effectiveness of two teaching strategies in an associate degree nursing program. *Teaching and Learning in Nursing, 4*(4), 133-138.

National Council of State Boards of Nursing (2016). A changing environment: 2016 NCSBN environmental scan. *Journal of Nursing Regulation, 6*(4), 4-37.

Oermann, M. H. (2015). Technology and teaching inno-vations in nursing education: Engaging the students. *Nurse Educator, 40*(2), 55-56.

Oller, C. (2012). *Paracentesis* [Video file]. Retrieved from https://youtu.be/6d-L6Hni6A4?t=4s

Paldo, A. (reporter). (2016, February 3:14:29 CST). *Parents worry about kid's lead exposure* [television news cast]. Peoria, IL: WMBD-Channel 31.

Pence, P. L. (2016). "Flipping a first-year medical-surgical associate degree registered nursing course: A 2-year pilot study. *Teaching and Learning in Nursing Journal, 11,* 52-57.

Rischer, K. (2015). *Clinical reasoning case studies*. Retrieved from http://keithrn.com

Towle, A., & Breda, K. (2014). Teaching the millennial nursing student: Using a "flipping the classroom" model. *Nursing and Health, 2*(6), 107-114.

Zerwekh, J., Claborn, J. C., & Miller, C. J. (2012). *Memory notebooks of nursing.* Chandler, AZ: Nursing Ed.com & Nursing Education Consultants, Inc.

18

"Pearls" from Classroom Educators

I solicited the feedback of nurse educators to share the creative strategies and tools they had developed to strengthen student learning in the classroom. Here are their classroom "pearls" that can also benefit and strengthen the learning of your students!

I use unfolding case studies and have students prepare for the concept BEFORE class by posting the case study online. Students download, and then complete the first five questions as a ticket to class. They must turn this in before class for two points (providing me with information to assess what my students may be lacking in comprehension for class discussion). Then the class material for active lecture is based on the case (with a few added personal touches); students are picked randomly to discuss the answer they have all prepared. I have student names on tongue blades in a bedpan that I randomly choose for individual participation. Later in small groups, the students finish the questions of the case study with discussion. The case's main concepts lead to other group activities such as ABG jeopardy or match the O2 delivery device with the clinical findings. The students have told me that they feel they know the patient by the time we are done!

—Jillann Grooms, RN, MSN, CNE
Assistant Professor
St. Catherine University
St. Paul, Minnesota

I incorporated your clinical reasoning case study on DKA (Diana Humphries) for an online assignment using Blackboard in my third semester class. This was a two-part assignment. The first half was designed to have students answer questions through interaction and collaboration on the discussion board. This approach varies from many projects in which students answer questions individually, and then combine them into one paper with many contributors. However, nursing revolves around collaboration, and this assignment format helped students learn to use a collaborative process to provide a perspective on the patient's care. I monitored the discussion board to ensure all students actively participated and addressed the assignment's questions.

The second portion was a peer-graded, in-class presentation in which the students provided solutions to the patient's problems. This could be a paper, PowerPoint, or skit. The groups each had ten minutes to present their solutions and rationales. This short time frame forced the students to focus on key points. Essentially, each group gave a SBAR shift report. Time was allotted for questions from their peers. This presentation was worth 50 percent of the total project score. The paper or PowerPoint was then submitted for an instructor grade, also worth 50 percent of the total project score. The entire assignment is valued at 3 percent of the total course grade.

At the completion of this exercise students demonstrated a strong understanding of DKA. They understood the pathophysiology, medications, and holistic care priorities of a complex patient. It made the lecture portion go by quickly and they clearly nailed it! This approach helped students understand HOW to integrate all aspects of care related to DKA and developed their ability to identify priorities and clinically reason.

To ensure that I am effective and meeting the learning needs of my students, I use a "start-stop-continue" strategy as a formative assessment tool midway through my theory class.

Asking "how's it going?" doesn't obtain needed feedback. Instead, ask focused questions. Ask students to tell you the following:

- What should you START doing?
- What should you STOP doing?
- What should you CONTINUE doing?
  (http://www.bu.edu/ctl/teaching-resources/start-stop-continue/)

I pass out a form in class with these three questions and give the students 15 minutes to complete. Students do not put their names on the form. I consolidate all answers and post them for all to see. If I am able to make changes based on majority opinion (eliminating all exams is not going to happen!) or if I can revise a portion of the class time, I do so immediately. The trade-off is that students have to commit to make changes as well. An added benefit of this is that it alerts the class to behaviors that drive other students crazy, without having to call them out on it. (FYI, I have the students create their own set of class rules during week one, so this reinforces the rules already out there.) This type of formative assessment helps me create a positive flow in the classroom, and demonstrates to the students that they are part of creating their own unique classroom and learning environment. This formative assessment could also be incorporated in a clinical course as well.

—Lin Rauch, MSN, RN, BSEd.
Nursing Instructor
Western Technical College
La Crosse, Wisconsin

This method was originally used by a major local teaching hospital to assess new graduates' ability to critically think and clinically reason. This method was adapted by myself and colleagues Melanie Benington, MSN, RN, Monica Losneck, MSN, RN, and Jennifer Sulzer, MSN, RN for second-semester ADN students. The group dynamics to facilitate learning are terrific. Three different scenarios related to diabetes were created as a collaborative effort among course instructors using the following:

Dot Method Step-by-Step
Split the students into groups (5–6 per group, if number of students allow)

1. Have the group pick a student to write on the board or paper
2. On the board or paper, the student should write the following titles:
   - Patient History
   - Signs and Symptoms
   - Possible Medical Problems (2–3 problems)
1. Priority Nursing Interventions (3 interventions)
2. Have the students read the individual scenario each group has been assigned
3. After reading, the students should identify items from the scenario to place under the titles (patient history and signs and symptoms, assessment findings)
4. The students should identify 2–3 medical problems that the patient could have with the given information
5. The students should assign a *different* color or symbol to each of the suspected medical problems
6. Taking one of the medical problems, students place another color dot or symbol next to each item under history and problem or assessment finding *that matches the problem colored dot or symbol*
7. This is repeated with each problem
8. Students then count the number of similar colored dots or symbols for each medical problem
9. The problem that has the most dots or symbols is the identified medical problem the patient is experiencing
10. Now, students identify 3 priority nursing interventions and rationales for the medical problem identified
11. Have each group present the case and their identification of the problem and discuss rationales
12. Instructor facilitates group interaction—redirects—clarifies and fills in gaps when students present
13. Each student has all 3 templates so they fill in as

other students present group findings and make a study guide in the process.

—Vykki Daus, DNP, CNM, MBA, RN
Assistant Professor of Nursing
Cuyahoga Community College
Westlake, Ohio

When I teach the stages of child growth and development, I found short cartoon strips from the comic section, or you could have the students search and bring them in. I asked students to identify the stages of growth and development represented by the cartoons and to discuss. Examples used were "Zits" and "Baby Blues."

—Debra Avery, RN, MSN
Nursing Faculty
Three Rivers College
Poplar Bluff, Missouri

For my classroom, I deleted A&P content from my theory classes since it had been already covered. But I noticed that students couldn't always connect the dots. So I use Jing, the free version of Screen Casting, to present voice-over-PowerPoint presentations. I break each segment of my lecture into multiple five-minute presentations that students may review at their convenience. I also use Jing for areas that some students want additional information on such as EKGs, pharmacology content, how to calculate certain math problems, etc. I post the links into my class site so that students can review this at any time. Students tell me that they listen to these over and over.

To encourage students to dig into their textbooks, I use online discussion boards for each book chapter. Students post three main concepts, physical assessment, or critical thinking questions. I select one of these questions to appear on the exams and I talk about their posts in class. It's a great way to see what they think about the material and helps them stay connected with it in between classes.

—Ruth Tamulonis, RN, MSN
Nursing Faculty
Yuba College
Marysville, California

When I first started teaching, I used PowerPoint and added games and activities, but I started running out of time to lecture to include them. I was stuck. I began incorporating case studies but having a separate case study

and patient scenario provided no continuity. I solved this dilemma by creating a series of case studies that evolved with ONE patient. Because I teach fundamentals, I would start the first week with one simple case study. This scenario provided contextualization of content that included bathing, vital signs, and nursing assessment. As the students progressed through the semester and the topics were higher in complexity, the patient developed complications that dovetailed with the classroom lecture. Students tell me that they preferred this active learning approach over the traditional passive classroom of having students just listening to me present. I have begun to record my lectures so students can review essential content anytime and especially before the next exam.

—Susan Growe, DNP, MSN/Ed, RN, COI
Nursing Faculty
Nevada State College
Henderson, Nevada

When I teach public/community health, my students love case studies and projects. My students have valued and enjoyed the following scenario:

I give them a disaster scenario of what to do with an anthrax exposure when delivered by a crop duster airplane. I have students work in groups to consider the following public health priorities:

- How to deliver ciprofloxacin to one million people within 72 hours
- Where they would deliver the medications
- How they will manage anxious crowds
- Who can pick up the medications
- What to do if someone asks for medication for their pet
- What if there are language barriers or allergic response to ciprofloxacin?
- How many and what health care professionals are needed?
- How to manage crowd control
- Where is the best location to set up

—Bonnie Copland, MSN, PHN
Adjunct Clinical Faculty
Azusa Pacific University
San Diego, California

I utilize numerous drawings in the classroom that engage kinesthetic and visual learners. In my maternal child course I have students draw either a normal newborn, a SGA newborn, a LGA newborn, or post-date newborn. But FIRST, they do the following to contextualize this important content and strengthen student learning:

- I have a list of features and assessment findings that are printed out on individual slips of paper that represent each of these infants
- Each student gets one of the slips.
- The students who get the slip that identifies the "type" of patient is the designated team leader.
- The rest of the students find their appropriate team leader. For example, if the assessment finding was that of a post-date infant, then they find the post-date team leader.
- I color-code the slips of paper to ensure everyone eventually makes it to the correct group.
- Each group has to draw the baby and include each specific finding in the drawing.
- They need to identify nursing diagnosis/priority, assessments, and cares that relates to the specific features of their identified newborn.
- Last, they explain their picture to their peers in front of the class.

—Laureen Turner, EdDc, MSN, RN, CNE
Assistant Professor
University of San Francisco
San Francisco, California

I have successfully used "Poll Everywhere," which is a website (polleverywhere.com) that allows the instructor to pose questions to students, either prior to class or during class that develops critical thinking and assesses student learning. Students can use their cell phones to answer questions provided and the website gathers the data for instructor review.

—Beverly Craig, RNC, MSN
Nursing Instructor
West Coast University
Irvine, California

To contextualize dehydration/fluids & electrolyte content I created the following scenario:

You received the following change of shift report. Craig Ferguson is an 87-year-old male who was admitted to the med/surg floor for dehydration last night. Past medical history includes hypertension and prostate can-

cer. His most recent vital signs were:

- T 99.8 F (37.7 C)
- P: 104
- BP:104/62
- RR: 24
- O2 sat: 96% room air

Mr. Ferguson lives alone and ambulates with a walker very slowly. He has not been out of bed since admission last night. He has dizziness and generalized weakness whenever he stands up. I then ask the following questions that I want students to answer:

- What do you want to ask the nurse during report to clarify Mr. Ferguson's fluid status (What else do you want to know?)
- List four subjective or objective assessment data that you will gather to assess Mr. Ferguson's fluid status to determine the status of his primary problem and current nursing priority.

—Jeannine Olson, RN, MSN
Nursing Faculty
California State University
Chico, California

In my classroom, I make it a priority to engage as many of the students senses as possible. I use numerous visuals, including models, which they can touch and ask questions that require students to reflect on what they have learned. I require pre-class reading assignments and utilize in-class quizzes derived from the reading. I do a test review at the end of the class by giving each student a white board and a dry erase marker. The students are paired and stand back to back. I ask a question and each student has ten seconds to write an answer or draw a frowning face. Then they show their partner their answers. Then I share the correct answer. I have found that this active learning strategy cements and connects student learning. When I use case studies, I divide my class into small groups. Each group presents its findings to the rest of the class.

—Gwen Reed MS, BS, RN, Paramedic, CEN
Nursing Instructor
Gillette College,
Gillette, Wyoming

We often hear the question, "Will this be on the test?" From my teaching experience, the key to facilitating more meaningful engagement with the content is to make it relevant. Begin class or clinical post-conference with a case study or an actual patient situation seen during a recent clinical experience. Then ask the students to explore concepts involved with the problems the patient experienced and nursing considerations that would help the students better understand the situation.

The development of concept maps, which enable students to visualize connections between the various mapped components also helps. Students are better able to recognize vital cues, make connections, and discover meanings. This technique, and applying theory to real patient situations enables students to better grasp the content and understand its relevance in clinical practice.

Another means to help make the content relevant is to give a pretest of the material at the beginning of class or conduct informal polling of students' current understanding of the concepts. The class ends with a brief, non-graded posttest that emphasizes the most salient points of the lecture content. Students learn from their errors made on both the pretest and posttest as much as they do from items marked correctly.

—Sandra O'Donnell, RN, MSN, CNE
Guest Lecturer
University of North Carolina at
Wilmington School of Nursing
Wilmington, North Carolina

I use the "divide and conquer" method to get students to participate and engage to think like a nurse in my classroom. First, I talk about creating a culture where everyone is here to learn and it is okay to not have the right answer. In order to solve a problem, it is the process, persistence, and work ethic that make it possible. I then ask Socratic questions to get students to think and do the problem solving for the nursing situations presented. I like to preplan my questions for the classroom environment and relate them to a patient care scenario. I can easily minimize content and teach primarily using case studies.

The second step is to direct each question to a small group of students. I can select a different row of students in the classroom each time a new question is posed. This process allows students to work together and to take their turn to "think like a nurse." The thinking aloud process mimics the conversations nurses have

with health care providers, patients, and families in the clinical environment.

It is liberating to eliminate content and put the students in action to learn through these questions. I took my content lecture and posted voice-over PowerPoints for the students to listen to prior to class. This allows class time for active learning, which does take time. Guiding student preparation prior to class is a major shift in faculty thinking, but well worth the effort. I have observed that students are more active and engaged with their learning and are more developed in their ability to "think like a nurse" with this constructive learning process. They own the knowledge, not the teacher.

—Barbara Hill, RN, MSN, CNE, CMSRN
Associate Professor
The Community College of Baltimore County
Baltimore, Maryland

I tie classroom theory, nursing skills lab, and the clinical experience together as much as possible. Our team maps out what the classroom theory instructor is going to teach that week, then we see if we can replicate/reinforce that in nursing lab and clinical assignments as much as possible. For example, if classroom theory content is going to cover hemodynamics and blood pressure, we discuss/demonstrate taking orthostatic blood pressures and practice that skill in nursing lab. At the clinical site, the students are expected to look at the patient's medical diagnosis, history, medications, and blood pressure history, and decide if they are at risk or are currently experiencing any problems with hemodynamics and intervene accordingly. This provides an opportunity to compare notes with the student, and discuss possible causes by applying classroom theory to the clinical context. This has been an effective strategy to integrate classroom theory with clinical realities.

—Susan A. Erlewine, MSN, RN-BC, HTCP, CHPN
Assistant Professor
Hocking College, Nelsonville, Ohio

I try to retain student engagement by mixing up formats for delivery. I may spend 20 to 30 minutes on lecture and conclude with a role play, game, or clinical scenario based on the material I just presented. I have also passed out 3" x 5" cards and stopped during lecture to ask the class to write down a question on the material that I just taught, which might be used as an item on the upcoming exam. Shifting formats requires them to re-engage, while reinforcing the lecture content.

—Becky Craig, RNC, MN, EdS, PhD
Nursing Instructor, Nursing Tutorial Lab
Perimeter College
Clarkston, Georgia

When teaching the Autonomic Nervous System, I teach students to remember the following: When in a lonely subway station late at night and someone is approaching you who looks strange and you sense that this person is a dangerous threat, you quickly run up two large flights of stairs to get to the street where there is a police officer. In order to make this physiologic response possible, what has to happen? Eyes dilate, heart rate increases, and the other physiologic effects of the sympathetic nervous system and how it impacts the rest of the body are present.

For the Parasympathetic Nervous System, I use the following scenario: You are in a quiet Italian restaurant, bright candle on the table, the aroma of garlic bread, and Andrea Bocelli music in the background. What is happening now to the body? Heart rate decreases, increase in saliva, peristalsis, etc. Students learn and love from this comparison because it is something that they can readily relate to.

—Frances Iacobellis, MS, RN
Assistant Professor
Long Island University
Brooklyn, New York

My goal is to create a nonthreatening and fun atmosphere to encourage learning. Humor is essential. On the more serious side, I stress that students will be on their own when taking the NCLEX, so it is paramount that they learn the concepts on their own. I also try to use everyday encounters to reflect more complicated concepts covered in our material.

• *Expect success.* Treat students as adults, and not students. When students ask me a question, I often respond back with a question. I may ask the student a question or two and then ask the remaining students in class to contribute. Allow for silence. Give them time to formulate a response. Assist students to reach their own conclusions with critical thinking through simple related questions that build on each other to

reach higher-level thinking and eventually, understanding.

• *Pick the student's brain.* Probe for the obvious by asking "Why?" or "How?" or "And then what happens?" I constantly ask students "Why" questions because I want to know if the students understand why something happens not just that it happens. "Why do we do this? What does it lead to? Why should we do this? What if we don't? What are the consequences? Are they serious? Will it result in negative consequences?" I find that students feel empowered when they are able to put simple concepts together.

—Lila Moersch, MSN, CNL
Nursing Faculty
Chamberlain College
St. Louis, Missouri

When HIPAA is first presented to students in the Fundamentals of Nursing course, students receive an index card and an envelope. They are asked to write a very private secret/notation on the index card about themselves, sign it, and then seal it in the envelope. The students are given reassurance that their secret will remain safe. (Also have students put some notation on the envelope so they know which envelop is their own.) Students are asked to pass their envelope to another student. They are not to open this envelop. Students are then asked, "How do you feel now that someone has some very private information about you?" Students share multiple answers such as embarrassed, worried, violated, nervous, etc. The students are then asked, "How do you think your patient feels when they tell you, the nurse, their most private information about themselves?" The whole room gets dead quiet. Someone always says, "I never thought of it like that." Then the students are asked, "Why do patients tell the nurse such private personal information?" Other students respond, "Because they trust us." This exercise is very powerful and students readily grasp the true meaning of confidentiality.

—Janice Eilerman, MSN, RN
Assistant Professor
Rhodes State College
Lima, Ohio

If classroom content is not relevant and will not be on

the test, I do not include this content in my PowerPoint or study guide. When I do a study session, nursing lab, or PowerPoint presentation I emphasize need to know content and then I challenge them to apply it to practice.
—Karen Flatt, RN, BSN, MSN
Practical Nursing Faculty
Northeast Technology Center
Claremore, Oklahoma

Reflect

What "pearls" will you incorporate into the classroom setting to strengthen the learning of students?

19

How to Transform Your Test Questions

Patricia Pence, EdD, MSN, RN

Testing and evaluation in nursing education is influenced by two major goals: to prepare students to be safe and effective nurses in clinical practice and to prepare nurse graduates to meet the minimum passing standard on their ultimate test, the National Council Licensure Examination (NCLEX). Nursing course exams and the NCLEX are both high-stakes tests that affect students' progression to graduation and entry into nursing practice (McDonald, 2014).

If you are a new nurse educator, you may feel overwhelmed about writing test questions. Sifting through the literature on test-item writing can be an even more daunting task. This chapter provides PRACTICAL strategies on what you NEED to know to begin transforming test questions for your nursing course exams. Nurse educators often enter academia with experience in clinical practice, but little knowledge about test development (Cooley & DeGagne, 2016). Your clinical experience and knowledge provides a strong foundation for designing your exams. Emphasize clinical reasoning and critical thinking in your test questions will make the test more relevant and meaningful for your students.

Equation for Successful Test Writing

To strengthen your ability to write test questions, the following equation will guide you:

Course content + objectives + NCLEX client needs + Bloom's Taxonomy of cognitive levels + Nursing Process = Improved quality of your test questions!

Practical Strategies to Transform Test Questions

Course Content and Objectives

Course content and objectives established in your course outline or syllabus guides your teaching, learning, and assessments (McDonald, 2014). Your course exams assess your nursing students' ability to APPLY the course content to the care of a patient in a clinical setting. Test questions should assess the essential nurse thinking skills and the student's ability to make a decision that will solve a clinical puzzle (Benner, et al., 2010). The course content and objectives are the primary source for building test questions that test your students' learning and ability to accomplish the objectives in the course (McDonald, 2014).

My teaching strategies and test questions are concentrated on the main course content and on what is necessary for safe nursing practice. Avoid testing on minor content (Oermann & Gaberson, 2014). The NCLEX does not expect nurse graduates to know or be able to test on minor details of nursing content (McDonald, 2014). Emphasize content that is clinically significant and NEED to know content. Research from the NCLEX practice analysis and detailed test plan can help you focus your teaching and learning on what is most relevant for entry-level real-world practice.

NCLEX Client Needs

The NCSBN outlines a "blueprint" for the NCLEX. A detailed list of activities for each client needs category and subcategory is in the test plan. The table below lists the client needs and subcategories with the percentages of the test items from each category or subcategory included in the test blueprint. See the detailed list of activities related to nursing practice of the client needs in the NCLEX Nurse Educator Version of the test plan at www.ncsbn.org. Integrated in the test items are the concepts of nursing process, caring, communication, documentation, teaching, learning, culture, and spirituality.

The NCLEX Nurse Educator Version of the test plan is a guide for nurse educators to use in writing NCLEX-style test questions. The categories in the NCLEX test plan provide an underlying framework to write test questions related to nursing course objectives and content.

I review my exams for test questions missing in any of the client needs categories, such as psychosocial integrity. For example, to address the psychosocial integrity category, a test question might be written on a clinical situation in which a nurse is assisting a patient coping with a new medical diagnosis.

Bloom's Taxonomy

The NCSBN integrates Bloom's Taxonomy of cognitive levels in test items written for the NCLEX examination. The 2001 revised version of Bloom's Taxonomy (Krathwohl, 2002) includes these cognitive levels with remembering at the lowest and creating at the highest cognitive level:

- Creating (highest level)
- Evaluating
- Analyzing
- Applying
- Understanding
- Remembering (lowest level)

Nursing is a profession that applies the knowledge, skills, and abilities to problem solve and critically think in nursing practice (McDonald, 2014). Therefore, the majority of test questions need to be written at an applying or higher cognitive level that requires students to APPLY learning to the care of a patient in a clinical situation (McDonald, 2014).

Coding your test questions by Bloom's cognitive level can reveal if this is a weakness in your exams. After reviewing the cognitive level of my test questions, I be-

NCLEX-RN client needs categories	Percentages
Safe and effective care environment	
Management of care	17–23%
Safety and infection control	9–15%
Health promotion and maintenance	6–12%
Psychosocial integrity	6–12%
Physiological integrity	
Basic care and comfort	6–12%
Pharmacological and parenteral therapies	12–18%
Reduction of risk potential	9–15%
Physiological adaptation	11–17%

(Source: NCLEX-RN Examination Detailed Test Plan retrieved at ncsbn.org website)

came aware of the need to increase the difficulty level of test questions and the questions that needed to be revised or removed. For example, test questions at the lower cognitive level of remembering were removed from my first-year fundamentals and medical-surgical nursing course. As a result, the majority of my test questions are at the applying or higher cognitive level. There are still some test questions at the understanding level, but these are kept to a minimum.

Nursing Process

Nursing process is one of the integrated concepts used in developing the NCLEX test plan and in writing test items. The nursing process *"is the fundamental blueprint for how to care for patients"* (Potter, Stockert, Griffin, & Hall, 2017, p. 209). The five steps in the nursing process—assessment, diagnosis, planning, implementation, and evaluation—require nurses to use critical thinking, clinical reasoning, and clinical judgment in nursing practice (Potter, et al., 2017).

Test items on the NCLEX test plan are written in the format of a nurse caring for a patient while performing one of the steps of nursing process. For example, test questions involve the nurse performing an assessment, planning care, implementing a nursing action, or evaluating nursing care provided for a patient. By coding my test questions using nursing process, I was able to recognize the need to add additional questions asking students to evaluate nursing care. Using the nursing process to guide test question development improves the quality of your exams, promotes test questions written at a higher cognitive level, and ensures your test questions address a nursing concern (McDonald, 2014).

Writing Test Questions

There are three parts to test questions:
1. Stem (question)
2. Distractors (incorrect answers)
3. Key (correct answer).

The terms *client, health care provider, and prescription* are used in NCLEX test items (NCSBN, 2016). Nursing test questions have traditionally used the terms *patient, physician or doctor, and orders.* Revising test questions to reflect current terminology of the NCLEX may help students adjust to these terms

before they take the NCLEX. Let's examine a test question I wrote using NCLEX terminology.

A nurse is caring for a client in the medical-surgical unit who was admitted with a pleural effusion. The nurse is assisting the health care provider who is performing a thoracentesis at the bedside. Which of these findings of the client is of **most** concern for the nurse? **(Stem)**
1. Reports a stinging sensation as the anesthetic is injected. **(Distractor)**
2. States, "I am having a pressure-like pain." **(Distractor)**
3. Begins to cough and deep breathe during the procedure. **(Key)**
4. Sits up leaning forward with arms on the bedside table. **(Distractor)**

The stem consists of two or more sentences that describe:
1. *A nurse caring for a client in a clinical setting.*
2. *A clinical problem that asks what the nurse would do.*
3. *Sufficient information within the stem so students are able to understand the purpose of the test question.*

The stem can be written as a question or an incomplete statement or sentence (Billings & Halstead, 2016; McDonald, 2014). Write stems as a question, since students will take additional test time rephrasing an incomplete statement as a question (McDonald, 2014). I typically allot 90 seconds per test question to determine how long students will have to take the exam. Sample test items listed in the NCLEX test plan are all written in a question format (NCSBN, 2016).

In the above question, the word most is highlighted in **bold.** Sample test items in the NCLEX test plan distinguish the word most in bold (NCSBN, 2016). McDonald (2014) cautions against highlighting words in the stem because students will overlook the emphasis placed on the highlighted words.

Common Errors in Writing Stems

Example stem: The client is undergoing a thoracentesis at the bedside.This is an example of an incomplete statement. However, there is not sufficient information in this stem for a student to understand the purpose of the test question. This stem would be very confusing for the student. There is no mention of the nurse, clinical setting, or what the nurse should do.

Example stem: A nurse is caring for a 35-year-old male client in the medical-surgical unit who was admitted with a pleural effusion. The client has a history of hypertension, bronchitis, smoking two packs per day, and drinking a beer every afternoon. The client's wife is in the waiting room. The nurse is assisting the health care provider who is performing a thoracentesis at the bedside. Which of these findings of the client is of most concern for the nurse?

Although the stem includes a nurse, a clinical setting, and asks what the nurse should do, there is too much information that will confuse the student and take longer to read. There is unnecessary information in this stem, such as the client's age, gender, past medical history, and wife. Avoid unnecessary information in the stem (Billings & Halstead, 2016; Oermann & Gaberson, 2014). Limit the information in your stem to what is NEEDED for the student to determine an answer. Be clear and concise when writing stems (McDonald, 2014).

Example stem: A nurse is caring for a client in the medical-surgical unit who was admitted with a pleural effusion. The nurse is assisting the health care provider who is performing a thoracentesis. The nurse will position the client to sit upright at the bedside. Which of these findings of the client is of most concern for the nurse?

Teaching is included in the stem (the nurse knows), which would lead a student to rule out the distractor: Sits up leaning forward with arms on the bedside table. Avoid teaching within the stem (McDonald, 2014).

Common Errors
The key is the correct or best answer. The key should be the same length as the distractors. Some test-taking strategies suggest students rule out other options by selecting the longest option as the correct answer.
1. Reports a stinging sensation.
2. States, "I have a pressure-like pain."
3. As the needle is inserted the client begins to cough and deep breathe. **(Key)**
4. Leans forward on the bedside table.

The key stands out as different because it is the longest option and attracts the student's attention (McDonald, 2014). All options should be the same length. Notice the key and distractors are numbered, not listed alphabetically. Numbering all options aligns with the format used in the sample items in the NCLEX test plan (NCSBN, 2016).

The **distractors** are the options that are not the correct answer. All distractors must be reasonable options, so that students will consider all the options (Billings & Halstead, 2016). Avoid writing distractors that are opposite options, such as increase or decrease, high or low, hypo or hyper (McDonald, 2014). Avoid using negative words in options, such as *not* or *never* (McDonald, 2014).

A nurse is caring for a client in the medical-surgical unit who was admitted with a pleural effusion. The nurse is assisting the health care provider, who is performing a thoracentesis at the bedside. Which of these findings of the client is of **most** concern for the nurse?
1. Shallow breaths noted during the procedure.
2. Reports he is not feeling any pain.
3. Deep breathing noted during the procedure. **(Key)**
4. Sits up leaning forward with arms on the bedside table.

Options 1 and 3 are opposite (shallow or deep breaths noted), which will attract the students to choose between these options and ignore options 2 and 4. Option 2 is a negative option using the term *not*, which would be ruled out by the students (McDonald, 2014).

The multiple-multiple-response question includes more than the four options typical in a multiple-choice question. Although this type of test question format has been used in nursing exams in the past, it should no longer be used. Avoid using "all of the above" or "none of the above" in the options (Billings & Halstead, 2016). See the example below. The multiple options would be confusing for students (McDonald, 2014).

A nurse is caring for a client in the medical-surgical unit who was admitted with a pleural effusion. The nurse is assisting the health care provider who is performing a thoracentesis at the bedside. Which of these findings of the client is a concern for the nurse?
1. Reports a stinging sensation as the anesthetic is injected.
2. States, "I am having a pressure-like pain."
3. Begins to cough and deep breathe. **(Key)**
4. Leans forward with arms on the bedside table.
a. 1, 2, 4

b. 1, 3, 4

c. 4 only

d. All of the above

Test Question Topics

Your clinical practice and experience in teaching nursing students is a place to begin thinking of the most common medical conditions treated, nursing tasks performed, or errors that you have observed in real-world practice. The textbooks I use for my nursing courses provide content for test question topics and key points for essential nurse thinking skills. Topics that can be developed into test questions include:

- Steps to perform procedures and rationales
- Clinical decision points
- Unexpected outcomes and related interventions
- Delegation considerations
- Nursing safety priority action or drug alerts
- Best practice charts
- Considerations for older adults
- Gender health and cultural considerations
- Health teaching
- Key features of a disease or drug therapy (Ignatavicius & Workman, 2016; Potter et al, 2017)

Sample Test Questions

My sample test questions include a rationale, textbook reference, objective, NCLEX client needs category/subcategory, Bloom's cognitive level, and the step in the nursing process. They are written as examples that apply content in my fundamentals and medical-surgical nursing courses. Students are able to view these categories as their "test review" after submitting their exam. I find that including these categories lessens the chance that my test questions are on trivial matter, outdated material, a lower cognitive level, or that my exams do not address the course objectives, NCLEX client needs categories, or steps in the nursing process.

Sample Question

A nurse is caring for a client in the medical-surgical unit who was admitted with a pleural effusion. The nurse is assisting the health care provider who is performing a thoracentesis at the bedside. Which of these findings of the client is of most concern for the nurse?

1. Reports, "I feel a stinging sensation."

2. States, "I am having a pressure-like pain."

3. Begins to cough and deep breathe. **(Key)**

4. Leans forward with arms on the bedside table.

- ***Rationale:*** The nurse should stress the importance of not moving, coughing, or deep breathing during the procedure to avoid puncture of the pleura or lung. The client may expect a stinging sensation from the local anesthetic and a feeling of pressure when the needle is pushed through the posterior chest. A thoracentesis is often performed at the bedside with the client sitting on the side of the bed, leaning forward, with arms resting on the bedside table.

- ***Textbook reference:*** Ignatavicius, D. D. & Workman, M.L. (2016). Medical-Surgical Nursing: Patient-Centered Collaborative Care, p. 511.

- ***Course objective:*** Demonstrate nursing judgment using the nursing process framework in order to address basic concepts of health conditions related to select body systems.

- ***NCLEX client needs:*** Physiological integrity/physiological adaptation

- ***Bloom's cognitive level:*** Applying

- ***Nursing process:*** Assessment

This sample test question requires students to APPLY learning about pleural effusion and the nursing responsibilities to prepare a client for the procedure and assist a health care provider during a thoracentesis. Assisting with an invasive procedure, such as a thoracentesis, is listed as the first related activity statement under Physiological Adaptation; a subcategory of Physiological Integrity in the NCLEX-RN educator version of the test plan (NCSBN, 2016). This sample question reflects the knowledge expected of an entry-level nurse who is assisting a health care provider during a thoracentesis.

Sample Question

A nurse is caring for a client in the medical-surgical unit who was diagnosed with a pulmonary embolism. The client states, "I do not think I can give myself a shot," when the nurse begins teaching self-administration of enoxaparin. Which of these statements is the best response by the nurse?

1. "Don't worry, the nurses can give your injections

while you are here."

2. "You will only need to be on the injections until the warfarin is effective."

3. "Why do you feel that you will not be able to give yourself the injections?"

4. "Tell me what concerns you about giving yourself the injections." **(Key)**

- *Rationale:* Clients with a pulmonary embolism may be fearful about self-administering anticoagulant injections. The best response is to address the client's concern about self-administering the injections. Telling the client that the nurses will give the injections does not address the client's concerns or promote self-care. Telling the client that the injections are only a temporary part of the plan of care does not address the client's concerns. Asking the client "why" is nontherapeutic and will block further communication.
- *Textbook reference:* Ignatavicius, D. D. & Workman, M.L. (2016). *Medical-Surgical Nursing: Patient-Centered Collaborative Care,* pp. 607–10.
- *Course objective:* Use therapeutic communication techniques to establish/maintain a nurse/client relationship in various community settings.
- *NCLEX client needs:* Psychosocial integrity/Physiological integrity
- *Bloom's cognitive level:* Applying
- *Nursing process:* Implementation

This sample question requires students to APPLY learning about pulmonary embolism and therapeutic communication while teaching a client about self-administration of anticoagulant injections. Listed under Psychosocial Integrity client needs is Therapeutic Communication in the NCLEX-RN educator version of the test plan (NCSBN, 2016). The nurse is expected to use therapeutic communication techniques to provide client support and encourage the client to verbalize feelings.

The subcategory of Pharmacological and Parenteral Therapies is in the Physiological Integrity category. In this subcategory, listed under Medication Administration, is the activity statement: Educate the client on medication self-administration procedures. The sample test question on a medication in the NCLEX test plan includes the generic name of the medication. This sample question reflects the knowledge expected of an entry-level nurse who is providing teaching for a client who has a pulmonary embolism and uses the generic name of the medication.

Sample Question

A nurse is caring for a client on a medical-surgical unit who requires a sterile dressing change. Which of the following techniques performed by the nurse best demonstrates maintaining sterile technique?

1. Allows fingers of sterile gloved hand to touch exposed hand and wrist.
2. Touches the inside surface of the first glove while pulling it onto the hand. (Key)
3. Holds the sterile gloved hands below the level of the waist after gloving.
4. Touches the edge of the sterile field with a sterile gloved hand.

- *Rationale:* Touching the inside surface of the first glove while pulling it onto the hand is the correct technique when applying sterile gloves. This prevents contamination of the outside of the glove, which must remain sterile. If sterile gloved hands fall below the waist, touch the edge of the sterile field, or touch exposed hand or wrist, they are considered to be unsterile.
- *Textbook reference:* Potter, P. A., Perry, A. G., Stockert, P. A., & Hall, A. M. (2017). *Fundamentals of Nursing* (9th ed.), pp. 481–82.
- *Course objective:* Quality and Safety: Recognize the importance of continuous quality and safety initiatives to improve client care and outcomes: Demonstrate 100% aseptic technique in applying sterile gloves.
- *NCLEX client needs:* Safe and effective care environment/Safety and infection control
- *Bloom's cognitive level:* Applying
- *Nursing process:* Implementation

This sample test question requires students to APPLY learning about asepsis while performing a sterile dressing change. This test question addresses the client needs category of Safe and Effective Care Environment and subcategory of Safety and Infection Control. Apply principles of infection control, such as sterile technique, is a related activity statement under the Safety and Infection Control subcategory (NCSBN, 2016). This sample test question reflects the knowledge expected of an entry-level nurse who is performing a procedure requiring sterile technique.

Alternate Test Item Formats

The NCLEX began introducing alternate test items in 2003. Alternate test items use technology, such as audio files, charts, tables, graphics, or videos, to test a student's higher cognitive levels or critical thinking (McDonald, 2014; NCSBN, 2016). Example of alternate test item formats may include multiple response, fill-in-the-blank calculations, ordered response, and hot spots (NCSBN, 2016).

For example, a test question in which audio files of abnormal breath sounds are embedded might ask students to determine how the nurse should respond after listening to the breath sound. A hot spot test question that shows a diagram of the chest and heart might ask students to identify the correct area for auscultating an apical pulse. An ordered response or "drag and drop" item might ask students to place in order the steps to draw up insulin from a vial, perform a catheterization, administer a heparin injection, or other procedure.

Based on prior experiences, I learned to anticipate technical difficulties when embedding technology in test questions. Test questions that involve the use of technology should be tested prior to administering your exam to students. Doing a pretest run of your exam can avoid any technical difficulties during the exam, which can lead to frustration and test anxiety among your students. Enlist support from technology staff in preparing test questions using pictures, audio or video files, charts, tables, or graphics, so that they are properly embedded in your test question.

Audio files, if played without using ear buds, can be disruptive during an exam. If audio files are used in a test question, students should be required to bring their own ear buds. A statement included in our course outline indicates the requirement for students to bring their own ear buds: There will be audio files on most tests. You will need to bring ear buds to each exam.

No more than three types of test item formats should be written in each exam (Oermann & Gaberson, 2014). The more complex the test question, the more time students

will need to answer the question. Provide specific instructions for each alternative format question, such as use of ear buds, referring to a table, picture, or graphic, before answering the test question.

Sample alternative test question: Medication calculation, Fill-in-the blank

A nurse is caring for a client in a pediatric unit who has a prescription for acetaminophen 15 mg/kg/dose PO every 4 hours as needed. The client weighs 48 lbs. (21.8 kg). Medication is available in 160 mg in 5 mL of oral suspension solution. How many mL should the nurse administer to the client with each dose?

Record your answer to the nearest tenth decimal point.

10.2 mL **(Key)**

- *Rationale:* Most pediatric medications are ordered in mg/kg. Identify the unit of measure needed to administer the medication. In this question the unit of measure is mL. Calculate the mg per kg for each dose. Estimate the answer. The medication order is about 2 times the unit dose in the oral suspension solution. Complete the calculation.

  15 mg/21.8 kg = 327 mg. 160 mg/5mL x 327 mg/X. X = 10.2mL.

- *Textbook reference:* Potter, P. A., Perry, A. G., Stockert, P. A., & Hall, A. M. (2017). *Fundamentals of Nursing,* p. 620.

- *Course objective:* Quality and Safety: Recognize the importance of continuous quality and safety initiatives to improve client care and outcomes: Demonstrate the correct steps in administering drugs.

- *NCLEX client needs:* Physiological integrity/Pharmacological and Parenteral Therapies

- *Bloom's cognitive level:* Applying

- *Nursing process:* Implementation

This sample test question requires students to APPLY learning about medication calculations. This question addresses the client needs category of Physiological Integrity and subcategory of Pharmacological and Parenteral Therapies. Listed in the related activity statements is the third activity: perform calculations for medication administration.

Provide clear directions for each alternative format question, such as how to indicate the answer for a fill-in-the blank medication calculation.

How to Review Exams with Students

A rationale written for the correct answer of each test question provides immediate feedback for my nursing students as they review their test results. Before I began adding rationales, test reviews were done in class after the exam. When students began to plan how to challenge my test questions, test reviews became chaotic and were not a productive use of class time. Including rationales has proven to be a useful tool to help students review the test questions and identify areas for remediation.

Our nursing policy states that students must provide three published sources to challenge the test question within one week of the exam. Requiring students to write a rationale to explain why they believe the test item is incorrect, and to cite three published resources to validate their reason for challenging the question has been recommended (Morrison, 2010). Students rarely challenge my test questions. Since I am revising my exams and piloting new test questions each year, students sometimes find errors or have a valid reason to challenge a question. Questions that are challenged are either deleted from the test bank or revised for future exams. Our course outlines also include statements about the requirements for testing and challenging test questions.

Sample Statements in my Course Outline for Test Review:

Test review will be available after submitting the exam and reviewing individual test results. Note taking or recording is not allowed during the test review. Students may make an appointment with the lecture instructor to individually review their test results.

If challenging test questions, the student must present written support from three professional sources. This must be given to the instructor for review within one week following the exam.

McDonald (2014) outlined advantages to writing a rationale and suggested a format for writing the rationale:

Advantages to writing a rationale:
• Improves the validity of your test
• Increases the quality of the test question
• Ensures correctness of the key or correct answer
• Serves as a resource for students to review the test

Format for writing a rationale:
• Include a textbook reference
• Explain why the correct answer is correct
• Explain why each of the distractors is incorrect

Including a textbook reference with each question provides support for the correct or best answer and deters students from challenging the other options in the test question.

Test Blueprinting

Oermann and Gaberson (2014) recommend a test blueprint or test plan to guide writing test questions. The test blueprint is a grid that includes the course content and objectives and the number or percentage of items in these categories (McDonald, 2014). Once the blueprint is developed, test item writing begins.

Here are examples of basic test blueprints that outline the number of questions for each unit exam and total points, and how each test item is categorized by course objectives for each unit exam. Blueprinting tests might seem to be time consuming and overwhelming when you have many other responsibilities. These examples can get you started with planning your course and test questions for your exams or examining your existing exams for revision if you have never blueprinted your course exams.

In this example for my medical-surgical course are six exams. There are five unit exams consisting of 60 questions. The final exam consists of 60 questions for the last unit and 15 questions from the previous units. This is a basic test plan. Some nurse educators may add columns for the number of lecture hours and percentage of lecture hours.

This second example would be used to list the questions written to meet the course objectives for each unit in my medical-surgical course. Nursing course exams test the students' mastery of the course content and objectives (McDonald, 2014).

Test blueprint	Questions
NUR 1211	
Unit 1 exam	60
Unit 2 exam	60
Unit 3 exam	60
Unit 4 exam	60
Unit 5 exam	60
Final exam	75
Total	375

Table 1

Test blueprint	Objective #1	Objective #2	Objective #3	Objective #4	Objective #5	Objective #6
Unit 1 exam						
Unit 2 exam						
Unit 3 exam						
Unit 4 exam						
Unit 5 exam						
Final exam						

Table 2

Each exam may not address all six course objectives for my course. This blueprint will identify whether all the objectives are addressed at some point in my course, or if an objective is NOT addressed at all.

Cross-referencing your exams

As discussed earlier, integrating the NCLEX client needs categories, Bloom's cognitive levels, and the nursing process in your course and test questions will help prepare students for the NCLEX and nursing practice. You can cross-reference your exams to identify the questions addressing the client needs, cognitive levels, and nursing process (McDonald, 2014).

The tables listed below are examples of cross-referencing by NCLEX client needs, nursing process, and Bloom's cognitive levels for my medical-surgical course.

You might choose to cross-reference by each unit when planning an individual exam. In the Bloom's cognitive level cross-reference worksheet are four cognitive levels that would typically be integrated in multiple-choice and alternate test questions.

McDonald (2014) recommends that all test questions should be written at the applying and analyzing cognitive levels. Students are learning critical thinking, clinical reasoning, and clinical judgment skills from the onset in your program. Test questions at the applying and analyzing level for a *fundamentals* nursing course are written for fundamentals nursing content. Likewise, by the time students are in the second year or advanced level of a nursing program, the test questions at the applying and analyzing level are written for the specific course content at that level in the nursing program.

NCLEX cross-reference worksheet Course NUR 1211				
Exams	Safe Effective Care	Health Promotion Maintenance	Psychosocial Integrity	Physiological Integrity
Unit 1				
Unit 2				
Unit 3				
Unit 4				
Unit 5				
Final				
Total				

Nursing process cross-reference worksheet Course NUR 1211					
Exams	Assessment	Diagnosis	Planning	Implementation	Evaluation
Unit 1					
Unit 2					
Unit 3					
Unit 4					
Unit 5					
Final					
Total					

Bloom's cognitive level cross-reference worksheet Course NUR 1211				
Exams	Remembering	Understanding	Applying	Analyzing
Unit 1				
Unit 2				
Unit 3				
Unit 4				
Unit 5				
Final				
Total				

This last table identified the number of test questions that were categorized at the remembering and understanding level in my exams for my first-year medical-surgical nursing course. Students have voiced concerns that first-year exams did not prepare them for the level of complex test questions in their second-year nursing course exams. This first-year medical-surgical nursing course, which is taught in the spring semester, is the "gateway" course that leads into the fall semester second-year nursing courses. By reviewing the cognitive level of my test questions, I realized the need to replace lower cognitive level test questions with higher cognitive level test questions.

Textbook Test Banks

Each nursing textbook publisher provides nurse educators with an online test bank. Some of the test banks list the same categories that I use with my test questions. Reviewing the test bank and using them as a "guide" will help you relate the course content and objectives to writing your own test questions. Use the test banks for ideas and change, or adapt them.

As a new nurse educator, I relied heavily on textbook test banks. But as I carefully reviewed the test banks, some of the test questions were written at the remembering or understanding level that emphasized recall and memorization of CONTENT, not the higher-level thinking that requires APPLICATION to pass the NCLEX. Textbook test banks may not have statistical testing or pilot testing with students (McDonald, 2014). Test bank questions provide a place to start and it was easier to revise a test bank question than create a new one from scratch.

Do not totally rely on test bank questions because there is a possibility that the test banks have been posted online for students or anyone else to purchase, without the publisher's authority. It is unfortunate that test bank "piracy" discredits test bank security. Better yet, use the principles from this chapter to create test questions that are unique to you and reflect what needs to be assessed from the content that you teach, then guard them with your life!

Preparing Students for the NCLEX

To keep up-to-date with testing on current nursing practice, the National Council of State Boards of Nursing (NCSBN) organization conducts a practice survey every three years on new nurse graduates' perspective about the frequency and importance of activities expected by their employers during the initial three months as they enter nursing practice (Wendt, 2010). The results of this practice survey are published in "Practice Analysis Report" and "NCLEX Test Plan, Nurse Educator Version" by the NCSBN that is available to view and download on the www.ncsbn.org website (National Council of State Boards of Nursing [NCSBN], 2016).

The client care activities in the NCLEX Test Plan can support and guide your curriculum and nursing

course exams. Although a common argument in academia is "not to teach to the test," using the client needs activities in the NCLEX test plan does not mean that you are "teaching to the test" (McDonald, 2014; Oermann & Gaberson, 2014). The NCSBN research reflects current expectations required of a graduate nurse entering clinical practice. Therefore, it is essential for nurse educators to review the current client care activities listed in the practice analysis and the educator's version of the detailed test plan to ensure that these activities are used to update course content. For example, intraoperative nursing care was recently deleted from the NCLEX Test Plan; subsequently, this topic was removed from our fundamentals course content.

The NCLEX

According to the NCSBN, "the NCLEX assesses the knowledge, skills, and abilities that are essential for the entry-level nurse to use in order to meet the needs of clients requiring the promotion, maintenance or restoration of health" (NCSBN, 2016). The majority of test items are written at Bloom's APPLYING or higher cognitive level. McDonald (2014) recommends all nursing test questions should be written at the applying and higher cognitive level, to best mirror the cognitive level of the NCLEX.

The same categories used to write items in the NCLEX are applied in my nursing course exams. Our nursing faculty uses the Blackboard Learning System for online testing. The Blackboard system allows the option to enter information for categories at the end of each test question. After my students submit their exam, they are able to view their results and the categories coded in each test question. Students are able to see how their test questions relate to the NCLEX client needs, Bloom's cognitive level, and the nursing process.

NCSBN Resources

Sample test questions are at the end of each client needs category section in the NCLEX detailed test plan. In the last section of the NCLEX, detailed test plan are item-writing exercises with scenarios and steps to item writing for nurse educators. Additional resources are available at www.ncsbn.org.

Item-writing experts from NCSBN lead several online courses for nurse educators: "Understanding the

NCLEX: A guide for nursing educators"; "Test development and item writing"; and "Assessment of critical thinking." A fee is required to enroll in the course. Contact hours are awarded upon successful completion. Information about enrolling for these courses is available at www.learningext.com.

Clinical Reasoning and the NCLEX®

Though teaching for the test should never be the ultimate objective of an educator, when clinical reasoning is emphasized and practically applied, this essential nurse thinking skill will prepare students for real-world practice, as well as the NCLEX.

The percentages of each of the client need categories are NOT equally weighted. The following categories, though they comprise half of the categories, can be weighted from 49–73 percent or almost three quarters of the NCLEX if weighted on the high side.

1. Management of care (17–23%)
2. Medication/IV therapies (12–18%)
3. Physiologic adaptation (11–17%)
4. Reduction of risk (9–15%)

These four categories represent the importance of possessing a deep understanding of the applied sciences and nurse thinking that situates clinical reasoning by emphasizing clinical priorities and identifying relevant data that may suggest a need to rescue. These four categories also reflect the needed mastery of the advanced level of nursing education.

In contrast, the remaining four client needs categories of the NCLEX represent 27–51 percent or about a quarter of the NCLEX if weighted on the low end.

5. Safety/infection control (9–15%)
6. Basic cares/comfort (6–12%)
7. Health promotion/maintenance (6–12%)
8. Psychosocial integrity (6–12%)

In comparison, these client needs categories are primarily fundamental level content areas as well as mental health. This does not diminish the importance of these topics to nursing education, but it serves to illustrate the content areas that must be emphasized and DEEPLY understood by students to ensure strong NCLEX passing rates.

To further understand the essence of the NCLEX, the following are the most important principles that will directly correlate to NCLEX success for students because they are the same priorities the NCLEX assesses throughout the examination:

1. Every question is a brief clinical scenario that is contextualized to the bedside.
2. Emphasis is on SAFETY, primarily safe clinical judgments.
3. No NANDA nursing diagnostic statements.
4. Emphasis on principles of clinical reasoning.
   - What is the best clinical judgment to make?
   - What is the nursing priority?
   - What is the rationale for every nursing intervention or physician order?
   - What is the expected outcome for any medication or physician order?
   - Within the context of the clinical scenario, what clinical data is significant and relevant?
   - What are the most common laboratory values and the nursing implications if they are abnormal?
   - Compare/contrast normal physical assessment findings with those that are abnormal, and then reflect and see if these abnormal findings are clinically significant.
   - Compare/contrast normal vital sign findings with those that are abnormal, and then reflect and see if these abnormal findings are clinically significant.

Practical Strategies to Strengthen Student Testing

These principles of HOW to take tests should be taught to help students choose the correct answers and not make simple errors on content that they know. These same principles of how to approach every test question will also prepare students for their ultimate test…the NCLEX (Kaplan, 2016).

- Carefully review the test question to determine what the question asks. Have students put this question in as few of their own words as possible to keep them from being distracted by too much information.
- If the topic is not clear, have students look at the question and review the answers for clues.
- Once the topic is identified, determine if there is enough data in the question to recognize a problem, if the nurse needs to ACT, or is there insufficient assessment data and the nurse needs to collect additional assessment data.

- Use the ABCs of airway, breathing, and circulation priorities to choose the correct answer. If there is a breathing problem response that makes sense as well as a circulatory problem that is also relevant, there are two correct answers, but when only ONE thing can be done, and ONE answer must be selected, a B-breathing priority, will always trump a C-circulatory priority in practice as well as in your tests and the NCLEX!
- There is no substitute for UNDERSTANDING content that is taught and how it will be evaluated. Just as in practice, if students do not know content they will not be able to APPLY it to the correct answer or the bedside. That is why educators need to emphasize deep learning of what is MOST important!

Reflect

Take time to carefully and thoughtfully review one of your course exams and answer the following questions:
1. How do you develop and write your test questions?

2. Do you use the NCLEX-test plan, nursing process, Bloom's taxonomy, and course content and objectives to write test questions?

3. Do you have clear expectations about testing in your course outline or syllabus?

4. What do you need to do differently to strengthen how you write test questions?

References

Benner, P. Sutphen, M., Leonard, V., & Day, L. (2010). *Educating nurses: A call for radical transformation.* San Francisco, CA: Jossey-Bass.

Billings, D. M., & Halstead, J. A. (2016). *Teaching in nursing: A guide for faculty* (5th ed.). St. Louis, MO: Elsevier.

Cooley, S. S., & DeGagne, J. C. (2016). Transformative experience: Developing competence in novice nursing faculty. *Journal of Nursing Education, 55*(2), 96-100.

Ignatavicius, D. D., & Workman, M. L. (2016). *Medical-surgical nursing: Patient-centered collaborative care* (8th ed.). St. Louis, MO: Elsevier.

Kaplan (2016). NCLEX-RN *Content review guide: Preparation for the NCLEX-RN examination* (4th ed.). New York, NY: Kaplan Publishing.

Krathwohl, D. R. (2002). A revision of Bloom's taxonomy: An overview. *Theory into Practice, 41*(4), 212-218.

McDonald, M. E. (2014). *The nurse educator's guide to assessing learning outcomes* (3rd ed.). Burlington, MA: Jones & Bartlett Learning.

Morrison, D. (2010). Test construction and item writing. In L. Caputi (Eds.), *Teaching nursing: The art and science* (Vol. 3, pp. 2-27). Glen Ellyn, IL: College of DuPage Press.

Oermann, M. H., & Gaberson, K. B. (2014). *Evaluation and testing in nursing education,* (4th ed.). New York, NY: Springer Publishing.

Potter, P. A., Perry, A. G., Stockert, P. A., & Hall, A. M. (2017). *Fundamentals of nursing,* (9th ed.). St. Louis, MO: Elsevier.

Wendt, A. (2010). The National Council Licensure Examinations. In L. Caputi (Eds.), *Teaching nursing: The art and science* (Vol. 3, pp. 65-81). Glen Ellyn, IL: College of DuPage Press.

PART FOUR

TRANSFORMING CLINICAL EDUCATION

Foundational Principles to Transform Clinical Learning

20

Keith Rischer, RN, MA, CEN, CCRN

"Experiential (clinical) learning depends on an environment where feedback on performance is rich and the opportunities for articulating and reflecting on the experiences are deliberately planned."

—*Educating Nurses: A Call for Radical Transformation,* p. 43

Clinical faculty may be expert clinicians, but this is no guarantee that they will be able to manage and effectively teach novice nursing students in the clinical setting. They must be adequately prepared to be successful in this role. Unfortunately, one-third of clinical educators have NO training whatsoever (Dunphy Suplee, Gardner, Jerome-D'Emilia, 2014). In order to teach students to think like a nurse, clinical faculty need to be better prepared.

As a new clinical adjunct, I had no formal training to prepare me. I was immediately overwhelmed as my students took to the floor and the clinical day began. How am I ever going to manage eight students with their patients at the same time? As an expert nurse in practice, I could easily manage three or four patients and unexpected curve balls, but this was something that orientation could not fully prepare me for. I took a deep breath, and used the principle of triage in the ED where I practiced to help get me through the day.

Which student has the most complex patient? Start there and see how she is doing. Good, the patient appears stable with no change. On to the next patient, quick check in and everything appears in order. Though I felt like a proverbial ping-pong ball bouncing from one student to the next, I began to relax slowly, looking for opportunities to teach and guide and let each student spread their wings and see how they would fly. Some launched, some struggled, but I survived that first clinical experi-

ence. Over time I tried new things and strategies. Some were successful, some failed.

This chapter will emphasize strategies and principles that are practical, others are transformational because they emphasize how to strengthen the THINKING of students by emphasizing clinical reasoning. These principles will also help you overcome difficulties you will eventually encounter and provide practical strategies to initiate needed change in your clinical to strengthen student learning. These principles will also help you be successful and strengthen student learning in the clinical setting. There are two different categories, principles that will transform clinical instruction, and those that will transform the clinical educator.

Principles to TRANSFORM clinical education:

1. Emphasize DEEP learning of MOST important
2. Emphasize THINKING, not the TASKS
3. QUALITY of clinical is more important than quantity

Each patient is a puzzle the nurse puts together

Principles to TRANSFORM the clinical educator:

1. The habits of highly effective clinical educators
2. Know YOUR strengths, weaknesses, and own progression in practice
3. Know your STUDENTS' strengths, weaknesses, and progression in practice

4. You are an educator FIRST, not a FRIEND to your students

Principles to Transform Clinical Education

Emphasize DEEP Learning of MOST Important

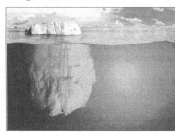

DEEP learning of what is MOST important is a transformational principle that must guide all that is taught in clinical as well as classroom settings. In order to USE and apply knowledge, this knowledge base needs to be guided by a sense of salience that recognizes what is most important (Benner, et al., 2010). Because students lack this sense of salience, it is the responsibility of educators to guide and identify what is most and least important. Clinical teaching and learning should emphasize essential knowledge, skills, and attitudes (Gaberson, Oermann, & Shellenbarger, 2015).

One practical strategy to deepen learning of what is most important is to have it repeated. The first time something is taught, this learning is temporary. REPETITION is essential to DEEPEN student learning. Neuronal networks become interconnected and developed in the brain with new learning when it is repeated over and over (Herman, Manning, & Zager, 2011). This is one reason experienced nurses are intuitive and can do complex skills without having to be intentional; it is ingrained and developed by repetition over time.

A metaphor for this principle of learning and neuroplasticity can be found on a motocross racing track. My son Levi is an amateur motocross racer who built a motocross track in our field. When it was first built, it was smooth from lack of use. To a motocross racer, the goal for a safe track is to have deep and wide ruts that are developed through multiple repetitions by going around the track over and over in the same place. In a similar manner, students need multiple "reps" to become proficient with any new skill; since it has not yet become ingrained with "deep and wide" neuronal "ruts".

Clinical learning is extremely stressful for novice student nurses, who are overwhelmed by not only the amount of content knowledge in the classroom they must learn, but also the sheer volume of information in a patient's chart. Because of a lack of experience, they tend to see EVERYTHING in the chart as equally relevant. Give a student three hours to prepare for clinical, and most will spend all 180 minutes reviewing the chart to make sure they did not miss anything. Recognize this tendency and simplify clinical learning. Make DEEP learning of the MOST important a priority before the first clinical. Use your lens of clinical practice to identify the clinical content that is most important in the clinical setting you are teaching.

DEEP Learning BEFORE the First Clinical

Students are anxious when they enter a new clinical setting. High levels of stress and anxiety are also a barrier to student learning. Help your students focus by identifying the most common medications, laboratory values, medical problems, most common complications, and nursing skills they are most likely to encounter in this clinical setting will help lessen stress and give them a sense of what to expect. It will also accomplish these essential objectives:

1. Decrease student anxiety by identifying what CONTENT is MOST important so application of content can be facilitated.
2. Provide DEEP learning of what is MOST important to that specific clinical setting.
3. Students will be better prepared and confident.

Use the following five questions to guide DEEP learning of what is most important in your clinical.

What are the most common medications (list 10–15)?

Primary care providers are creatures of habit. Though there are more than 5,000 medications in a drug handbook, if a nurse has a DEEP understanding of around 100 medications, she/he will be well prepared for clinical practice after graduation. Make it a priority to identify and list the 10–15 most commonly used medications in your clinical setting, and expect students to know what is MOST important about these medications, including the mechanism of action, in their own words!

What labs are most relevant (5–10)?

Though the most common lab panels have several labs

per panel, clarify for students that not every lab is equally important to nurses. This was discussed at length earlier in the book. For example, on a basic metabolic panel (BMP) there are typically ten chemistries, but from my perspective, the MOST important labs that are ALWAYS relevant and must be noted are the sodium, potassium, glucose, and creatinine.

Assess student mastery of fluids and electrolytes by asking students WHY sodium, potassium, glucose, and creatinine are most important and how they relate to physiologic functioning and homeostasis. Then you will know if they really know and understand this content. Do the same thing with a CBC, LFT, or other lab panels most commonly seen in your clinical area.

What are the most common medical/surgical presentations (list 3-5)?

Identify the most common medical problems or surgeries performed on patients on your unit so students can review this content before the very first clinical. This will DEEPEN student learning two ways.

1. Provide a review of NEED to know textbook content. Emphasize the importance of UNDER-STANDING the pathophysiology of the primary problem for every patient. When this is understood, the most relevant labs to identify and TREND will be recognized as well as nursing priorities and most common complications. For online resources, Medscape.com is a professional data base that provides needed background and information not found in a traditional nursing textbook.

2. Compare/contrast textbook content with how each patient actually presented. This is a principle that novice nurses who are "concrete" or textbook learners struggle with. Not every patient will present with textbook symptoms, but may have variances or ambiguity. Determining acceptable ambiguity is an essential nurse thinking skill that needs to be developed.

What are the most common complications patients may experience?

Teach your students to be PROACTIVE by anticipating the most common complications and EARLY signs to recognize a problem before it is too late. By identifying the most common complications, you will encourage

nurse vigilance and prevent failure to rescue, which will ensure safety in practice.

Examples of complications for an acute care medical-surgical unit include

- Hypoxia
- Fluid overload
- Hypoglycemia
- Sepsis
- Exacerbation of COPD
- Bowel obstructions
- Post-surgical pneumonia
- Post-surgical ileus

What nursing skills will be consistently used?

Depending on the clinical setting and level of students, certain nursing skills will be utilized more consistently than others. Though medication administration is a given in any clinical setting, besides PO, are subcutaneous, IV push, IV piggyback, or IM injections typically ordered? If students will be caring for patients with NG tubes, gastrostomy tubes, Foley catheters, chest tubes, or even ventilated patients with ET or tracheostomy tubes in the critical care settings, these will require specific skills that students must be prepared to use if this is a clinical expectation. By identifying these skills, students will be expected to come to clinical prepared and responsible to practice those skills in the nursing skills lab to ensure that they are proficient in the clinical setting.

Integrate DEEP Learning across the Program

Start by initiating these strategies to deepen student learning in the clinical setting. But to bring needed change and transformation to your program, have the entire department and all clinical settings level this information by semester using this principle of DEEP learning of what is MOST important in the program.

For example, the following are typical clinical rotations in most nursing programs:

- Fundamentals
- Basic med/surg
- Advanced med/surg
- OB
- Peds
- Mental health

If each clinical rotation in your program identified the

most important medications (10–15 each) and labs (5–10), by the end of the nursing program, students would have a DEEP mastery and understanding of 90–100 medications and 30-plus labs! This knowledge would be supported by what they have seen in practice, which will contextualize learning of this essential content, a paradigm shift that can transform nursing education (Benner, et al., 2010). This DEEP mastery of pharmacology and lab values will also be needed to pass the NCLEX.

Emphasize THINKING, not the TASKS

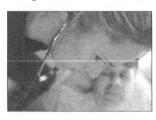

As I look back at my professional progression as a nurse educator, my approach to clinical education validates the findings found in Benner's Novice to Expert theory. I was TASK-oriented as a novice nurse educator, also a defining characteristic of a novice nurse (Benner, 1984). My primary objective each clinical was to see how many meds could be passed and how many procedures my students could participate in each clinical day.

If every student was able to pass medications, and some were able to insert a Foley catheter or an NG tube, it was a good clinical day! Though I was exhausted at the end of a typical clinical, bouncing like a ping-pong ball from one task to the next, I was confident that my students were learning because they were able to acquire experience by performing the TASKS of the professional nurse.

Though tasks are important and students must be proficient to be safe in practice, developing the ability to clinically reason will transform nursing education and help students think in action as a clinical situation changes (Benner, et al., 2010). To make this paradigm shift in your clinical setting, make it a priority to DECREASE time spent on tasks, and INCREASE the time developing critical and clinical thinking. I will share some practical tools and strategies that clinical faculty can use to realize this essential objective later in this book.

QUALITY of Clinical Is More Important Than Quantity

Nursing programs emphasize the amount of hours of clinical instruction that students receive in the clinical setting or simulation. But the amount of time that students have in these settings is no guarantee that mean-

ingful, quality learning takes place. In order to maximize the hours spent in the clinical setting and ensure quality learning, instruction needs to be individualized to the student. This is why it is so important to provide supplemental tools and resources in the clinical setting (Gaberson, Oermann, & Shellenbarger, 2015).

A supplemental tool or concise clinical paperwork that emphasizes critical thinking and clinical reasoning can be more valuable than several hours in the clinical setting that emphasizes repetition of skills and ten pages of clinical paperwork. Make it a priority as a clinical educator to make the most out of each clinical to enhance the QUALITY of time spent in the clinical setting by developing nurse THINKING, not on the total amount of hours or pages of clinical prep.

Each Patient Is a Puzzle the Nurse Puts Together

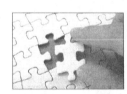

In order to put a puzzle of any size together, it is important to first find the pieces that are similar in shape or color, or have a RELATIONSHIP. Once these relationships are identified, test them to see if they "fit" or are related and then fit together. Once the first two pieces are fitted together, the puzzle just got a little bit smaller and will be easier to complete. In the same way, guide your students to see that every patient they care for is in essence a clinical "puzzle" that has multiple pieces of clinical data that also has a "fit".

Guide students to recognize that though there are significant amounts of clinical data that includes the present problem, lab values, vital signs, physician/nursing assessments, past medical history, current medications, this clinical data is NOT isolated, but has a RELATIONSHIP to each another. When the nurse observes these relationships and the "fit" is recognized, the critical thinking that is required for practice is developed. The clinical puzzle is assembled and the essence of the patient's needs and priorities become evident to the nurse.

Principles to Transform the Clinical Educator

The Habits of Highly Effective Clinical Educators

Like a new nurse in practice, new clinical faculty require a mentor to develop and guide their learning so they will successfully transition from bedside nurse to clinical educator. Clinical educators need to be confident in the clinical setting. Teacher confidence will enhance the learning of your students. If you are lacking in confidence, a distance between you and the students will be created (Billings & Halstead, 2016). If you are new to clinical education, you have what it takes to prepare students for real-world practice, but there is a learning curve that needs to be recognized.

To identify what makes a clinical educator effective, students were asked to identify what traits and habits they valued (Nehring, 1990). Seven habits or traits were identified. The thread that ties these seven habits together is the quality of the RELATIONSHIP between the educator and student. To cultivate a healthy relationship, support, encourage, and respect students, be honest and direct, and communicate caring (Gaberson, Oermann, & Shellenbarger, 2015).

As you review these seven habits, reflect and determine which habits are a strength and which are a weakness for you. Resolve to do what is needed to make any weakness a needed strength, and you will be well on your way to be a highly effective nurse educator!

Habit #1. Good role model. What does your example communicate? Are you living out the values and ethics of the nursing profession that include caring, compassion, and respect consistently in all that you do? If there is a lack of integrity demonstrated by faculty due to an inconsistency between what is taught and lived out, students will recognize the inconsistency and will be more likely to model what they see.

Habit #2. Enjoys nursing and teaching. As I look back at nurse educators who influenced me as a student in nursing education, it was those that had an obvious passion and love for nursing as a profession and clearly enjoyed working with students and teaching. This passion is contagious. Be sure to pass it on!

Habit #3. Well prepared. Step back and observe this habit from a student's perspective. What is communicated when an educator comes to class or clinical NOT prepared? They can appear incompetent and unprofessional. This tends to decrease student confidence in the ability of an educator especially if it is a pattern. Make it a priority to do what is needed to come to class or clinical always prepared.

Habit #4. Clinically excellent. When you model excellence in clinical practice, you live out the example you want your students to become. Make it a priority to maintain currency in clinical practice any way you can once you transition to academia full-time. Students do notice the difference. If you are full-time in academia and unable to remain current in clinical practice, make it a priority to remain current in the literature and best practices in your setting so that this excellence and knowledge is still communicated to students.

Habit #5. Approachable. Do everything possible to be approachable to students so they are comfortable coming to you with questions. This is why it is so important to create a safe environment for students to ask questions in the clinical setting. When this is intentionally demonstrated and communicated by faculty, student learning will increase and stress will decrease!

Habit #6. Encourages mutual respect. When respect is given to students, respect will be reciprocated to the educator. But if an educator is rigid, antagonistic or demonstrates other attitudes of disrespect to students, disrespect will be returned. Clark (2008) identified this lived reality as a "dance" where one attitude leads and the same will readily follow. The spirit and attitudes that you sow into the lives of others will return back to you. What seed are you currently planting?

Habit #7. Provides support and encouragement. Students are consistently stressed and need continual encouragement. Most students are high achievers who feel the burn of nursing education and over time begin to feel like a failure if they are unable to maintain the high GPA they have been accustomed to. Think of students as sponges. They will readily soak up the knowledge that you impart and share in the clinical setting as well as your praise and encouragement! Look for the good, be generous with praise and your students will receive the encouragement and validation they need to regain confidence as a student nurse.

Know YOUR Strengths, Weaknesses, and Own Progression in Practice

In order to be an effective clinical educator, you need to determine your level of professional progression and how it compares to the students you are teaching. Use Benner's Novice to Expert theory to guide you (Benner, 1982). For example, if you are a newer nurse (< 3 years) in practice and are now a clinical educator, according to Benner, you are currently in the competent level or third stage of development as a nurse. This stage is only one level from a student who has graduated (advanced beginner).

If you are a nurse educator who is in the competent stage as a practicing nurse, recognize the limitations and struggles you will likely have that are related to your professional development as a nurse. In your new role as an educator, you will take a step or two back from your current level of proficiency and expertise in the clinical setting. Expect to feel like a "novice" for a season. This, too, will pass and you will continue in your clinical progression as a nurse educator who gets better and more proficient over time.

Educator Strengths vs. Weaknesses

If you are a new clinical educator, conduct an inventory of your personal and professional strengths and weaknesses and how they translate to being an instructor in your particular clinical setting. The personal strengths/weaknesses are relevant to the personal dispositions and how this translates to clinical education. A clinical educator must be able to be flexible, multitask, handle stress appropriately, communicate effectively, and most importantly, love to teach! If this is your disposition, you have a strong foundation that will translate well to clinical education.

Reflect on each aspect from the list below that has relevance to you as a nurse educator. Determine if they are currently a strength or a weakness. Your objective is to identify any weaknesses and make them your strength.

PERSONAL Strengths/Weaknesses

- Do I enjoy teaching and transferring my knowledge to others?
- Am I able to effectively communicate with others as well as with those who are of a different gender or ethnic background?
- Do I easily make judgments or assumptions about others?
- Am I a flexible person who has the ability to multitask?

- Am I easily stressed when things do not go as planned in the clinical setting?
- Am I able to handle the stress that is inherent in the clinical setting?

PROFESSIONAL Strengths/Weaknesses

- Does my current clinical practice translate to this setting?
- Do I have practice-based knowledge of the most common medications, treatments, and lab values used in this setting?
- Do I have a DEEP knowledge of the mechanism of action of the most common medications used in this setting?
- Do I have a DEEP knowledge of the most common labs and the physiology that causes the most common derangements in this setting?
- Do I know the most common presentations on this unit and possess a DEEP understanding of the pathophysiology of these problems?
- Do I know the worst possible/most likely complications to expect in this setting?

Know Your STUDENTS' Strengths, Weaknesses, and Progression in Practice

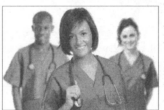

The EXPECTATIONS that you have for students must be based on what is REALISTIC for novice or advanced beginner students. Realistic expectations are foundational for a successful clinical experience! When some nurse educators communicate their greatest struggle with students, they state, "They are unable to put the clinical picture together" and "They are not able to think like a nurse." Though these are common concerns, they also represent the typical struggles that Benner (1982) identified that novice and advanced beginner students have because of their lack of clinical experience.

New nurse educators learn the job of clinical instruction primarily from other educators. I had to learn that there is a difference between clinical INSTRUCTION and supervision/evaluation. Nursing students are novice beginners who will make mistakes and will not demonstrate skills perfectly from the start. The clinical nurse educator needs to *guide* students in their clinical learning and provide opportunities for students to practice skills and become more proficient. Although supervision and evaluation is a part of the process of clinical instruction, it is not the main purpose or goal of clinical instruction. Rich, experiential clinical learning requires feedback on performance and allows students to reflect on their practice (Benner, et al., 2010).

My greatest challenge as I transitioned to the role of a clinical educator was that I was a clinical expert in practice for more than 20 years in critical care and ED. My knowledge level was advanced, and I assumed that students had a similar knowledge base because of their current education and what they had been taught. Unfortunately, there was a clear gap between my expectations and their ability to live up to them. This gap led to frustration and increased stress for both students and myself.

A metaphor that has helped keep me grounded is to visualize fundamental students as literally "wet cement." Like wet cement that was just mixed in a wheelbarrow, it is sloppy and goes everywhere! But after a year of fundamentals, just like wet cement in a posthole, it begins to firm up and take some shape. This is the second year/level student. If you are teaching advanced level clinical, affirm your fundamental faculty and all the hard work that was needed to "firm up" your students so that you can continue to see them "harden" as they take final shape by the end of the program!

Student Strengths/Weaknesses

Every clinical group that you will teach is unique. No two are alike! They come to you as individuals who are unique. Each group has its own personality. Therefore, make it a priority to see what makes each individual student "tick." What are their personal or professional strengths and weaknesses? How can you best support each student to promote her/his learning? It is important to get to know each student personally so you can tailor your educational approach with each student without crushing their spirit. Do NOT incorporate a "one-size-fits-all" approach to teaching your students. As a male educator, I was at times more blunt and direct with male students who sometimes needed to be pushed because I sensed they were coasting. But I was hesitant to use this same approach with female students because it may have the opposite effect.

Students are responsive to a clinical educator who gives freely and will "soak up" all that you have to pour into them. This is one reason why clinical education is so emotionally and physically exhausting. You literally pour out of yourself all that you have to offer to students to promote their learning. This is why it is also imperative to follow the self-care recommendations addressed earlier.

Students are also hard on themselves and many do not see clearly how well they are doing as a student learner. A student's self-talk tends to be primarily negative and this influences their perception of their ability as a nursing student. I have seen my top students see themselves as failures and doing poorly when nothing could be farther from the truth! Therefore, AFFIRM and ENCOURAGE each student in clinical. Look for the good and what was done well and openly communicate this. I am not advocating baseless praise or the "everyone gets a ribbon" for showing up mentality. In order for praise to be effective, it must be sincere and earned. When it is warranted, do not let it go unrecognized.

Students Are Either Novice or Advanced Beginner Nurses

Patricia Benner is best known for her early nursing research that led to her first *book, From Novice to Expert: Clinical Excellence and Power in Clinical Practice.* This work detailed how nurses progress, develop skills and understanding of patient care over time. The five levels of nurse proficiency in practice that Benner identified are:
1. Novice
2. Advanced beginner
3. Competent
4. Proficient
5. Expert (Benner, 1984)

Every nursing student begins as a NOVICE nurse with no clinical experience. By the time they enter the advanced level of nursing education and graduate, they are typically ADVANCED BEGINNERS. The next level is COMPETENT. Competency takes an additional two to three years to attain once in practice. What each of these five levels have in common is that to progress from one level to the next requires TIME and clinical EXPERIENCE. There are no shortcuts to professional progression!

A student novice nurse with little to no clinical experience will be a concrete/textbook learner who also sees EVERYTHING as relevant and important to know in both the classroom and clinical settings. Students at this level are TASK-oriented (Benner, 1984). If they have completed the tasks of charting the vital signs, nursing assessment, and administered scheduled medications, they have had a good clinical day! Because of this lack of clinical experience, they struggle to recognize variations from textbook content in practice and identify nursing priorities.

As a student progresses through the final year of the program, they are now an advanced beginner who will begin to recognize exceptions to concrete textbook content, and see certain clinical data as relevant. However, they continue to have difficulty recognizing nursing and clinical priorities (Benner, 1984). The relevance of Benner's framework is that it defines definite steps and levels of clinical progression and the characteristics of nursing practice at each level. It is important to review the essence of Novice to Expert so that expectations for students are REALISTIC.

How a Novice Nurse Thinks

There are predictable patterns that represent how a new student nurse thinks and processes clinical data while providing patient care. Have you witnessed any of these characteristics of a novice nursing student in your clinical?

- Experiences anxiety and lack of self-confidence in the clinical setting
- Relies heavily on textbooks and other resources
- Tends to be a concrete learner whose knowledge is organized as facts and follows policies and standards by rote
- Is comforted by clear-cut rules of what to do and does NOT appreciate clinical ambiguity
- Focuses on the tasks that need to be done and struggles to see the holistic needs of the patient. As a result, tends to forget to assess thoroughly before doing an intervention.
- Relies on step-by-step procedures and is TASK oriented (Alfaro-LeFevre, 2013)

Based on the application of this theory to practice, nursing students will struggle to recognize the clinical data that is most RELEVANT and determine the resultant nursing PRIORITIES. There are two questions that nurse educators can integrate in the clinical setting to facilitate student progression in practice:

- What clinical data did you collect or review from the chart is RELEVANT? WHY?
- What is your nursing PRIORITY? WHY?

Additional Points to Consider

- Encourage your students to consistently give their best effort to be the best nurse possible. Benner's theory confirms that time alone will not make a nurse an expert clinician. Just because a nurse has been in practice for 20, 30, or even 40 years is NOT a guarantee that they are also expert clinicians. To progress through all five stages and become an expert nurse, a student must be motivated and guided by the desire to be EXCELLENT in all that they do. Expert practice at its very root is SELF-MOTIVATING (Benner, Hooper-Kyriakidis, & Stannard, 2011).
- Students who are passive, not highly engaged, and want to be spoon-fed content are more likely to be marginal nurses once in practice. This mindset can be changed by providing activities and exercises in the clinical setting that will "stretch" them enough to recognize what they do not know, so they are motivated to learn what is needed to be a safe nurse in practice. One practical way to encourage an ongoing desire for excellence is to encourage your students to pursue certification in their desired nursing specialty after graduation. This will lay the foundation for professional growth and knowledge development that will likely lead to expert practice over time.
- Caring remains foundational for the nurse to progress and develop to become an expert practitioner. The heightened level of involvement that caring represents is foundational to expert nursing practice (Benner & Wrubel, 1989). Caring is the motivation that helps the nurse notice the most effective interventions as well as identify subtle signs of improvement or deterioration.
- Nursing practice can also regress or go backward over time. If the nurse is engaged and motivated in practice, he/she will progress with time and experience. But what happens if that same nurse experiences depression, the stress of a divorce, or burnout in her current position? Is it realistic to maintain the same level of motivation and engagement under these circumstances? For most it is not, and regression to a lower level of proficiency may occur.

You Are an Educator FIRST, Not a FRIEND to Your Students

Is the nurse educator a friend to the student who wants to be liked, or is the nurse an educator, and friendship is optional? I struggled with this dichotomy. Being new, I wanted to be the "nice" educator students liked. This is a natural tendency that seems harmless, but in reality, is dangerous and must be recognized as an unhealthy paradigm to guide educational practice. Think about the implications of this paradigm. What are the consequences and impact when an educator wants to be liked? The educator will give students what they WANT, not what they NEED.

For example, students NEED active learning that makes them think and work hard to practice clinical reasoning. But they WANT passive lectures that package the content in content-heavy slides so they can be spoon-fed by willing faculty. But spoon feeding adult learners is unhealthy and counterproductive. You may be liked, but your students will suffer because they will not have the skill set to be prepared to think like a nurse. As a result, they may be more likely after graduation to fail to recognize problems and complications until it is too late.

Embrace your responsibility to be an EDUCATOR, whose primary responsibility is to PREPARE students for professional practice and do what is needed, not expedient, to accomplish this objective. Let students feel the warmth of your passion for nursing, teaching, and for them as students. Learning flourishes when there is an authentic relationship present with your students. Though you may be hard by doing what is needed, most students will inherently respect you for it.

Reflect

1. Identify the three most common presentations on your clinical unit that your students should be prepared to care for?

    1.

    2.

    3.

2. Identify the three most common complications (Jason's) that patients are most likely to experience in your clinical setting?

    1.

    2.

    3.

3. What principle (s) will you incorporate to increase your effectiveness as a clinical educator?

4. What is one action step you can do today to strengthen student learning by integrating this principle in the clinical?

References

Alfaro-LeFevre, R. (2013). *Critical thinking, clinical reasoning, and clinical judgment: A practical approach.* (5th ed.). St. Louis, MO: Elsevier–Saunders.

Benner, P. (1982). From novice to expert. *American Journal of Nursing, 82*(3), 402–407.

Benner, P. (1984). *From novice to expert: Excellence and power in clinical nursing practice.* Upper Saddle River, NJ: Prentice Hall.

Benner, P., & Wrubel, J. (1989). *Primacy of caring: Stress and coping in health and illness.* Menlo Park, CA: Addison-Wesley Publishing Company.

Benner, P., Sutphen, M., Leonard, V., & Day, L. (2010). *Educating nurses: A call for radical transformation.* San Francisco, CA: Jossey-Bass.

Benner, P., Hooper-Kyriakidis, P., & Stannard, D. (2011). *Clinical wisdom and interventions in acute and critical care: A thinking-in-action approach.* (2nd ed.). New York, NY: Springer.

Billings, D.M., & Halstead, J.A. (2016). *Teaching in nursing: A guide for faculty* (5th ed.). St. Louis: MO, Elsevier.

Clark, C. M. (2008). The dance of incivility in nursing education as described by nursing faculty and students. *Advances in Nursing Science, 31,* E37–E54.

Dunphy Suplee, P., Gardner, M, & Jerome-D'Emilia. (2014). Nursing faculty preparedness for clinical teaching. *Journal of Nursing Education, 53*(3), S38-S41.

Gaberson, K. B., & Oermann, M. H. (2010). *Clinical teaching strategies in nursing* (3rd ed.). New York: Springer Publishing Company.

Ignatavicius, D. D., & Workman, M. L. (2016). *Medical-surgical nursing* (8th ed.). St. Louis, MO: Elsevier.

Nehring, V. (1990). Nursing clinical teacher effectiveness inventory: A replication study of 'best' and 'worst' clinical teachers as perceived by nursing faculty and students, *Journal of Advanced Nursing, 15,* 934-940.

Potter, P. A., Perry, A. G., Stockert, P. A., & Hall, A. M. (2017). *Fundamentals of nursing* (9th ed.). St. Louis, MO: Elsevier.

21

Clinical Education that Prepares Students for Professional Practice

Keith Rischer, RN, MA, CEN, CCRN

"Overall we found little formal instruction on HOW to set priorities...The bulk
of the teaching and learning about selecting the most important priorities
occurred in specific clinical settings and referred to particular patients"

—*Educating Nurses: A Call for Radical Transformation*, p. 52

Though all aspects of nursing education are important, the clinical setting is where everything that has been taught in the classroom and skills lab must come together and be applied at the bedside. Clinical education must be the greatest strength of any program in order to maximize students' learning and prepare them for professional practice. This chapter will provide practical strategies and skills that may not be directly addressed and utilized in the clinical setting, but are needed to help students successfully transition to real-world practice.

This includes an emphasis on:

- Preparing to assume care
- Clinical communication
- Patient education
- Problem solving
- Priority setting
- Time management

Preparing to Assume Care

Once in clinical practice, students will not have as much time to prepare for care with multiple patients. They will need to quickly, concisely, and systematically collect relevant clinical data on each patient. To teach students how to efficiently gather clinical data, the "big picture" or the essence of the primary problem and what brought the patient to the clinical setting must first be identified. Once the big picture is understood, the nurse can identify REL-

EVANT clinical data that will help put the current picture in context. This is another reason why students must be able to APPLY classroom content and clinical reasoning, so this transference to the clinical setting can be realized.

Though this can be a struggle, guide students to become proficient in accessing the most important clinical data in the medical record. Electronic medical records (EMRs) are becoming the standard for reviewing and documenting in acute care. Just as you want students to have a systematic approach to giving report and an SBAR, a consistent approach to collecting clinical data will prepare students for real-world practice.

In order to identify relevant clinical data from the medical record and time-map the clinical day, be sure that your clinical paperwork is SHORT and well designed to facilitate the collection of clinical data. In my experience, clinical paperwork is another area where there is TMI in nursing education. It can overwhelm novice students with numerous pages. Make it a priority to embrace the paradigm "LESS IS MORE" and apply this to the clinical prep and paperwork required in your clinical setting!

Big Picture Clinical Data

In order to quickly identify the essence of the patient's story, have students go to the admitting history and physical (H&P) and/or the primary care provider's most recent progress note. This is an excellent place to start and note what is most relevant to visualize the big picture and put the clinical puzzle together. The nurse can quickly gather the following data and note it on the patient preparation worksheet.

Primary Care Provider's Progress Note

- Patient name, age, primary medical problem, day of admission
- RELEVANT past medical history that is related to primary medical problem. The patient may have ten medical problems, but focus on the one or two that are influencing the current problem.
- Concise summary of this admission and any problems as well as progress toward the current plan of care from the physician's perspective. What circumstances brought the patient to the doctor office/ED and led to being admitted?

Specific Clinical Data

Once the big picture or essence of the current clinical situation is identified, RELEVANT specific clinical data can be collected. Use the following sections of the chart or EMR to access and note:

- **Lab Values.** Identify RELEVANT lab values based on student knowledge of the primary problem. TREND these most important lab values, even if they are normal, because they have clinical significance. Note the direction of the trended labs. Determine if they are improving or reflect a possible problem.
- **Vital Sign Flowsheet.** Note and write down the last set of vital signs and any clinical TRENDS that may be significant over the last shift. Identify patient ambiguity for vital signs that may be outside textbook norms.
- **Nursing Assessment.** Highlight head-to-toe nursing assessment with data that includes an emphasis on the most relevant body system based on primary problem as well as abnormal assessment findings.
- **Medication Administration Record (MAR).** What PRN medications were given in the past shift or 24 hours? Clarify with the nurse in report which PRN medications are working and what needs to be done differently based on evaluation (pain meds/pain control, etc.).

- **Kardex**. Focus on Kardex data that includes code status, contact precautions, primary physician/group, location of IVs and any infusions, new orders, activity, labs to be drawn on next shift. This also includes allergies, diet orders, and diagnostic tests for the shift.
- **Intake and Output (I&O).** Note if I&O is relevant by documenting the output over the last 8/24 hours and trend of daily weights.
- **Your Evaluation.** Once this clinical data is assimilated, you will begin to get a sense of the nursing priorities for your patient. Begin to formulate these priorities and when you obtain a nurse-to-nurse report, you will be able to clarify your thoughts as needed with the nurse. Once the essence of the current nursing priority is identified, the plan of care follows with resultant interventions and outcomes that will advance the plan of care on your shift.
  - Sometimes students do not complete a nursing assessment until much later in the shift. They have no concept of how important it is to have a baseline. This must be done within the first hour of the shift! Clearly communicate this expectation to students because it is common to hear students explain, "I do not want to wake the patient," or "I was planning on getting that later," etc.

Clinical Communication

Safety is the unifying thread for everything that is done by the professional nurse. Though safety is traditionally applied to patient care and medication administration, patient safety can be compromised if there is inadequate communication with other nurses or care providers. Every time a nurse communicates a clinical concern or gives report to the oncoming nurse, this is a HIGH RISK encounter that will directly impact patient care one way or another. Most graduate nurses struggle with this essential skill and as a result do not feel well prepared to communicate effectively with members of the health care team (Neal-Boylan, 2013).

Collaborative Communication

Remind students that every interaction with another member of the health care team is akin to a baton handoff in a track and field race. Each runner in the relay is part of the team. In order to successfully complete the race, there must be a smooth and seamless handoff of the baton from one runner to another. If the baton is inadvertently

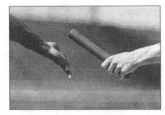

dropped during the handoff, it is disastrous and results in failure. In the same way, if the nurse is unable to concisely and effectively communicate with any member of the health care team, disastrous consequences can follow that ultimately impact the patient.

Respectful and effective communication between all members of the health care team not only advances the plan of care but also ensures and guards patient SAFETY. Since nurses most often communicate with other nurses and primary care providers such as physicians, I will discuss ways that I have found most effective to communicate with these two groups within the health care team. These principles are also universal and translate to any member of the team with whom the nurse needs to communicate.

Students struggle to see themselves as part of the health care team. I call it the "I'm just a student" complex. It doesn't help that staff nurses tend to also regard them as "just a student." In order to overcome this barrier, the educator needs to embrace the role and responsibility of being a cheerleader for each student. Encourage and affirm their significance as a member of the health care team from fundamentals through the end of the program. By the end of the program, this "just a student" complex will likely be overcome as they begin to anticipate and embrace the transition from nursing student to a professional nurse in practice after graduation.

SBAR to I-SBAR-R

Situation, Background, Assessment, and Recommendation (SBAR) is the Joint Commission's recommendation for best practice of standardized communication in health care. SBAR promotes quality and patient safety because it helps members of the health care team communicate patient information in a clear, complete, concise, and structured format; improving communication efficiency and accuracy. In addition to S-B-A-R, an additional "I" for identification and additional "R" for repeat-read back are now recommended.

The general components of I-SBAR-R include the following:

- **I: Identification.** Identification of yourself including name, title, and the name of your patient.
- **S: Situation.** What is the primary problem or concern?
- **B: Background.** What background information is RELEVANT? (keep concise)
- **A: Assessment.** What assessment data is RELEVANT?
- **R: Recommend.** What does the nurse recommend to advance the plan of care?
- **R: Repeat-Read back.** Repeat and read back the plan of care and new orders that may have been obtained from the primary care provider.

Communication Must Be Practiced

Students require numerous opportunities to concisely give end-of-shift report or communicate concerns directly to the primary nurse. But like any skill, if is not practiced, it does not become fluent and well developed. With a little bit of creativity, nurse educators can create many opportunities to weave the SBAR throughout the nursing program

- **Clinical**. Integrate SBAR in your clinical paperwork throughout the program. The consistency and repeated use will strengthen the safety and skill of communication with your students.
- **Clinical post-conference.** Have students share the SBAR on their patient that they gave to their nurse. Constructively provide feedback.
- **Classroom.** Develop scenarios that reflect a change of status and then have students practice the SBAR together when the nurse needs to contact the care provider. Have each portion of the class take an S-B-A-R and share with the class. My UNFOLDING Reasoning case studies come with the SBAR already integrated as a change of status or end-of-shift report.
- **Simulation.** Use simulation with a patient who develops a clinical concern and requires an SBAR.

How to Teach Students to Communicate with Physicians

Students will have little to no opportunities to communicate directly with physicians or primary care providers in the clinical setting. But students need to be prepared for this eventual reality. The following insightful points come from a physician colleague who communicated the following principles that nurses need to keep in mind when communicating with physicians or primary care providers:

1. Most physicians are by nature very competitive. Do not challenge this competitive spirit by provoking them with a hint of/or obvious challenge. If this is sensed, the nurse will quickly lose.
2. Keep all communication simple and on point.
3. Communicate a spirit of collaboration if a physician is being difficult. State your concern, but preface it with, "I need your help."
4. Do not DEMAND your recommendation—COLLABORATE. For example, communicate your concern for additional pain meds, recommend a higher dose, but then state, "What do you think?" This approach promotes collaboration and a team approach to meeting the needs of the patient.

Practical Application

When the time comes to make that phone call to a direct care provider, the following will guide a collaborative dialogue to ensure that the patient is advocated for.

1. Know the patient's story well enough so that you are able to answer basic questions related to your clinical concern.
2. When calling because of a patient concern, make it a priority to give just enough information to allow the provider to visualize what is going on. Don't give too little information and don't give too much that is not directly relevant to the primary concern. Make it "just right"!
3. Dialogue and have a voice in any interaction. When requesting a pain medication and you suggest morphine and the physician agrees or suggests hydromorphone but states a dose that is likely too low, don't be afraid to share your concern that it may not be enough. Suggest a slightly higher dose range or more frequent PRN schedule and you will likely get what your patient needs.
4. If you do not understand the rationale for an order or medication the doctor wants to order, be humble and do not hesitate to ask for clarification. Don't fake it! Remember that this is also a patient safety issue.
5. If you have a serious concern, be specific with clinical data that supports your concern and if possible, be clear about what you want.

Patient Education

Nursing students are reluctant to embrace the responsibility of educating their patients. They are aware of what they do and do not know as a novice nursing student and need encouragement to integrate patient education each clinical day. If patient education is done well, students can improve patient outcomes by empowering patients and their families by helping them to understand their illness and take responsibility to do their part to promote and maintain their health. But in order for patients to DEEPLY understand the primary problem that will require them to make needed change, they must understand the essence of the PATHOPHYSIOLOGY of the primary problem at their level of understanding. This is another reason that students must also UNDERSTAND pathophysiology; so they can teach it!

An example of a patient I cared for in the ED illustrates this principle. Hank, a 65-year-old, presented to the emergency department with increasing shortness of breath that began the day before. He was diagnosed with hypertension three years before and was started on both an ACE inhibitor and a beta blocker. He stopped taking all his medications three months prior to the ED visit because he ran out and felt fine.

He was now diaphoretic and having difficulty breathing with bibasilar crackles. He had an initial BP of 240/140. A chest X-ray revealed that he was in acute pulmonary edema due to a hypertensive crisis. He was stabilized in the ED with nitroglycerin sublingual and a nitroglycerin IV gtt that brought his BP down to 150/94 when he arrived to the floor and I assumed care. As I was completing the admission and had time to discuss the events that led to this hypertensive and possibly life-threatening crisis, it became apparent that this crisis and admission could have been prevented. He admitted that he did not have a clear understanding of hypertension and the importance of taking his medications.

Hank was a retired plumber and he understood pipes. Using his frame of reference, I likened his arteries to pipes. The buildup of pressure has no obvious symptoms until the pressure becomes too high and the pipes burst. Though he fortunately did not have a stroke with debilitating consequences, it was a real possibility that he needed to understand. I then likened his heart to a sump pump that was being overwhelmed with too much pressure to pump against and was unable to keep up. The back pressure and overload on the heart was causing fluid to fill up in his lungs, causing the shortness of breath and current problem of pulmonary edema. The lightbulb went on and he remarked, "If someone had simply explained this to me three years ago, I would've understood what hypertension is and would have known why it is so important to take my medications!"

To empower students and strengthen their ability to provide patient education, the following are practical strategies to give students needed confidence:

1. **Individualize to patient.** Make it a priority to make all education (and care plans!) INDIVIDUALIZED to the patient and family needs. Use metaphors or principles the patient readily understands. Get inside the lived experience and story of your patient and family by determining
   - Education level and profession/career experience
   - Age
   - Mastery of English language, particularly if patients are immigrants
   - Once this relevant information is known, the nurse can communicate effectively in order to teach effectively.

2. **Keep it simple.** Keep teaching as simple as possible to ensure that it will be understood. Teach the simple concepts about a topic first, and then move to the more complex. Be sure to use language that your patient can understand and avoid medical terminology whenever possible (Freda, 2004).

3. **Reinforce everything that is taught.** Use the following principles to reinforce what is taught:
   - Teach the one concept you want your patient to learn FIRST.
   - Ask your patient to restate in their OWN words what you have taught, so you can be sure he understood. Engage in dialogue to determine effectiveness of education, not just yes or no answers. If any knowledge gaps are identified, address them immediately.
   - Use visual aids for teaching; identify the preferred learning style of those you are teaching and adapt your teaching to accommodate.

- Always use written educational materials for the client to take home, if available. (Freda, 2004)

4. **Integrate education while providing care.** Teach students to make education a natural part of nursing practice while providing care. Clearly communicate to the patient everything that is done and why they are doing it throughout the shift. This includes the plan of care simply stated and the rationale for nursing interventions, the data from vital signs, nursing assessment, and the administration of any medications or treatments. For example, if a student's patient is postoperative and needs to use the incentive spirometer (IS), do not just tell the patient to do this five to ten times an hour and a superficial reason for its use. Go a little deeper into the rationale and explain WHY. Explain that the alveoli are miniature deflated balloons that need to be re-inflated after surgery to prevent pneumonia and other complications. Through proper and consistent use of the IS, these balloons can be re-inflated and ensure an uneventful and timely discharge!

When patients as well as families are educated well, this can reduce the number of readmissions for chronic health problems and promote patient positive health and outcomes. Teach students to utilize these principles consistently to ensure that each patient and their family not only have their immediate care needs met, but empower them to remain healthy and ensure long-term health stability and wellness.

The nurse needs to determine what the patient and/or family NEEDS to know. Are they willing or ready to learn? What do they currently know? What do they want to know? How do they learn best—written, hands-on, verbal instruction? What is the best time to teach? (Avoid teaching when in pain or any other discomfort.) Additional principles that will help students be confident educators include:

- Keep education patient-centered.
- Assess physical capability and developmental level.
- Provide quiet and private area for teaching.
- Engage patient in learning—make it active learning.
- Collaborate teaching and goals with patient/family.
- Assess retention of teaching by teach back method.
- Document teaching and patient response.
- Apply the nursing process to patient teaching: assessment, etc. (Potter, et al., 2017)

Problem Solving

Problem solving is a nurse thinking skill that needs to be developed and practiced in the clinical setting. Problem solving is the ability of the nurse to recognize and define the problem, gather relevant data to clarify the problem, generate alternative responses, and choose the best approach considering the patient needs and response (Oermann & Gaberson, 2014). Problem solving can be developed through clinical experience with patients, but can also be strengthened without hands-on care through tools such as case studies. Case studies expose students to clinical scenarios that they may not typically encounter and allow them to practice problem solving and clinical reasoning (Gaberson, Oermann, & Shellenbarger, 2015).

Using Case Studies

Case studies can be integrated in the clinical setting in the post-conference setting. At the fundamental level, faculty can develop cases that present simple problems that identify and require basic nursing interventions. The goal at this level is for students to learn how to APPLY concepts to clinical situations, think through problems, and solve them. Students can work together as a group to problem solve by exploring different perspectives of the case, the relevant clinical data that was noticed, interpretation of data, and the clinical judgment that was made as a result. As students progress through the program, case studies can become more complex, with additional problems that unfold with a change of status that needs to be recognized by the nurse (Gaberson, et al, 2015).

Student-Developed Case Studies

To strengthen student learning in the clinical setting, have students create a case study based on an actual patient that students care for and the objectives relevant to the clinical setting. This strategy can effectively supplement the learning in specialty areas such as pediatrics when the number of patients may be limited, but can be used in any clinical setting.

For example in a pediatric setting, case study elements that students can address and develop could include:

- Explain health issues that brought the child into clinical setting.
- Identify the developmental stage of the child and traits of this stage.

- Identify nursing priorities, interventions, and plan of care.
- Describe influences of culture, school (peer groups), and the family on the development of the child.
- Identify and explain the role of the school nurse with this child.
- Include health and well-being trends that are relevant to this population, such as childhood obesity or teen parenting. (Schreiner & Murray, 2012)

After the case study has been completed, ask students to reflect and evaluate their learning. In one study that used this strategy, student evaluations were overwhelmingly positive (Schreiner & Murray, 2012).

Priority Setting

Inexperienced nursing students struggle with setting priorities (Benner, 1984). Teach students that the essence of setting priorities is determined by differentiating between problems that need immediate attention and problems that can wait (Alfaro-LeFevre, 2013). Patient priority setting is like a deck of cards that is continually being shuffled. The top card represents the highest priority. Once this priority task is done, it goes to the bottom of the deck and the next important priority now needs to be completed.

Practical priority setting using the principle of triage depends on the nurse's ability to recognize which patient concern/task needs immediate attention, what interventions need to be done FIRST, and what can wait. Proper priority setting is also a component of clinical reasoning. Review the earlier chapter on this foundational concept to develop not only nurse thinking but priority setting in practice.

Triage and setting priorities correctly in the clinical setting require time and clinical experience. Students lack this needed experience. This skill will be further developed after graduation as students acquire additional clinical experience. With a multiple patient assignment, in order to recognize which patient is the highest priority, one key aspect of clinical reasoning is required: RECOGNIZE the RELEVANCE or significance of clinical data that is in the chart or collected by the nurse and INTERPRET it to determine if a clinical problem is present. If relevant clinical data is not recognized or acted upon, the priority patient or concern is not recognized. This can contribute to a delay of care for a patient who may have a critical concern and result in failure to rescue.

Listen to Your Gut!

Teach students to listen when their gut instinct tells them something is not quite right with their patient. Though they may not be able to put their finger on the specific problem, pay close attention to this feeling and investigate and assess further to delineate a concern. Even if students are not able to identify a concrete assessment finding that confirms the feeling, there is a reason for why it is there and it could represent a potential problem.

Subtle assessment findings that may represent a change in status such as skin that was dry but is now slightly moist or a slight increase in heart rate are subtle signs that may represent a much larger problem. When the nurse is able to recognize the significance and the rationale for assessment findings that are slightly abnormal, this provides context to recognize the significance of the initial observations.

For example, sympathetic nervous system stimulation is not expected in a patient who is recovering from surgery. Tachycardia, subtle change in skin color, moist or diaphoretic skin with normal blood pressure due to the compensatory response of an elevated heart rate are all EARLY signs of any shock state. But if students recognize and understand the significance of these findings, they will be able to accurately INTERPRET this clinical data, which is an essential component of clinical judgment making.

Emphasize the importance of being proactive not Reactive in practice. Proactive will mean that students can be in control of the situation with early intervention, or avoid an emergency by anticipating a potential problem BEFORE it develops. Reactive means that they wait too long to intervene and can possibly find themselves doing compressions with their patient's life at stake. I ask them, "How do you want to run YOUR practice? Do you want to be proactive or reactive?" The answer is obvious.

To help develop students' ability to recognize and establish proper priorities and the priority patient, the following principles of priority setting will prepare them for professional practice as well as for the NCLEX!

Priority Patient

If students have more than one patient in the clinical setting, who will be seen first and why? The following principles will guide the development of this essential nurse thinking skill.

- **How old is the patient?** The older the patient, the higher risk they are to develop complications. Therefore, if all considerations are equal, see the oldest patient FIRST.
- **When were they admitted?** The more recent the day of admission, the more likely the patient is higher acuity and at risk for a change of status. Therefore, if all considerations are equal, see the most recently admitted patient FIRST.
- **When did they have surgery?** The more recent the day of surgery, the higher the acuity and risk for a change of status. Therefore, if all considerations are equal, see the most recent surgical patient FIRST
- **How many body systems are involved?** Chronic renal failure patients are an excellent example of patients who typically have multiple body system derangements because of systemic metabolic changes influenced by renal disease. If medical complexity is present and all other considerations are equal, this patient should be seen FIRST.

Priority Assessments

Though a head-to-toe assessment is done on every patient, do your students know when to modify this assessment based on the patient's primary problem? For example, a patient admitted with COPD exacerbation will require a much more thorough and detailed respiratory assessment. Less attention can be paid to the GI system.

Nursing Priority

The ABCs of priority setting are always relevant and must remain in this order. If a patient has airway, breathing, or circulatory priorities, set priorities in the sequence of alphabetical order! Encourage nurse vigilance with an awareness of the most likely or worst possible complication for your patient as a means to establish a care priority. This was discussed earlier in the prior chapter. Encourage students to identify the worst possible complication while in report at the beginning of clinical. What interventions are required for EARLY intervention?

Priority Interventions

Priority interventions are implemented once the nursing process has correctly identified the priority patient, correct priority assessments, and nursing priority. If the nursing priority is NOT correctly identified, the interventions that follow will not benefit the patient and advance the plan of care.

Time Management

As inexperienced nurses, students may also struggle with time management, even if they have one patient. Here are practical principles to help them see the big picture of managing time in the clinical setting and help them successfully multitask.

- Determine what must be done right now vs. what can wait (example: pain meds).
- Determine what must be done in a specific time frame to ensure patient safety (example: blood glucose before meals) and what interventions can wait.
- Document vital signs and nursing assessment in the chart as soon as possible, preferably before going to your next patient.
- Group patient care tasks together as much as possible.
- If doing a procedure or providing care, visualize what you need and bring all that is needed into the room the first time.
- Complete one task before starting another.

Reflect

1. What aspects of this chapter do you need to incorporate in your clinical to practically prepare students for professional practice?

2. What is one action step you can do today to integrate this in the clinical setting to strengthen student learning?

References

Alfaro-LeFevre, R. (2013). *Critical thinking, clinical reasoning, and clinical judgment: A practical approach.* (5th ed.). St. Louis, MO: Elsevier–Saunders.

Benner, P. (1984). *From novice to expert: Excellence and power in clinical nursing practice.* Upper Saddle River, NJ: Prentice Hall.

Gaberson, K. B., & Oermann, M. H. (2010). *Clinical teaching strategies in nursing* (3rd ed.). New York: Springer Publishing Company.

Gaberson, K. B., Oermann, M. H., & Shellenbarger, T. (2015). *Clinical teaching strategies in nursing* (4th ed.). New York: Springer Publishing Company.

Ignatavicius, D. D., & Workman, M. L. (2016). *Medical-surgical nursing* (8th ed.). St. Louis, MO: Elsevier.

Potter, P. A., Perry, A. G., Stockert, P. A., & Hall, A. M. (2017). *Fundamentals of nursing* (9th ed.). St. Louis, MO: Elsevier.

Gaberson, K. B., Oermann, M. H., & Shellenbarger, T. (2015). *Clinical teaching strategies in nursing* (4th ed.). New York: Springer Publishing Company.

Neal-Boylan, L. (2013). *The nurse's reality gap: Overcoming barriers between academic achievement and clinical success.* Indianapolis, IN: Sigma Theta Tau International.

Oermann, M. H. & Gaberson, K. B. (2014). *Evaluation and testing in nursing education,* (4th ed.). New York, NY: Springer Publishing.

Schreiner, L. & Murray, J. (2012). Student-developed case studies. *Journal of Nursing Education, 51*(12), 719-720.

22

Nuts and Bolts of Clinical Education

Keith Rischer, RN, MA, CEN, CCRN

*"To transform clinical education) "Faculty will help students progress
in their development, with experiences designed to encourage them to, first,
think like nurses, then care like nurses, act like nurses, and finally be nurses."*

—Christine A. Tanner, PhD, RN, FAAN

It is now time to put everything together in a practical-framework to create a clinical experience to structure the clinical day and develop clinical reasoning in students. The overall goal of clinical instruction is to lead and guide students to discover knowledge for themselves. Your instruction must involve the student as an active participant in their learning.

Clinical instruction must be supported by mutual TRUST and RESPECT. This is essential to support learning and student growth. Educators need to desire to see students succeed and partner with them in achieving success. These values are lived out when the educator is (a):

- Competent guide
- Supports students
- Stimulates students to be the best they can be
- Facilitates learning by planning and providing appropriate activities (Gaberson, et al., 2015)

This chapter will detail practical strategies that will maximize student learning and faculty sanity in the high stakes arena of the clinical setting. It also provides strategies to develop the nurse thinking skill of clinical reasoning. To get started, let's start at the very beginning of clinical education, which is faculty and student orientation to the clinical site.

Faculty Clinical Orientation

Preparing to enter a new clinical setting is like starting a new job. You may have little to no experience, but are expected to be fully functional once you are on the floor. The clinical educator represents the educational institution coming as a guest to the clinical setting. Since clinical sites are at a premium, it is imperative that a positive relationship and partnership is established. Orientation to the facility, clinical site, and review of policies and procedures will smooth out expected bumps, but will take time so plan accordingly.

Spend time preparing clinical staff and explaining expectations for the students in your clinical rotation. Explain what level of students, learning goals for this clinical rotation, and what the focus will be. Depending on the setting, staff may have had advanced students who have two to three patients and a student who is team leader. Staff may be under the assumption that first-year nursing students are ready for complex assignments or multiple patients. This is why it is so important to clarify student expectations during each clinical course and provide a copy of clinical guidelines to the nursing staff as well as charge nurse and nursing manager.

In addition to meeting all policy and computer documentation requirements of the institution, faculty orientation should include a "shadow" shift, where the clinical educator follows and observes a nurse from the unit to get a firsthand perspective on patient care in this setting. Be sure to provide contact information and meet personally with the following members of unit leadership:

- Nurse manager
- Clinical educator
- Charge nurse(s)

Because each clinical setting is different, use a basic orientation checklist that covers the most important aspects that will prepare you to enter the clinical setting with confidence. At a minimum, be sure that your orientation covers the following key points:

Institutional

- Review of essential/mandatory unit policies and procedures
- Parking for students
- Documentation

Specific Unit Setting

- Names, titles, roles of those staff will be working with students consistently (charge nurses)
- Expectations for student documentation
- Where to gather for pre/post-conferences
- Where students can collect data (units want to avoid being overrun at once with students!)
- Medication system and access codes
- Location of charts, supplies, and equipment relevant to patient care
- Primary nurse expectations for communication and delegation to students
- Clinical guidelines that include clinical expectations, contact information, facility policies, and any other information that you find necessary. Have students sign a form that indicates they received and reviewed your clinical guidelines. Keep the signed form in their student file with their final clinical evaluation.

If you are a part-time clinical adjunct, obtain the schedule for past as well as upcoming content that will be taught in the classroom and nursing skills that students will be responsible for that semester. This will help guide student expectations as well as hold students accountable. Some have been known to say, "I don't know that. We haven't covered…in our program" when in fact it was! If you are a new clinical adjunct, before beginning a clinical rotation, the following aspects of your role as part of the teaching team should be addressed, clarified, and clearly communicated:

- Access or obtain a copy of syllabus and student handbook
- Learn how to communicate student concerns and process for remediation
- Learn expectations for attending team meetings and channels to provide input and communicate concerns personally
- Obtain contact for teaching team lead and expectations for frequency of communication

Student Clinical Orientation

Once you have been oriented to the clinical setting, you will be prepared to orient students in the first week of clinical. Reviewing hospital policies and procedures, paperwork, and charting expectations are a standard for any clinical orientation and some of this content may be done ahead of time. The stress and anxiety of students can be palpable at times. Do what is needed to encourage, support, and answer all questions so students will be prepared to care for patients.

Have students do a scavenger hunt to find most needed equipment, etc. This is an excellent idea that also keeps clinical orientation learning ACTIVE! Steps to incorporate a scavenger hunt include the following:

- Create a list of essential items, supplies, equipment that students must know where to find them
- Have students work in groups of 2–3 to locate these items and write down location on list provided
- Set a time limit of 15–30 minutes depending on the length of the list

Communicate expectations to students that include the importance of teamwork. Students who are no longer busy are expected to check in with other students and help as needed. Teamwork also needs to be extended to the entire floor by answering call lights and making themselves available to the nurses on the unit. Communicate expectations for documentation and how quickly students need to document data in the medical record if they are allowed to do so. If students can document in the EMR, expectations need to mirror clinical practice.

Print copies of facility policies and protocols for students to review, such as blood glucose procedure, wound care, diabetic, blood transfusion, etc. Determine the resources you expect students to bring to clinical. Could you keep a copy of essential textbooks somewhere on the unit as a resource so students do not need to bring them each week?

Identify specific content areas to include in your clinical orientation that emphasize DEEP learning of the MOST important information. Identify the following at orientation or better yet BEFORE orientation.

1. Most common medications administered in this setting (top 10-15)
2. List of medication knowledge questions that students will be asked
3. Most common labs (top 10)
4. Most common clinical presentations/medical problems (3-5)
5. Nursing skills that will be used

Clinical Paperwork

The amount of clinical paperwork that students are required to complete each week is another area where TMI tends to prevail in nursing education. Clinical paperwork, including the written care plan, can be several pages or more in length. Students do not know what to focus on and every aspect of clinical paperwork is seen as equally important.

Emphasize DEEP learning of what is most important and the paperwork must reflect this priority as well. Developing the ability to THINK like a nurse using clinical reasoning is the primary objective of clinical education. Use this standard to evaluate the strength of current clinical paperwork. If you have recommendations to change clinical prep, go through the department chain of command to determine if clinical paperwork can be changed by faculty based on the principle of academic freedom or if paperwork is standardized throughout the level and needs to be reviewed by the team. Numerous tools are included in this book that can be adapted to strengthen the application of clinical reasoning in your clinical paperwork.

Crucial Components of Clinical

The following are key aspects of the clinical day with practical recommendations to structure the clinical day:

• Patient assignments

• Student preparation
• Pre-conference
• Patient care begins: FIRST half of clinical
• Patient care begins: SECOND half of clinical
• Post-conference

Patient Assignments

When making patient assignments, consider the level that you are teaching to guide the type and number of patients that students are assigned. At the fundamental level, most students should be assigned one patient. But using the guideline that the advanced level clinical experience needs to mirror real-world practice, the skills of multitasking and priority setting for more than one patient can only be developed by having multiple patient assignments. As much as possible, assign advanced nursing students two patients within your clinical setting. It may not be practical for every student to have a two-patient assignment, but create a schedule so that at least two to three students each advanced clinical have a multiple patient assignment.

I have had advanced students take up to three patients in the past. As I look back, this burden was excessive for most students to handle successfully, and have since limited multiple assignments to two patients. Patricia Benner and the coauthors of *Educating Nurses* (2010) also advocate for no more than two patients to be assigned to students in the clinical setting.

The patients who are assigned are also an indirect responsibility shared by the instructor. This is one reason why it is reasonable for students to receive a one-patient assignment in acute care. With the increasing acuity of patients and the supervision that students need with tasks, having students take additional patients in an acute care setting can be difficult. If your clinical site is in long-term care, patients are stable, making it much easier for each student to care for two patients.

To make a two-patient assignment doable for students, I assign a simple patient who may be going home in the next day and a middle-of-the-road patient with multiple medications who is not too demanding. I make the student responsible for all aspects of care for both patients, including medications and treatments. I save the most complex patients on the unit for students who have a single-patient assignment to maximize their learning.

How to Make Assignments

Deciding on the number of patients that students will care for is simple. Making actual assignments is a bit more difficult. The following are some practical tips to guide you in making assignments for your students (Billings & Halstead, 2016).

- Get input from the charge nurse to determine suitable patients. This also helps to build a trusting, supportive relationship between you, the program, and the staff of the facility where you have clinical.
- Quickly make rounds and talk to each patient to obtain a quick overview and receive permission for a student to assist in providing care that day.
- Expect the unexpected! Have an extra one or two patients in addition to what your students will require in case a patient goes home early, or something else changes.

Student Preparation

Guide student learning by helping them recognize the aspects of the medical record that are most important to the nurse for their level. Depending on the clinical setting, students may come in the night before to complete patient preparation. If this is the case, limit the length of time students spend collecting data so that they are able to spend adequate time preparing for their patient the night before. It is also important to communicate a time limit regarding how much time they spend preparing for their patient the night before and get needed rest. I found this out the hard way when a student who appeared excessively tired admitted that she had been up all night preparing for her patient and had gotten no sleep!

In programs I taught clinical, student preparation was the night before for the first year of the program. The advanced level of the program typically had students come in the same day. If possible, this is an arrangement that is well suited for the development of students at their respective levels. Fundamental students benefit from the security of additional time to situate their knowledge to the bedside and have a higher degree of confidence coming in as prepared as possible.

At the advanced level, everything needs to mirror real-world clinical practice as much as possible. Therefore, have your advanced students prepare the same day, which is what they will do in practice. I have found about an hour to be adequate for students at this level to prepare for patient care, though even this amount of time is not reflective of real-world practice. I developed a simple, one-page patient preparation sheet that is an adaptation of what I use in clinical practice. It is best suited for advanced students and allows them to complete patient preparation in about 15 minutes per patient. This tool will be presented in the next chapter.

Pre-conference

Pre-conference is a valuable exercise that benefits the clinical educator as well as students. It provides an opportunity to validate student safety BEFORE clinical begins, as well as an opportunity for students to express concerns and seek clarification about the plan of care (Billings & Halstead, 2016). I keep pre-conference short, less than 15 minutes. I begin by sharing any updates and clarifying any questions that students may have. I validate student safety by having each student provide a brief summary of their patient to the clinical group based on the first eight questions from the clinical reasoning template. Since each student has only about one minute, each student uses the following structure to present their patient to the clinical group:

- Age/gender/primary medical problem.
- Based on the data collected, what is your nursing priority?
- What is the plan of care, including nursing priority/nursing interventions? (Have students ask this same question of the primary nurse when receiving report to ensure consistency and collaboration).
- What body system will you most thoroughly assess based on the primary problem of your patient?
- What is the most likely/worst possible complication to anticipate?
- What nursing assessment(s) will identify this complication if it develops?

By using a consistent structure as well as an emphasis on clinical reasoning, these questions provide another opportunity for students to practice nurse thinking that will prepare them for professional practice. Pre-conference also provides an opportunity to decrease student stress by being able to ask any clarifying questions before assuming care. Depending on the responses of students to these questions, I can quickly determine if students are prepared or unsafe to assume care at the BE-GINNING of clinical.

Patient Care Begins: FIRST Half of Clinical

The first two hours are always the busiest and start with a bang! Between the initial set of vital signs, nursing assessment, and medications that need to be passed, there is no shortage of things that need to be done. Once I receive the nurse report from the prior shift, I set priorities based on the acuity of the patients, just as I would do in practice. Once a student has collected the first set of vital signs and nursing assessment within the first hour, I ask the following clinical reasoning questions of each student:

• What clinical assessment data did you just collect is RELEVANT and needs to be TRENDED because it is clinically significant?

• Does your nursing priority or plan of care need to be modified in any way after assessing your patient?

Because medication administration will make me unavailable for up to an hour or more, I keep this initial student contact brief and no more than a couple minutes in length. Once this brief collaboration has taken place with each student and there have been no significant changes that require an intervention, I can focus on assisting students with medication administration or any treatments that need to be done, knowing that there are no fires to put out, at least not yet!

Medication Administration

Though medication administration is a basic skill, do NOT allow this to be the emphasis or consume most of your time in the clinical setting. Your primary objective as a clinical educator is to develop the THINKING of each student and have the time to develop this each clinical. Depending on the level of your clinical, there are two practical approaches that can be implemented to make this possible.

• Have fewer students pass medications each clinical

• Another option for fundamental students is to have them pair up for the first few weeks to manage a single patient. One student passes meds, and the other does clinical paperwork. Both are involved in assessment and documentation. They have to work together as a team and collaborate. When I am not helping students with meds, I check in with students'

progress on their clinical paperwork and making sure students are correctly documenting in the medical record.

• If a student has successfully "tested out" with you and is safe to administer medications, if possible in your setting, have the students administer medications with the nurse to whom they are assigned. This will allow you to focus your time and attention on students who require additional mentoring and guidance in the clinical setting with medication administration or any other aspects of care. Let the nurse know your expectations for medication administration and what questions should still be asked!

Have a predetermined list of questions that you expect students to answer before administering medications. The five questions that I would use for the most common medications include the following:

1. What is the pharmacologic class? What is it for?
2. Why is your patient receiving it?
3. What is the expected patient response based on the mechanism of action?
4. What assessments do you need to know before you administer and then follow up afterward?
5. Is this a safe dose? Is the dose range low–mid–high?

Patient Care Begins: SECOND Half of Clinical

Once the dust settles after the first half of clinical, my priority is to spend time with EVERY student to develop the thinking that is required by the professional nurse. The following are some practical strategies that emphasize clinical reasoning that I have found successful to develop nurse thinking:

1. Identify relevant data
2. Recognize clinical relationships
3. Review chart together
4. Questions to promote learning

Identify Relevant Data

As you review clinical paperwork and data they have collected from the chart, ask students to identify relevant clinical data that can include lab values, vital signs, and assessment data. Students must be able to verbalize the clinical significance, or WHY this data is relevant. When a student is able to do both, the foundation of critical and clinical thinking is strengthened and established.

Recognize Clinical Relationships

The ability to identify and recognize relationships or patterns of clinical data is a thinking skill that nurses develop as they acquire experience in practice. Clinical educators have the ability to develop real-world nurse thinking skills by guiding students to recognize these six clinical relationships with each patient in their care.

1. What is the RELATIONSHIP of the past medical history and current medications?
2. What is the RELATIONSHIP between RELEVANT present problem data and the primary medical problem?
3. What is RELATIONSHIP between RELEVANT clinical data and the primary problem?
4. What is RELATIONSHIP between the primary medical problem and nursing priority?
5. What is RELATIONSHIP between the primary care provider's orders and primary problem?
6. What is RELATIONSHIP between diseases in PMH that may have contributed to the development of the current problem?

As you review each student's clinical paperwork or the medical record, reinforce these clinical relationships by asking them as a question.

Review Chart Together

There is nothing more powerful than the patient medical record to make clinical realities and classroom content come alive. Use the chart to promote your students' learning in the clinical setting. As an experienced nurse, it is easy to take for granted the fluidity and ease that you are able to navigate through a chart to obtain essential information to prepare for patient care. Novice student nurses do not have this experience and need intentional guidance to develop the skills required to access what is most important from the medical record. Be sure to review this essential skill in clinical orientation and reinforce it in the clinical setting as you briefly review the medical record together.

Though I may only have a few minutes with each student, I personally highlight and review these aspects of the medical record:

History of present problem
- What was the chief complaint that brought your patient to the hospital or current care setting? This can

be found in the emergency department record, or in the H&P of the admitting physician.
- Determine if the patient presentation was textbook or had variances to expected norms. Because novice nurses are concrete learners, the textbook is the standard, and students do not readily recognize the variances or ambiguity that is often seen with presenting symptoms of any illness. When presenting symptoms are different than textbook norms, this contextualization to practice will maximize learning because students have the clinical "hook" of their own patient's case to illustrate this reality.

Labs/diagnostic tests
- Briefly review the current labs with an emphasis on RELEVANCE and the current TREND of the most important lab values. If your clinical is in acute care, the EMR has revolutionized the ease of not only having all lab values on one screen, but the most recent lab is underneath the current. This facilitates the identification of current trends to help nurses determine if their patient is improving based on these physiological markers.
- Situate the clinical relationship of relevant abnormal lab values to the primary problem to integrate this relationship to promote student learning.

Primary care provider note
- Though reviewing the most recent nursing documentation is a given, the most recent primary care provider's note allows the nurse to see the BIG PICTURE of where this patient has been and where the patient is going. This note must be reviewed by students as part of their clinical prep. However, students will require guidance to UNDERSTAND the rationale or the WHY of the primary care provider's plan of care.
- Once this aspect of care is understood and the relationship of new orders based on the primary problem is understood, essential pieces of the clinical puzzle are recognized and the picture begins to come together!

Questions to Promote Learning

Asking questions is the single most effective strategy in the clinical setting to develop the critical and clinical thinking required for practice, yet schools of nursing do not adequately utilize pedagogies of inquiry (Benner, et al., 2010). The pedagogy of inquiry is not unique to nursing education, but goes back over 2,500 years to the Greek philosopher Socrates and his approach to learning that is referred to as Socratic questioning. In order to maximize the effectiveness of this pedagogy in your clinical, it is imperative that the nurse educator create a safe environment for students to learn and to make mistakes.

To ask questions and guide learning effectively, the educator must balance promoting and developing thinking without it coming across like an interrogation!

Avoid any hint of confrontation or nonverbal communication that could be interpreted as demeaning. Ask questions in a positive and supportive manner; this will promote the safe environment students need to maximize their learning. Reinforce that their responses will not influence their clinical grade.

Start with lower-level comprehension questions to assess what students know (remember the definition of critical thinking...unless students KNOW they will be unable to APPLY) and then build to higher-level application and analysis questions. If a student is unable to answer a clinical question, do not offer the answer but instead ask another question that is at the student's knowledge or comprehension level to draw out the correct answer from the student.

Ask a student what a beta blocker is blocking. Many are unable to answer this question. Back up and ask a simple knowledge/comprehension question. "Which nervous system is a beta blocker blocking, parasympathetic or sympathetic?" Most students recognize that it is the sympathetic nervous system and the resultant fight or flight response. Another approach that the clinical educator can use when a student does not have an answer to a question is to give time to respond by allowing silence. This will allow the student to regroup and draw the response out on their own if they are able to do so.

To use questions to develop nurse thinking, I have found the following questions to be the most effective.

General Questions
- What is the ONE thing you can do today to advance the plan of care?
- What additional information do you need to review in the chart to help you advance the plan of care?
- What will be the most important things that need to

be included in your end of shift report to ensure that the plan of care continues to be advanced?
- What examples of BEST nursing practice did you observe from your primary nurse?
- What examples of POOR nursing practice did you observe from your primary nurse? What contributing factors may have influenced poor practice that was observed? (these questions may be best suited for clinical post-conference and discussed as a group together)

"What If" Questions
This series of questions effectively situates the most likely/worst possible complication. Use the most common complications in your clinical setting to promote this proactive nurse thinking skill. Expect students to not only identify the nursing assessments but also the interventions if any of these complications develop. Create your own "what if" questions based on your clinical setting.
What if your patient...
- Develops chest pain?
- Develops a temp of 101?
- BP drops to 90/50?
- Develops acute confusion on patient controlled analgesia?
- Develops rapid irregular heart rate of 140?
- Develops sudden onset of shortness of breath?

Why?
This one-word question is relevant and needs to be asked because the nurse must not only be able to DO the right thing, but know the WHY or rationale of EVERYTHING that is done in clinical practice to be safe.
- WHY is your patient receiving this medication?
- HOW will you know it was effective?
- WHY did the physician order this treatment/medication?
- HOW will it benefit the patient?
- WHY would this nursing intervention be effective to advance the plan of care?

What Are Your Priorities?
Since priority setting is a struggle for novice/advanced beginner nursing students, be intentional to address priority setting by asking students:
- Does your nursing priority or plan of care need to be modified in any way after assessing your patient?

• What educational priorities have you identified and how will you address them?

Clinical Reasoning Questions to Develop Nurse Thinking

Use my 12 clinical reasoning questions that capture the essence of how a nurse thinks in practice. Better yet, incorporate them into your clinical paperwork. I have had faculty successfully use the following 12 questions as the basis for advanced clinical paperwork.

Formulate and reflect on the following BEFORE providing care:

1. What is the primary problem and what is its underlying cause or pathophysiology?
2. What clinical data from the chart are RELEVANT and need to be trended because they are clinically significant?
3. List all relevant nursing priorities. Which nursing priority captures the "essence" of your patient's current status and will guide your plan of care?
4. What nursing interventions will you initiate based on this priority and what are the desired outcomes?
5. What body system(s), key assessments, and psychosocial needs will you focus on based on your patient's primary problem or nursing care priority?
6. What is the worst possible/most likely complication(s) to anticipate based on the primary problem?
7. What nursing assessments will identify this complication EARLY if it develops?
8. What nursing interventions will you initiate if this complication develops?

Formulate and reflect on the following WHILE providing care:

1. What clinical assessment data did you just collect that are RELEVANT and need to be TRENDED because they are clinically significant to detect a change in status?
2. Does your nursing priority or plan of care need to be modified in any way after assessing your patient?
3. After reviewing the primary care provider's note, what is the rationale for any new orders or changes made?
4. What educational priorities have you identified and how will you address them?

Socratic Questions

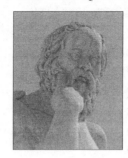

Socratic questioning is similar but different than clinical reasoning. Clinical reasoning is the essence of nurse thinking and is a construct unique to practice-based professions such as nursing. Once RELEVANT clinical data is identified by a student, use Socratic questions to assess and probe student thinking further, to determine the extent of student knowledge related to patient care or to analyze understanding of an essential concept or line of reasoning.

This is the higher level of analysis and understanding nursing students require to reason through the nuances and ambiguities often present in patient care. It teaches students to dig beneath the surface of what they think and cultivate deep learning. Using Socratic questions will help develop active, independent learners.

Five Types of Socratic Questions

To get the wheels turning and make an ancient Greek philosopher practical, here are categories of Socratic questions and the types of questions nurse educators can ask to evaluate the critical thinking of nursing students in the clinical setting (Oermann, 1997):

Clarification Questions

• Tell me about your client's condition/problems/needs
• What are the most important client/family/community problems? Why?

Questions to Probe Assumptions

• You seem to be assuming that your client's responses are due to _____. Tell me more about your thinking here.
• On what data have you based your decisions? Why?
• Your decisions about this client/family/community are based on your assumptions that _____. Is this always the case? Why or why not?

Questions to Probe Reasons

• What are other possible reasons for ____?
• Tell me why?
• What would do if ____? Why?

Questions on Differing Perspectives

• What are other possibilities? Alternatives?

- How might the client/family view this situation?
- Tell me about different interventions that might be possible and why each one would be appropriate?

Questions on Consequences

- If this occurs, what would you expect to happen next? Why?
- What are the consequences of each of these possible approaches?
- What would you do in this situation and why?

Caring Questions

These two questions were discussed earlier and emphasize the importance and relevance of caring and the art of nursing.

1. What is the patient likely experiencing/feeling right now in this situation?
2. What can I do to engage myself with this patient's experience and show that they matter to me as a person?

Validating Student Documentation

Before you can start post-conference and call it a clinical day, there is one last thing that must be reviewed and evaluated: student documentation. One of the benefits of carefully reviewing student documentation is that it reflects the abilities, weaknesses, and strengths of the student. Students who are sloppy and minimal in their documentation may carry this trait into their practice and will need to be watched and assessed more closely, while those who are incredibly detailed and thorough will be likely to carry this into their practice.

If the clinical site allows students to chart in the electronic medical record, this facilitates reviewing the documentation for all students. Simply make notes, and then review your feedback with each student and have them make corrections as needed. I communicated that the final hour of clinical was when I expected student documentation to be completed so it could be reviewed, adjustments made if needed, and students would still have plenty of time to complete clinical paperwork and be prepared for post-conference.

Post-conference

Although it is tempting to shorten post-conference at the end of a busy clinical day, I have found that this is one of the richest opportunities for students to learn and reflect from not only their clinical experience, but also from the patient care experiences of other students. Encourage student participation in all aspects of post-conference. The faculty role is to facilitate and guide student discussion on the clinical experience, identify problems, or ventilate feelings (Billings & Halstead, 2016). Commit at least 45-60 minutes for post-conference discussion.

Post-conference provides the opportunity to instill the professional behavior of reflection. Student learning and connections to classroom theory can be enhanced during post-conference by asking high-level questions that require students to think critically (Oermann, 2008). This can be facilitated by asking any or all of the following reflection questions.

- What went well today in clinical and why? (HIGH point)
- What would you do differently today and why? (LOW point)
- What did you learn today that you can apply to future patients you care for?

Developing Nurse Thinking

To develop clinical reasoning, each student needs to share specific events of the clinical experience and replay it (Nielson, Stragnell, & Jester, 2007). Sharing clinical experiences with group discussion can expand and strengthen student learning (Benner, et al., 2010). As students reflect and share, faculty need to put these clinical narratives into context, question assumptions, identify knowledge gaps, and help students discover insights (Ironside & Hayden-Miles, 2012). This requires faculty to remain fully engaged as student's share, despite being emotionally and physically exhausted at the end of the clinical day! This level of reflection will facilitate the development of clinical reasoning and judgment (Kuiper, 2013).

Use Tanner's model of clinical judgment to further guide reflection. This includes having students reflect on the following (Wheeler, Butell, Epeneter, Langford, & Doughty Taylor, 2016):

Noticing

- What did you notice about this situation in clinical?
- What was your initial grasp of the situation? Did this change as the situation unfolded?
- Be thorough in describing what you noticed as being important to the story of this situation.

Interpreting

- Describe what you thought about the situation.
- Have you had previous experiences that helped guide you during the situation?
- How did your formal knowledge from your nursing and liberal arts education help you in this situation?

Responding

- As you proceeded through this situation, what were your goals?
- How did you help in the situation?

Reflection-in-action

- What were the key issues happening in the situation? What was the outcome?
- Were you engaged in the situation and did you fully understand what was happening during the situation?
- Were there others who helped you in the situation? What did you learn from them?

Reflection-on-action and clinical learning

- What occurred as a result of your nursing actions? Were you satisfied with these results?
- Were there particular actions you were proud of? Or, were there actions you wished you could do over and improve?
- Were there things that you would do differently if you encountered this situation again?
- How will you prepare yourself for similar situations in the future?

Connecting Classroom and Clinical Learning

Another strategy that connects classroom and clinical content is having full-time faculty develop open-ended questions directly related to what has been taught recently in the classroom. This is helpful when clinical adjunct faculty are utilized who do not typically have firsthand knowledge of what is being taught on campus (Harvey, 2015).

An example of open-ended questions that were developed in one study was related to nursing ethics and alterations in the respiratory system. One of the course objectives was to "discuss the ethical values within the Code of Ethics for Registered Nurses which are most applicable to the care you provided to your patient this week." This led to developing the following questions that were utilized in post-conference (Harvey, 2015):

- Discuss the ethical considerations in providing care to your patient with end-stage respiratory disease.
- What are the physical and psychological manifestations of a patient with end-stage respiratory disease?
- Define the term "aggressive treatment"
- How might the ethical considerations vary with a patient receiving aggressive treatment versus end-stage aspects of the disease?

Make post-conference a place where it is safe to share mistakes and learn from errors in clinical judgment. Students have the opportunity to learn from other students' mistakes so that they are not as likely to repeat them in practice. Though a high bar is necessary for excellence in nursing education, it is important to remember that every nursing student is also human and will likely make a mistake at some point in the program. Therefore, emphasize that a student is not defined by their mistakes, but by their response to them. Any error or missed assessment, when shared in the context of post-conference reflection, is a clinical take-away that will not be forgotten by that student or by the entire clinical group.

In addition to reflection, post-conference is also an opportunity to discuss the highs and lows of what students have observed by the actions of nurses on the unit. Examples of "lows" may include unsafe practice or disrespectful and uncivil behavior experienced or witnessed by a student. These "lows" and influencing factors that may contribute to their existence must be openly addressed. By acknowledging the pressing demands of real-world clinical practice, but offering practical strategies to maintain a high bar of patient safety and a culture of respect, you will prepare students for what they will soon experience after they graduate and encourage the highest level of professionalism in all they do.

Another topic to have students reflect on in post-conference is caring. If I did not have time to discuss caring with students during clinical, the two caring questions I have formulated provide a basis for each student to share their reflections.

In addition to reflection, post-conference an effective forum to discuss relevant topics in nursing. This is an opportunity where the clinical nurse educator has the freedom to share what is important to them as a practicing nurse. Though I did not have a topic for every post-conference clinical, I made it a priority to discuss subjects such as men in nursing, incivility in the nursing profession, and the importance of caring before the end of the clinical rotation.

Clinical Journals

Do you ever wonder what students are thinking? There is an easy way to get inside the mind and lived experience of your students each week. An indispensable exercise that will strengthen and develop nurse thinking is the use of a weekly clinical journal. When students reflect and share their highs and lows of the clinical day, how they applied classroom learning in the clinical setting, and the emotions they experienced while caring, these insights give a window to the souls of your students and evaluate their current level of clinical thinking.

To successfully use journaling to strengthen reflection, identify the clinical objectives that are met, determine the length and content that needs to be included each week. I did not grade journals, so students were encouraged to be real and have the freedom to share their insights without it impacting their clinical grade. However, I did provide feedback and encouragement when and where needed!

Components for clinical journaling can include the following:
- Reflect on what you learned
- Reflect on the feelings you experienced
- Reflect on what could have been differently to obtain a desired outcome

Specific questions that educators can use to facilitate student journaling include the following (Billings & Halstead, 2016):
- How do you feel about your clinical day?
- What was the best part of your clinical day?
- What did you feel most confident about?
- If you could do your clinical day over, what would you do differently?
- What did you learn today that you can apply to future patients with similar problems?
- What do you need to learn more about?
- What went well with the interactions that you had with your primary nurse?
- Did you have any patient quality or safety issues that needed to be addressed?

Requiring students to use focused reflection by using specific questions with journaling and post-conference discussion was found to be an effective strategy to integrate classroom and clinical learning and strengthen the development of clinical reasoning (Murphy, 2004). To accomplish this objective in nursing education, I created two tools to structure student reflection based on Tanner's model of clinical judgment making. They are "Reflection-IN-Action" and "Reflection-ON-Action" that are explained in depth later in the book and included in the Transformation Toolbox.

Traits of Unsuccessful Students

Just as there are clinical indicators of patients who are at higher risk to develop complications due to age and pre-existing medical problems and at risk to require "rescue" by the nurse, there are traits that at-risk students demonstrate that need to be recognized by clinical educators. Just as EARLY identification of a patient complication will likely result in successful "rescue" with a change of status, EARLY identification of at-risk students can help them be successful.

In one study, the following traits and examples of behavior were identified in unsuccessful students (Lewallen & DeBrew, 2012):

Unable to function in fast-paced clinical environment
- Unmotivated
- Disinterested
- Unable to think critically
- Lacks basic skills
- Tries to fly under the radar (tries to avoid being noticed)

Jeopardizes patient safety and commits legal/ethical violations
- Unsafe behaviors
- Legal/ethical issues
- Overconfident

Unprepared for clinical and does not show improvement
- Patterns of negative behaviors do not improve
- Unprepared for clinical
- Consistently tardy

- Does not take responsibility for learning
- Makes excuses
- Poorly written work
- Immature

Difficulty communicating with patients, faculty, peers, and clinical staff

- Poor communication skills with patients
- Poor professional communication
- Receives complaints
- Does not demonstrate caring behaviors

Successful Students

In contrast, students who were successful demonstrated the following traits and examples of behavior (Lewallen & DeBrew, 2012):

Prepared for clinical setting

- Brings needed resources
- Professional in dress and manner
- Researched medications and patient pathophysiology
- Prompt with attendance and paperwork
- Organized

Able to think critically by transferring knowledge from the classroom to the clinical setting

- Strong knowledge base that is applied in clinical setting
- Attentive and makes clinical connections
- Critical thinker and problem solver

Able to develop appropriate plan of care and provides safe care

- Understands and can use nursing process
- Prioritizes care

Builds relationships and communicates effectively with faculty, staff, patients, and peers

- Effective communicator
- Demonstrates respect
- Works well with others
- Asks appropriate questions

Has a positive attitude and is willing to learn

- Seeks out learning opportunities
- Eager to learn
- Positive attitude
- Self-motivated
- Caring
- Open to learning
- Engaged
- Honest

Demonstrates progress, accepts feedback and adapts to clinical experience

- Receives constructive feedback and uses to demonstrate progress and growth
- Flexible in the clinical setting

Identifying the traits of successful as well as unsuccessful nursing students is relevant not only for educators but also for students. Faculty should describe what is expected and communicate these expectations and characteristics that successful students represent. If both students and faculty are aware of what comprises unsatisfactory performance, this can help remove some of the ambiguity that is inherently present in clinical evaluation of students. Use these traits to guide clinical evaluation. These characteristics are easily measurable to determine if the student is performing according to these expectations. It can simplify clinical evaluation by making it more concrete and removing as much subjectivity as possible. Incorporate these traits in your clinical evaluation form if they are not already present. This is a practical way to integrate educational best practices into the evaluation of students in your program

How to Evaluate Student Performance

When I was a new clinical adjunct, evaluating student performance was one of the most difficult responsibilities I had. Because I was new to this role, I was uncertain and unsure of my clinical judgments of students and tended to err on being overwhelmingly positive with most students. But objectively evaluating student performance is one of the most important responsibilities of a clinical educator.

Student evaluation is inherently subjective. It is your interpretation of student performance. This can lead to accusations of being biased or unfair. If there are performance issues that must be addressed, depending on the maturity of the student, they may or may not take responsibility and may instead blame you as the instructor or even file a complaint.

Carefully review the syllabus, student handbook, and clinical performance rubric that guide expectations for safe student performance and make sure it is well understood by students as well as yourself. Ensure that the rubric is concrete and each aspect of performance is clearly defined and able to be understood by both students and faculty. This will remove as much subjectivity as possible. It is important to clarify how your program defines unsafe practice and what will result in remediation and what could result in immediate course failure.

Another way to evaluate students is to provide a copy of the clinical evaluation form for students to review (this should also be done in orientation) and ask them to verbalize how they met the goal of health promotion, patient teaching, etc. Use your observations to validate the accuracy of this assessment by the student. This can be an effective strategy to use in clinical evaluation.

Evaluating SAFETY

The following questions need to be answered to provide guidance and clarity for standards of unsafe practice in your clinical:

- How many incidents equal unsafe clinical practice?
- Is one incident a concern, or does there need to be a pattern of unsafe practice?
- What type of incident is unsafe that can be remediated, compared with examples that may constitute a course failure? (Scanlan, Dean Care, & Gessler, 2001)

Student behaviors that violate patient safety standards can include (Herman, Manning, Zager, 2011):

- Failure to follow the Rights of medication administration
- The number and nature of medication errors that will be allowed as part of the learning process
- Failure to follow infection control standards (hand washing/isolation precautions)
- Failure to follow patient safety standards (patient was put at risk)
- Failure to adhere to HIPPA laws
- Failure to report RELEVANT clinical data to nurse or clinical instructor
- Failure to document nursing assessments, interventions, evaluation of care, or documentation that was inaccurate
- Performing nursing interventions without supervision when supervision is required
- Failure to ensure emotional safety of patient. Patient/family expressed concerns regarding lack of caring or inappropriate conduct/communication

Evaluating THINKING

Educators evaluate the thinking and problem-solving ability of students to determine safety in the clinical setting. Faculty tend to focus on evaluating task completion and observing skills. Evaluating student thinking can be more difficult, yet it is something that also must be determined. Student journals can be one tool that educators can use, but this provides an indirect measure of nurse thinking. What educators require are tools that can directly evaluate clinical reasoning and clinical judgment making of students.

There are four distinct aspects of nurse thinking that need to be assessed in the clinical setting:

- Nursing process
- Critical thinking
- Pattern recognition or clinical relationships
- Clinical reasoning

The traditional written care plan emphasizes only one aspect of how a nurse thinks, which is nursing process. Critical thinking, pattern recognition, and clinical reasoning also need to be evaluated by the clinical educator. I have developed tools that can help develop and evaluate these additional nurse thinking skills and will be discussed in the next chapter.

Teaching vs. Evaluation

The clinical educator must strike a balance between the two sometimes competing roles and responsibilities of a TEACHER and EVALUATOR of a student's performance. This is an area I struggled with as a clinical expert who worked with fundamental students in the clinical setting. As a new clinical adjunct, my pendulum swung in the direction of being an evaluator of almost everything a student did in the clinical setting. If problems were identified, I wanted to be sure they were recognized and addressed and needed remediation initiated.

As I look back, there was a mindset that would have helped me be more effective as a clinical educator. I needed to have realistic expectations. This is one reason why I have now adopted a "mulligan" system with my students in the clinical setting. If you are a golfer, you know that a mulligan is an agreement to have ONE "do over" if a bad shot was made during the round; it does not count. You get another chance to do better and hit another ball. In the same way, I have seen that students also need a "mulligan," but it needs to be done with wisdom, because patient care is involved, not a game of golf!

If an error was made that would not have caused patient harm, it is addressed and needed learning and expectations are clearly communicated. Because students, as in golf, are allowed only ONE mulligan, the problem behavior must be addressed and successfully remediated. If this or a similar problem does not resurface again during the clinical rotation, it is treated as a successful "do over" and NO adverse effects are reflected in the summative clinical grade. On the flip side, if a mulligan is given and the same or similar problem resurfaces, this is now a pattern that must be treated as a problem that warrants attention and remediation.

Formative vs. Summative Evaluation

The example I just gave with a mulligan illustrates the essence of FORMATIVE evaluation. The goal of formative assessment is to gather feedback that can be used by the instructor and student so improvement can be made. The purpose of formative evaluation is to help students develop clinical knowledge, skills, and indicate areas where additional learning and practice are needed so that performance can be improved. It is diagnostic and should NOT be graded. In contrast, SUMMATIVE assessment is graded and is the summary or measure of the level of proficiency that has been demonstrated at mid-clinical and final evaluation. It summarizes student competency to determine if students have achieved the clinical outcomes and competencies (Gaberson, Oermann, & Shellenbarger, 2015).

Because fundamental students are novice nurses, a greater emphasis must be placed on teaching, with evaluation being secondary. At the advanced level, evaluation should be weighted higher because of the increased amount of clinical experience that leads to expectations for higher levels of clinical performance. When advanced students are unable to translate basic fundamental content to the bedside, it is a RED FLAG that requires fur-

ther assessment to determine if other clinical deficiencies may also be present.

Ensuring Fairness

To be as objective as possible with clinical evaluation, it is imperative to AVOID ASSUMPTIONS about any student. This is also a caring intervention with Swanson's caring theory discussed earlier, and has relevance in this context. Each of us has some degree of bias or assumptions about students based on our past experiences. These assumptions may be based on age, gender, ethnicity, sexual orientation, or even the presence of tattoos and body piercings. Be aware where your assumptions tend to lie and do what is needed to give every student a level playing field in your clinical.

Additional principles to ensure fairness in clinical evaluation include the following (Gaberson, et al., 2015):

1. **Reflect and identify values, attitudes, and beliefs that may influence the evaluation process.** Remember that students also have their own sets of values and attitudes that influence how they receive evaluation of performance. You may need to guide students to become more self-aware and accepting of any weaknesses so they can be addressed and remedied.

2. **Clinical evaluation is based on course outcomes or competencies.** Identify the specific clinical objectives that must be met and criteria to determine if they were met. This removes all subjectivity related to evaluation.

3. **Develop a supportive clinical learning environment.** The educator must develop a healthy culture where students are supported so learning and development of clinical competencies take place. Students need to feel safe and comfortable asking questions and seeking guidance rather than avoiding them as well as you in the clinical setting. Students need to know that your feedback is intended to help them IMPROVE performance and not REMOVE them from the program!

4. **Provide enough learning time BEFORE performance is evaluated.** Since students need to focus on learning and practice skills, provide enough time to allow students to demonstrate that they are able to meet course objectives before formal evaluation.

How to Provide Feedback

Feedback is the cornerstone of effective clinical teaching and improves students' clinical performance (Cantillon & Sargant, 2008). Feedback can be defined as providing specific information that compares the student's observed performance against the standard that has been taught. To be effective, feedback must be given with the intent to improve the student's performance and presented in a way that allows the student to comprehend and accept it so that feedback can be applied in practice (Cantillon & Sargant, 2008).

One of the most important responsibilities that an educator has in the clinical setting is to provide honest, ONGOING feedback on students' strengths as well as weaknesses and what they need to do to improve. Do not wait until scheduled times (mid-term, etc.) to provide this feedback, but do so in a timely manner. To create a culture where student feedback will be well received regardless of the content, consistently AFFIRM students and what they are doing well. Nursing students tend to be high-performing achievers and can feel like failures because of the rigors of nursing school when constructive feedback is given.

To provide feedback that enhances student learning, the majority of students valued feedback that was both positive and constructive. When students are engaged in learning, feedback will be more effective. When feedback is absent, ambiguous, and inconsistent, this is a barrier to student learning (Giles, Gilbert, McNeill, 2014). To provide feedback well, both students and educators need to be engaged and consistent to strengthen student learning.

When feedback needs to be given, use the following principles to provide needed feedback that same clinical day (Herman, Manning, Zager, 2011):

- Be concrete and specific with your concerns.
- Guide students so they can improve performance. Continue to observe and assess to determine if improvement has been made and provide feedback (positive or constructive).
- Be timely. Be sure to address the concern before the student leaves the clinical site.
- Always give feedback in PRIVATE, never in front of others, including the patient.

In one study, providing feedback using the following steps enhanced teamwork and collaboration in the clinical setting (Motley & Dolansky, 2015):

1. **Create a culture of feedback.** Educators must communicate to students that feedback is a normal, everyday occurrence in the clinical setting.
2. **Use structured communication tools.** Use pre-conference and post-conference to ask consistent questions each clinical.
3. **Encourage dialogue.** In order to develop the higher-level thinking skills of problem solving, analyzing situations, and applying knowledge, dialogue and questioning with students is required each clinical. Dialogue also teaches the professional skill of collaboration.
4. **Acknowledge the human factor.** Know each student well enough so that feedback is given that considers the personality and temperament as well as the student's perspective and rationale for clinical judgments.
5. **Embrace a leadership role.** Embrace the responsibility to be a leader and model this to students. Use your passion for nursing to inspire, motivate, advocate, and support students, and use a variety of learning activities including unfolding case studies to prepare students for practice.

Be aware of any nonverbal messaging and communication when you are under stress that can adversely impact the student-faculty relationship that makes it difficult for students to learn from you. Just as in a personal relationship, the time it took to develop a healthy trust relationship can be destroyed in seconds when any of the following faculty behaviors are evident:

- **Negative body language.** Be aware of what your body language, facial expressions communicate to students.
- **Harsh tone of voice.** Choose your words carefully when providing feedback or interacting with students. What you say and HOW you communicate and provide feedback will not be quickly forgotten. Put as much effort into determining what you will say as you did in carefully documenting the concern.
- **Judgmental attitude.** Be careful not to make negative assumptions or judgments with words that could wound your students.

Providing Negative Feedback

Sharing negative feedback to students is difficult and challenging, but is essential to help students be successful (McGregor, 2007). In order to provide negative feedback effectively, the following steps guided faculty to communicate negative feedback that was well received by students (Meyer & Peters, 2010):

1. **Faculty's written description of the situation.** Before meeting with the student, write a concise, factual account of the situation that is free of judgments or assumptions.

2. **Student's verbal explanation of the situation.** Have the student read what faculty wrote and encourage the student to share their perception of the event.

3. **Student's written summary of the situation.** Allowing the student to write out their observations and perception creates an environment where the student feels heard and respected. This reflection can provide valuable insight to the educator.

4. **Mutual discussion to understand the issue and review options for addressing the issue.**

5. **Faculty's written plan of action based.** Once all information has been assimilated by faculty, next steps can be determined.

Be a Coach

Be a coach to your students in the clinical setting. Instead of looking for deficiencies and what students are struggling with, address student learning from a strengths-based approach. A strengths-based approach creates a partnership with the clinical instructor, which focuses on exploring the student's capabilities, initiative, and skills (Kalkebrenner & Brandt, 2011).

Coaching uses role modeling and regular meetings with students to review performance and new skills, or encourage and enhance decision making. The coaching process relies on regular and clear, direct feedback from clinical faculty on student performance. The educator must be aware how each student is doing and if they meet clinical outcomes. Setting goals at the beginning of the clinical rotation can help define the direction and needs for each student. This coaching approach also encourages partnership with each student (Kalkebrenner & Brandt, 2011).

How to Manage the Struggling or Unsafe Student

The clinical setting stresses students the most (Mahut, 1998)! In one program, 10-20 percent of students had documented struggles in the clinical setting (Lynn & Twigg, 2011). The clinical educator has the solemn responsibility to protect the public from a student who is not safe to practice despite attempts to remediate. If a student has persistent struggles or has made an error, determine if they have insight. I am much more concerned about a student who has little to no insight or becomes defensive when concerns about clinical performance are discussed than the student who acknowledges the error and need to remediate. Depending on the severity of the concern, you may choose to address it immediately or it could wait until the end of clinical. It is essential to frame student performance as much as possible in the positive and use the program's definition for safe clinical practice as the bar that defines acceptable/unacceptable behavior.

Evaluating Emotional Safety

Unsafe student practice that may meet terms of dismissal from the program with no remediation allowed can usually be determined by identifying the end outcome to the patient had this incident been allowed to progress. Would patient harm have been likely or possible? If so, this would meet criteria for possible dismissal and failure of the clinical component. Though the majority of student concerns are the result of violations of PHYSICAL safety, educators need to also evaluate any concerns related to EMOTIONAL safety.

This is more difficult to ascertain, but is another aspect of safety that needs to be assessed. Emotional safety concerns may include a student who demonstrates a lack of sensitivity or caring toward the patient or any verbal or nonverbal behavior including communication that was harsh, abrupt, rude, or said in a way that was perceived as disrespectful and caused anxiety or stress to the patient.

To evaluate the emotional safety of students' care requires the educator to incorporate a simple routine at the end of each clinical. Quickly round on all patients at the end of the clinical day. Ask each patient or family member, "How was your experience of being cared for by… .today?" By using an open-ended question, you are providing the opportunity for the patient to share not only any possible concerns, but also affirm a positive experience the patient had with the student.

This same question also needs to be asked of the primary nurse assigned to work with the student that day. Whether documenting a clinical concern or evaluating student performance, anecdotal feedback by patients, family, and primary nurse can support faculty observations, especially if a student concern is present.

From my clinical experience, these are the most common student concerns and examples that I have witnessed. I have classified them as struggling or unsafe.

Struggling (remediation possible)

Inability to complete head-to-toe assessment fluently or correctly

- Unable to correctly identify valvular landmarks (aortic, pulmonic, tricuspid, mitral)
- Unable to properly complete respiratory assessment by not auscultating side to side, or not auscultating each landmark with a complete inspiration/expiration

Inability to correctly administer oral, subcutaneous, intramuscular, or intravenous medication

- Forgetting one of the "rights" of safe administration
- Unable to identify correct landmarks for injection
- Poor technique related to injection, not following procedures that were taught in skills lab

Breaking of sterile technique

- Dressing change
- Foley catheterization
- Spiking IV bag

Emotionally unsafe

- Lack of caring or mannerisms/actions that caused patient or family to feel anxious or caused emotional distress

Unsafe (no remediation)

Violation of medication "rights"

- Wrong medication
- Wrong dosage
- Wrong patient

Patient fall or close call due to inability to maintain basic safety

- Bed in high position
- Incorrect use/lack of waist belt

Because it is inevitable that remediation will be needed at some point in the clinical setting, familiarize yourself with the proper procedures and protocols regarding students so that you are proactive and one step ahead when any problem arises. Communicate student concerns directly with full-time faculty as soon as possible. Just as in clinical practice, documentation of a student concern must be factual, objective, detailed, and relevant to the current problem.

Once a struggling or potentially unsafe student has been identified, an inherent challenge will be the additional time commitment that will be required to document as well as manage this student in the clinical setting. Because additional monitoring will be needed to determine if remediation has been successful, the time that is needed to develop and promote the learning of other students can be impacted. It is important to recognize this reality and make needed adjustments in your clinical group.

Four-Step Clinical Remediation Process

In one study, clinical failures decreased by 4 to 6 percent when a four-step process was implemented. Consider adapting the following steps to strengthen your remediation process and increase student success in your program once a struggling student is identified (Lynn & Twigg, 2011).

- **Step one.** Identify the student's specific learning needs that need to be addressed to successfully remediate
- **Step two.** Develop a lesson plan or a mutual contract between the student and faculty of record in the clinical setting.
- **Step three.** Complete the lesson plan. This includes meeting with faculty of record in the nursing skills lab, work with human patient simulator to assist with clinical application, and synthesis of clinical knowledge and prioritization of patient needs. Skills lab faculty utilize the clinical grading rubric as a basis for evaluation during the simulation exercise.
- **Step four.** Successfully complete a clinical readiness test that incorporates nursing process to evaluate the student's clinical knowledge, application and synthesis of knowledge, and prioritization of patient needs. Clinical grading rubric is used for this testing. The student will return to the clinical setting or meet with the coordinator to determine options for continuing the course, depending on the outcome

If a student has a documented concern that is successfully remediated in the skills lab, what happens if the same problem reoccurs in the patient care setting? Refer to your student handbook or department policies. Clinical failure can best serve the needs of the struggling student and benefit them in the long run if they choose to continue in the nursing program. I have seen students who failed clinical come back, work hard to make needed changes, and be a stronger and better student as a result.

Always have a copy of nursing program policy handbook, nursing department phone tree, and copy of your clinical guidelines at the clinical site. At end of day, when a concern must be addressed, meet privately with student to go over the situation and the follow-up needed (completing incident form, remediation, etc.). Documentation is essential, so email the student and appropriate nursing faculty about what was discussed, what needs to be done, and set a follow-up meeting. This creates a paper trail to prevent "I was not told that." Make sure that you follow and complete the college policy within the specified time frame for clinical concerns. Students may have an option to appeal.

Provide careful documentation and feedback when unsafe behavior occurs. Take notes on a worksheet or copy of nursing program evaluation shortly after the occurrence to ensure accuracy of the details of unsafe behavior. Documentation identifies if the unsafe behavior is an isolated incident or a pattern of repetitive errors (Chunta, 2016).

Reflect

1. Do you tend to emphasize tasks or thinking as a clinical educator?

2. How do you develop the THINKING of students in the clinical setting?

3. Based on applying Benner's Novice to Expert theory to the level of students that you teach, are your clinical expectations of performance realistic? Do they need to be adjusted in any way?

4. What struggles do you have evaluating student clinical performance?

5. What did you learn from this chapter to strengthen your effectiveness as a clinical educator?

6. What is one action step you can do today to strengthen student learning in the clinical setting?

References

Benner, P., Sutphen, M., Leonard, V., & Day, L. (2010). *Educating nurses: A call for radical transformation.* San Francisco, CA: Jossey-Bass.

Billings, D. M., & Halstead, J. A. (2016). *Teaching in nursing: A guide for faculty* (5th ed.). *St. Louis, MO: El*sevier.

Cantillon, P., & Sargeant, J. (2008). Giving feedback in clinical settings. *BMJ (Clinical Research Education), 337.*

Chunta, K. (2016). Ensuring safety in clinical: Faculty role for managing students with unsafe behaviors. *Teaching and Learning in Nursing, 11*(3), 86-91.

Gaberson, K. B., & Oermann, M. H. (2010). *Clinical teaching strategies in nursing* (3rd ed.). New York: Springer Publishing Company.

Gaberson, K. B., Oermann, M. H., & Shellenbarger, T. (2015). *Clinical teaching strategies in nursing* (4th ed.). New York: Springer Publishing Company.

Giles, T.M., Gilbert, S., & McNeill, L. (2014). Nursing students' perceptions regarding the amount and type of written feedback required to enhance their learning. *Journal of Nursing Education, 53*(1), 23-30.

Harvey, G. (2015). Connecting theory to practice: Using guided questions to standardize clinical post=conference. *Journal of Nursing Education, 54*(11), 655-658.

Herman, J., Manning, L.S., & Zager, L.R. (2011). The eight-step approach to teaching clinical nursing. Duluth, GA: I CAN Publishing.

Ignatavicius, D. D., & Workman, M. L. (2016). *Medical-surgical nursing* (8th ed.). St. Louis, MO: Elsevier.

Ironside, P.M., & Hayden-Miles, M. (2012). Narrative pedagogy: Co-creating engaging learning experiences with students. In G.W Sherwood & S. Horton-Deutsch (Eds.), *Reflective practice: Transforming education and improving outcomes* (132-148). Indianapolis, IN: Sigma Theta Tau International.

Kalkebrenner, A.C., & Brandt, P.A. (2012). Coaching strategies for clinical learning: A strengths-based approach to student development. *Nurse Educator, 37*(5), 185-186.

Kuiper, R.A. (2013). Integration of innovative clinical reasoning pedagogies into a baccalaureate nursing curriculum. *Creative Nursing, 19*, 128-139.

Lewallen, L.P., & DeBrew, J.K. (2012). Successful and unsuccessful clinical nursing students. *Journal of Nursing Education, 51*(7), 389-395.

Lynn, M.C., & Twigg, R.D. (2011). A new approach to clinical remediation. *Journal of Nursing Education, 50*(3), 172-175.

McGregor, A. (2007). Academic success, clinical failure: academic success, clinical failure: struggling practices of a failing student. *Journal of Nursing Education, 46*(11), 504-511.

Mahat, G. (1998). Stress and coping: Junior baccalaureate nursing students in clinical settings. *Nursing Forum, 33,* 11-19.

Meyers, B., & Peters, J. (2010). An understanding approach to managing student issues. *Nurse Educator, 35*(2), 54-55.

Motley, C.L., & Dolansky, M.A. (2015). Five steps to providing effective feedback in the clinical setting: A new approach to promote teamwork and collaboration. *Journal of Nursing Education, 54*(7), 399-403.

Murphy, J.I. (2004). Using focused reflection and articulation to promote clinical reasoning: An evidence-based approach. *Nurse Education Perspectives, 25*(5), 226-231.

Nielsen, A., Stragnell, S., & Jester, P. (2007). Guide for reflection using the clinical judgment model. *Journal of Nursing Education, 46,* 513-516.

Oermann, M. (1997). Evaluating critical thinking in clinical practice. *Nurse Educator, 22*(5), 25-28.

Oermann, M.H. (2008). Ideas for post-clinical conferences. T*eaching and Learning in Nursing, 3,* 90-93.

Oermann, M. H., & Gaberson, K. B. (2014). *Evaluation and testing in nursing education,* (4th ed.). New York, NY: Springer Publishing.

Potter, P. A., Perry, A. G., Stockert, P. A., & Hall, A. M. (2017). *Fundamentals of nursing* (9th ed.). St. Louis, MO: Elsevier.

Scanlon, J. M., Care, W. D., & Gessler, S. (2001). Dealing with the unsafe student in clinical practice, *Nurse Educator, 26*(1), 23–27.

Wheeler, P.L., Butell, S.S., Epeneter, B.J., Langford, C.A., & Doughty Taylor, J. (2016). Storytelling: A guided reflection activity. *Journal of Nursing Education, 55*(3), 172-176.

23

Tools to Transform Clinical Education

Keith Rischer, RN, MA, CEN, CCRN

"To transform nursing education and meet the current and future needs of the clinical environment, innovative methods of teaching and learning are required now."

–Marsha Howell Adams, President of the National League for Nursing

There is a supplement to this book, a "Transformation Tool-box," in the appendix with handouts and worksheets for both the classroom and clinical settings to facilitate trans-formational change. These tools contextualize clinical rea-soning and will save hours of time and empower you to implement a "clinical reasoning curriculum" that will help your students to think more like a nurse. Each of these tools have been successfully "road tested" by educators across the country to bring transformational change. You may make copies of these tools as long as they are used only for your students in the program where you teach.

Tool #1:
DEEP Learning of MOST Important Clinical Template

This tool is a Word doc template that identifies the MOST important content and skills that students will use and apply in clinical BEFORE they start to practice in this setting. This content was discussed at length earlier. Use this template to list for students the following con-tent areas so they are well prepared to USE and APPLY this knowledge in your next clinical!

1. Top ten medications
2. Top ten labs
3. Most common illnesses/surgeries
4. Most common complications
5. Nursing skills

Tool #2:
Patient Preparation Worksheet

If you teach advanced students or have Capstone students who need a simple, yet practical patient preparation worksheet that will help them transition to real-world practice, this tool that can be adapted for this objective. Though patient prep worksheets can be as individual and unique, this Word doc worksheet lays an excellent foun-dation that can also be modified to fit your needs because it is a Word doc.

This worksheet contains four main components.

1. **Schedule day.** Provides an hour-by-hour planning of the day, with the larger spaces for even hours which tend to be busier with medication adminis-tration and treatments.

2. **Nursing assessment comparison table.** The table below the schedule has two rows of body system assessment data. The first row is what the nurse col-lects from the chart as part of patient prep or writes down from the nurse-to-nurse report. The row below is what the nurse writes down after assessing the patient. This provides for a quick comparison of data to identify any TRENDS that may be a clin-ical concern.

3. **Kardex data.** The bottom section contains basic Kardex data to ensure safe practice.

4. **Clinical reasoning questions.** On the reverse side

of this worksheet are the 12 clinical reasoning questions that provide the essence of what a nurse needs to know and how to think to provide safe care.

Reflect

1. How do you emphasize DEEP learning of what is most important in your clinical setting?

2. What tools can you incorporate in the clinical setting to develop the THINKING of nursing students?

3. Is it possible in your clinical setting to have students do an alternative assignment to decrease the number of students who provide direct patient care?

References

Benner, P. (1982). From novice to expert. *American Journal of Nursing, 82*(3), 402–407.

Koharchik, L., Caputi, L., Robb, M., & Culleiton, A.L. (2015). *American Journal of Nursing, 115*(1), 58-61.

Mahaffey Harmon, M., & Thompson, C. (2015). Clinical reasoning in pre-licensure nursing students. T*eaching and Learning in Nursing, 10,* 63-70.

Tanner, C. A. (2004). The meaning of curriculum: Content to be covered or stories to be heard? *Journal of Nursing Education, 43*(1), 3–4.

Tanner, C. A. (2006). Thinking like a nurse: A research-based model of clinical judgment in nursing. *Journal of Nursing Education, 45*(6), 204–211.

"Pearls" from Clinical Educators

24

Nurse educators are gifted with creativity. Nurse educators across the country were willing to share their creative strategies and tools they had developed and successfully used to strengthen student learning in the clinical setting. In this chapter, I share their clinical "pearls" so you can benefit and strengthen the learning of students in your clinical setting.

I attempt to teach my students to anticipate situations and events. I use the book *Left of Bang: How the Marine Corps' Combat Hunter Program Can Save Your Life* (Van Horne & Riley, 2014) to emphasize this concept. This book discusses how the Marine Corps use situational awareness training to anticipate threats, read behavioral and environmental changes, and use "gut instinct." Left of bang is an anticipatory mode, such as evaluating a patient, checking your car before getting into it when it is parked in a dark area, or noticing environmental changes such as an equipment malfunction, or a change in a patient's behavior. Bang is the event that we do not want to occur. Right of bang is the reaction and repair of an event outcome. We want to stay left of bang to anticipate dire threats to patients and ourselves.

This anticipatory thinking is exactly what we do as practicing nurses and try to instill in students. Anticipatory evaluation is used to avoid an event. I use the term "left of bang" frequently in my classes, and ask the students for ex-

amples that they have witnessed in their clinical rotations. It is surprising how much they notice without realizing it, and this reflective exercise demonstrates and reinforces, through their own examples, how anticipation (or lack of it) made a difference in patient outcomes.

Instinct is something that is commonly believed to be developed only through years of experience. I beg to differ. I think we can teach our students to develop nursing instincts from the first day of nursing school by teaching anticipatory and situational awareness. Once they have learned the essentials of a baseline assessment, we can expand that knowledge to look for anomalies. Even if they cannot immediately pinpoint *what is wrong,* knowing *something is wrong* can mean alerting a nurse or their instructor to a potential "bang" situation. Students fear being made to look foolish and hesitate to alert others in case they are wrong. I believe this "left of bang" concept helps to alleviate those fears.

Isn't this exactly what we want nursing students to learn and use?

• Reference: Van Horne, P., & Riley, J. A. (2014). *Left of Bang: How the Marine Corps' Hunter Program can save your life.* New York, New York: Black Irish Entertainment LLC.

—Lin Rauch, MSN, RN, BSEd.
Nursing Instructor
Western Technical College
La Crosse, Wisconsin

I created the Quick Medication Guide (download included in Appendix C) after teaching pharmacology in nursing for three years. I noted that many generic medication classes shared prefixes, suffixes, or maybe a few letters in the middle that were common. I had tried to point these out to students during lecture, but students preferred only to notice the brand names because they were usually much easier to pronounce. Then, NCLEX changed testing patterns and now test only generic names of medications. After 20 years of clinical experience, I did not know every drug, much less every generic. How could I prepare students for practice? What I did know was that about 90 percent (my own guesstimate) of generic classes shared commonalities. If I could get students to recognize these commonalities, relate them to the class, and then know the vital information for pharmacologic classifications to safely administer, I knew pharmacology would not be so overwhelming for students.

With that insight, I started developing the Quick Medication Guide. I gave it to students at the beginning of the pharmacology class as a reference for didactic and clinical coursework. I went to the clinical site to oversee my clinical adjuncts and used the opportunity to "quiz" students on this content. We would pull up an EMR and get started. Students would read the brand and not always know. For example, a patient was taking Januvia (sitagliptin). The student would look at the brand name and not be able to remember anything about the medication, but I reminded them to look at the generic name. They would look closely and see the "gli" remembering that "gli" means to lower blood glucose. So the student can transfer this knowledge of blood glucose lowering agents from class to clinical. Many students have told me they posted my Quick Medication Guide in the med rooms at their units or clinics after graduation. Pharmacology used to be one of the toughest subjects for my students, now it is one of their favorites!

—Nancy Delmont, MSN, RN
Department Chair
Southwest Baptist University,
Bolivar, Missouri

I developed a patient assessment form (included in Appendix C) to help first-semester nursing students strengthen and develop their assessment skills. The first page provides a template to address each body system assessment when providing patient care. For the second and third pages of this tool, I would later assign students in groups of two to assess two residents who had a similar medical diagnosis and ask them to compare their findings and plan of care. Students reported their assessment findings and plan of care during post-conference. My students valued this exercise and shared that this form guided them as well as helped them think about the specific needs of each patient and what data was essential to document regarding the assessment and plan of care.

—Patricia Pence, EdD, MSN, RN
Nursing Professor
Illinois Valley Community College
Oglesby, Illinois

The "Care Web" (included in Appendix C) is an innova-tive clinical teaching-learning strategy that can be used by the student as a transitional step in the development of basic clinical reasoning prior to moving toward complex concept mapping. With this simplified approach, the novice student engages in an un-crowded learning process, which decreases confusion and frustration when planning patient care. With the use of the "Care Web," the novice student will analyze patient data gathered, identify the issues and concerns and follow through with the remaining steps of the nursing process. The de-crowded format allows students to "untangle the web," connect links, and determine relationships of issues/concerns when planning care, which serves as a foundation for continued clinical reasoning development.

The following is a step by step guide for the use of the "care web." The student will:

1. Gather all patient data: health history, labs, diagnostics, current status/progress notes, etc.
2. Analyze the data in order to identify the patient issues/concerns NOT to include medical diagnosis unless it is attributed to the patient's history.
3. Make an issues/concerns list.
4. Follow the nursing process as outlined in the template (always to keep in mind that it is at the "time of care by the student" for all outcomes, interventions, and describing supportive rationale.

—Claudette Abounader, MS, ANP
Assistant Professor of Nursing
Utica College
Utica, New York

A prepared clinical instructor needs a "toolbox." This "toolbox" should contain the following components:

- Focus for the day
- Plan for post-conference Worksheets with specific questions and activities to promote learning

Develop your activity/worksheets based upon themes where you see your students struggling in the clinical setting, or content weaknesses that need to become a strength! The activities are intended to be completed during the clinical day, not done as "homework." If a student doesn't finish the activity, students can finish them prior to post-conference while waiting for everyone to assemble. It helps students download the day and make some well-thought-out contributions to post-conference. This also helps students chunk their learning into smaller pieces.

It is more effective to chunk than trying to learn about medication administration, being a caring nurse, communication, safety, time management, setting priorities, etc., all in one day. It goes without saying that leveling the activities correctly is essential. I would recommend that there be a correlation between their theory and clinical learning. Here are some examples: What should be written in a nurse's note? What can I learn from interviewing patients about their illness? How can I communicate with a health care provider about a change in a patient's condition? What are some apparent safety issues, etc.?

I also teach the last med/surg course prior to graduation. At this level, students must be prepared to integrate into a health care environment where they will dialogue with many other professional disciplines. Therefore, the nurse must be able to speak and understand these languages including medical diagnosis, problem lists, symptomatology, etc. In the clinical area, I allow my advanced students to come to me with an "old-fashioned" problem list. I tell them to "call it something and name the problem." Then I have them tell me about it. As they progress, they are able to better organize their thoughts based upon who the audience is that they are addressing (i.e., patient, family, primary care provider, case manager). It frees the student to think outside the box instead of only being allowed to use NANDA to identify care priorities especially when communicating with other disciplines. I do allow them to use NANDA terminology on the problem list because

it does help the student to think conceptually. It is just not the only game in town to guide nurse thinking.

—Barb Hill, RN, MSN, CNE, CMSRN
Associate Professor,
The Community College of Baltimore County
Baltimore, Maryland

When I teach in the clinical setting students frequently ask, "What do I write in a nurse's note, nothing really happened today?" I developed several questions to jump-start students' thinking in what to address in a nursing progress note. These questions include the following:

- *Any changes in the patient's condition and what was done about it?*
- *How well did the patient perform ADL's?*
- *Pain management trend, frequency of pain meds, and what adjunctive therapies work to control pain.*
- *Document anytime you or the primary RN call primary care provider.*
- *If you held a medication, document why it was not given.*

Instead of repeating myself for each student who has similar questions, these questions helped students initiate their progress note and save me valuable time in the clinical setting!

—Barbara Hill, RN, MSN, CNE, CMSRN
Associate Professor
The Community College of Baltimore County
Baltimore, Maryland

Teaching students how to critically reason is paramount to successful preparation for professional practice. Students will tell you that my mantra is that they be proactive rather than reactive in providing safe patient care. The more they know about their patients, the more proactive they will be! I encourage students to see the patient and his/her medical record as a puzzle, and that students need to put the puzzle pieces together to create a cohesive picture that will help them predict potential issues or problems that might impact the patient or the care that needs to be provided.

To enhance the student's ability to develop the skills needed to become that proactive thinker, I provide a series of exercises to build reasoning and analysis. These include written guidelines for preparation and pre-conference presentations and on-campus practice, mining important information from data-packed case studies. One of the most important strategies I use occurs one-on-one in the acute care clinical setting.

Early in my teaching career, I realized that students struggled to review the medical record. Students would open a chart and start reading from the beginning and move through the chart from "front to back," typically reading physician orders first without fully knowing the history or other pertinent data. This strategy creates no context in understanding the patient, hospital course, or appropriate nursing implications. Now with electronic medical records, nurses have access to significant amounts of data and it becomes even more important to have a workable strategy to build a cohesive view of the patient.

I now spend time with each student helping him or her develop successful strategies to interact with the patient's medical record and glean the significant data, the puzzle pieces that will put the clinical puzzle together. **Helpful strategies:**

1. Start with the parts of the record that explore the reason for hospitalization and pertinent patient history.
2. Review admission data including laboratory and diagnostic testing, then chronologically plot out assessment data, including laboratory and diagnostic testing.
3. Look for reasons why a laboratory result might have changed. For example, did the patient have a surgical procedure? A blood transfusion? Consider the impact of results on the patient, nursing implications that need to be considered, and problems that could be synthesized.

—Isabel N. Ososki, RN, BSN, MSN, MBA, CNE
Associate Professor of Nursing
Millikin University School of Nursing
Decatur, Illinois

When teaching fundamental psychomotor skills, I have students video record themselves performing the skill. The student immediately reflects on their performance afterward and again after watching their video. The reflection tool I have students use is based upon Debriefing for Meaningful Learning developed by Dr. Kristina Dreifuerst. I have successfully used this strategy teaching basic and advanced skills for associate degree nursing and practical nursing students. This approach helps stu-

dents develop metacognitive skills such as reflection, increase proficiency in completing the skills safely, and improving communication with the patient. See references at the end of this chapter for more on this strategy to develop clinical reasoning skills with simulation.

—Lisa M Beals, RN, MSN
Simulation and Skills Lab Coordinator
Bolivar Technical College
Bolivar, Missouri

To increase student engagement in the classroom I have an activity I use each time in class. Students are required to read what has been assigned in order to participate and understand the content taught that day. There is no way to cover everything in pediatrics in the five weeks I have with my students. To address what is most important with my content, I review the patient population that we have in our hospital and community and base my material on those disorders or diseases. The students do not feel as overwhelmed with the amount of material to read. I have observed that students retain the material longer if they participate actively in the learning process.

—Linda A. Strong, MSN, RN, CPNP, CNE
Associate Professor, Pediatric Nursing
Cuyahoga Community College
Cleveland, Ohio

To teach civility, I dress up as a pickle (adopted from "The Pickle Pledge"). My character is named Patti Pickle and I use a scenario that illustrates incivility between two nurses. This strategy teaches students how to deal with conflict. It is essential to provide relevant conflict resolution tools so students are well prepared to deal with incivility once in practice. The educator role plays Rose, a new graduate nurse on a postpartum unit, night shift. Patti Pickle is a seasoned nurse who is uncivil and consistently gives nurses—especially new nurses—a hard time during shift report.

This is the incivility scenario that I developed:

The new graduate nurse was not able to ambulate her Cesarean section patient because she was nauseated and vomiting. She is concerned about communicating this to Patti Pickle. Rose gives shift report and Patti states in a condescending voice, "I can't believe you did not get the patient up. You had all night and this morning. You are never going to make it as a nurse! This is unacceptable.

I am going to report this to the nurse manager!" Rose apologizes and explains that she asked the other nurses if she should get the patient up and they said absolutely not. The patient was too ill. After report, Patti Pickle storms off toward the nurse manager's office.

After the scenario, I turn to the students and ask how they would handle this situation. We discuss Joe Tye's "Pickle Pledge" and the definition of incivility and civility. Dressing up as a Patti Pickle and role playing helps the students understand how incivility is unprofessional, disrespectful, and causes high levels of conflict and stress. This exercise prepares students to address conflict and face the Patti Pickles in nursing practice using conflict resolution techniques.

—Mary Bowman, MSN, RN
Assistant Professor of Nursing
Concordia University
Irvine, California

To bring meaningful active learning to my classroom or nursing skills lab, I set up several stations. Students are divided up into groups of three to four and given 10-15 minutes at each station. For example, when teaching a respiratory unit for first-semester fundamental students I developed the following stations:

1. Patient education with selected respiratory medications to a patient and their family. I include questions such as "What is important for them to know and what is not?" "How will they remember that information once they get home?"

2. Teaching a patient how to properly use an inhaler. I have several practice inhalers so this skill can be demonstrated.

3. Listening to different lung sounds on the high fidelity manikin and identifying what they are and WHY they are present (applied pathophysiology)

4. Complete a worksheet of dosage calculations related to respiratory medications

5. Complete a worksheet of NCLEX-style questions on respiratory medications or med-surg questions on the respiratory system

6. Assemble and disassemble a handheld nebulizer. (I find that students don't know how to put them together when they are required to use one in a simulation scenario.)

7. Read a short medical history on a patient along with

additional information provided since the patient arrived in the ED and then give a hand-off report to the oncoming nurse.

—Rebecca Ellingson, MSN, RN, BA
Department Head of Nursing
Indian Hills Community College
Ottumwa, Iowa

I emphasize the importance of identifying priorities in the clinical setting. Though there may appear to be numerous priorities, I guide my students to select the TOP nursing priority and develop a plan of care. I then help them see how the other priorities they identified are related to the top priority to see the bigger picture. Priorities in acute care can quickly change and sometimes be short lived. I help students to see the importance of comprehensive discharge planning and making sure the appropriate education, resources, and health promotion are in place to prevent future problems related to the original problem and/or priority. I have used Keith's RAPID Reasoning template (included in the Transformation Toolbox) to facilitate student learning. Another question I ask my students is to identify ancillary services needed to implement interventions in the plan of care. This approach gives students permission to focus on the top nursing priority, but also accomplish other goals (i.e., education, health promotion, psychosocial, spiritual support) through the use of leadership and delegation.

—Kala Streibel, RN, MSN
Nursing Faculty
Red Deer College
Red Deer, Alberta, Canada

In clinical, with the nurse's permission, I had students pull the nurse's meds from the med carts and set them up in the patient drawers. The labels were still intact so there were no safety issues and the nurse and I supervised and double-checked medications to ensure safety. Students had to choose the correct syringe to put in the drawer if it was injectable, and anticipate any medication-related supplies and place them in the drawer that the nurse might need. The students felt that they learned a lot about medications as they did this activity. I posed questions about medications as they worked. Students learned how to use a medication administration record and use the computer-based medication administration system as well. I realize these are simple activities but sometimes simple is best.

—Debra Avery, RN, MSN
Nursing Faculty
Three Rivers College
Poplar Bluff, Missouri

For clinical, I switched to concept mapping vs. long papers and care plans. I ask students to complete a quick concept map that we all discuss in post-conference. Students draw their maps on the board so others can review, make suggestions, ask for more information, etc. It's a great way to practice SBAR, see linkages between concepts, etc. It allows us to review theory information in the clinical setting in a way that is relevant for students. Twice each semester students take this quick map using their peers' input, and convert it into a more complete one. They add a care planning section based on one or more acute problems and submit it for grading. I've seen such an uptick in critical thinking—students can identify nursing priorities, see connections, incorporate labs, treatments, etc.

One final clinical item I've tried is patient rounding. When we are working on heart sounds, students may care for a patient with a particular murmur. They invite their peers in to listen, and then discuss what they've just heard. Of course, they obtain patient consent first. This is a way for all ten students to hear a murmur, see a chest tube, etc., versus just the one student who is caring for that individual patient.

—Ruth Tamulonis, RN, MSN
Nursing Faculty
Yuba College
Marysville, California

Each week in clinical, I already know what has been covered recently within the classroom setting. I also know the diagnoses and problems of the weekly assigned patients. During post conferences, I call upon students whose patients present with medical diagnoses and clinical manifestations that have recently been discussed in the classroom. The discussions regarding significant concepts related to these situations are insightful and thought-provoking. These post-conference dialogs make the classroom concepts come alive for the students and thus more relevant to the clinical presentations.

—Sandra O'Donnell, RN, MSN, CNE
Guest Lecturer
University of North Carolina at
Wilmington School of Nursing
Wilmington, North Carolina

Mental health nursing students are often blinded by anxiety, especially in the beginning of clinical. Based on my experience and student feedback, here are some things that have helped to decrease student stress in this setting:

• What to wear during psych-mental health clinical is always a difficult topic. "Business casual" translates differently among the generations of aging nursing faculty and young students. When I explain how clothing serves as a form of nonverbal communication, I use the story about a group home resident who believed that pretty young female students wearing their version of "business casual" were government-supplied prostitutes. "Pump up the frump," I say when selecting business casual wear. "I don't want to see any cleavage on the top or bottom. No butt cracks or whale tales allowed when bending over taking a blood pressure." One student borrowed her mother's clothing for psychiatric clinical. Another came in a suit and tie. I finally gave up on the "business casual" dress code. Uniform scrubs work best in most settings. Safety first!

• Remember that the anxiety students feel is just a fraction of that experienced by your mental health patients.

• As a student, you may be the most important person in your patient's life today. You can have more impact than even professional staff. Just by receiving students' undivided attention today for a few hours, patients' self-esteem can be bolstered, interpersonal communication can be improved, and some hope may be restored.

• Nobody chooses to have a severe mental illness. Children do not develop the dream of "Someday, I'm going to become a drug-abusing, anxiety-ridden, suicidal, and depressed person. I'll lose jobs, housing, friends, and family while getting kicked around by the mental health system. Yeah, that's what I want to be when I grow up. Everyone will be so proud of me."

• I tell many stories about my previous students. One

former student was obviously anxious and wide-eyed with panic written all over her face when she walked onto a locked psychiatric unit for the first time. She was greeted by a patient who rushed up to her saying, "Don't be afraid, we will help you." Always gets a laugh from students. This example illustrates the importance of maintaining neutrality, both in verbal and nonverbal communication.

- Reflection is said to be the most neglected aspect of the learning process. Reflective journaling is an invaluable component of the clinical paperwork assignment. Differentiating thoughts and feelings as part of the assignment helps students assess their own cognitive and emotional processes. One student wrote about her sadness as she sat in her car crying for half an hour after leaving the mental health unit. "I never realized the amount of suffering mentally ill people endure. I've been so insensitive until now." Other stories about students' tearfulness in post-conference can be helpful. Sometimes after working with an adolescent with a long and unbelievable history of loss, neglect, abuse, or sexual torture, a student becomes tearful relating the experience to peers and apologizes for "being so emotional." I tell them that those tears are appropriate. I'm more worried about the student who does not respond emotionally to such experiences.

—Peggy Hernandez, EdD, APRN, PMHCNS-BC, CNE
Assistant Professor
Wichita State University
Wichita, Kansas

I have changed many things over the last five years of clinical and classroom teaching. I think my greatest revelation at clinical is the power of using questions using real-world challenges my students experience regarding what to do after report is finished and patient care begins. At a long-term care unit clinical after report, I routinely ask my students:

- Which patient from report would you go see first, second, third and why in that order?
- What relevant clinical data would you need to pass on to your team such as the nursing assistant or supervisor?
- I quiz them about the most important assessments

with a patient with diabetes and what the symptoms of a complication are.

- If you were the nurse today after report, what would you do first?

My expectations are different depending on what level the students are in our program. I no longer emphasize how much my students do, but rather can they rescue their client. I tell them what they need to know and cut out all of the fluff (as much as possible).

I do not focus on NANDA nursing diagnostic statements (I teach LPNs). I focus more on the problem and the outcome and emphasize the importance of evaluation.

—Karen Flatt, RN, BSN, MSN
Practical Nursing Faculty
Northeast Technology Center
Claremore, Oklahoma

The use of the M-W acronym provides the student nurse with a method to recall the basic physical assessment data of the patient and the ability to transfer this information to various types of documentation systems. The acronym that I developed provides a "sticky" method to recall information and prevent omission of patient assessment data, affecting the plan of care.

M-W Acronym

M–Musculoskeletal: General mobility and strength of extremities, general ROM, strength of hand grasps

N–Neuro: Response to stimuli, alert and oriented to person, place, time, and situation

O–Oh my: What has happened to you lately: details (location, type, size, etc.) of tubes, drains, IV sites, wounds, sutures, staples, dressings

P–Pain: Location, duration, intensity, related signs of pain, and recall of most recent medication with effectiveness

Q–Cardiac: Quality of heart tones, rhythm, amplitude, radial and pedal pulses bilaterally, presence of edema

R–Respiratory: Depth, auscultation of upper/ lower, anterior and posterior lung fields, nail bed and lip color, cap refill, presence of cough

S–Skin: General skin temp and moisture, assess overall skin integrity and pressure points

T–Tummy: Bowel sounds, palpation of abdomen, nausea or level of appetite, ask about most recent BM with characteristics

U–Urinary: Assess urinary catheter or ask about last urination, color, clarity, amount, and ease of elimination

V–Vital signs: Temp (assessment device utilized), B/P with position, pulse rate (identify if apical or radial or A/R), respiratory rate, pulse ox and use of oxygen with delivery of type and percentage of oxygen

W–We will be Safe: Top side rails up, call light in reach, phone at bedside, personal alarm on, etc.

—Cynthia Stoerzbach, RN, MS, CNE
Nursing Faculty
Carl Sandberg College
Galesburg, Illinois

Place a student with the same RN as much as possible during the clinical rotation. I interviewed the charge nurse of the unit to look at the available nurses on the assigned clinical day of the weeks ahead. RNs who worked at least 80 percent of the time on clinical days were evaluated for their interest and ability to work with the same nursing student. Overall this approach was a huge success and a win-win for everyone. The students stated that they never felt more supported. The RNs stated that they enjoyed mentoring the same student and enjoyed participating in the student's professional development. The hospital appreciated the development of a supportive relationship based on trust. They felt that this type of relationship would decrease potential errors and increase patient satisfaction by utilizing QSEN principles in a collaborative relationship.

—Katie Kruse, RN, MSN
Professor of Nursing
Cypress College
Cypress, California

Clinical Orientation Information Packet:
An orientation packet is given to each student that lists the day's agenda. This packet serves as a concrete reference that will outline "what will happen today." It can include basic information that the student needs for the duration of the clinical rotation, e.g., instructor's phone numbers and email, hospital number, cell phone policy, where to store valuables, etc., and how the students' families should contact them during clinical in case of an emergency. Most nursing programs have student handbooks and clinical guidelines that are given to all students.

This orientation packet, specific to the instructor, al-

lows the instructor to include any other pertinent information for the site, faculty, or clinical.

Self-assessment and Reflection:
Have students answer questions about their career or educational experiences, perceived clinical strengths or weaknesses, or what they want to accomplish during this specific clinical.

Decrease Student Stress!
Do what is possible to decrease stress during orientation and try to alleviate it by providing a welcoming environment. Simple gestures like providing doughnuts or snacks can aid in establishing a sense of bonding and community. Faculty may also consider bringing useful tools to distribute to the students such as charting guides or medical abbreviation lists.

Student Feedback and Evaluation
One of the instructor's responsibilities is to provide feedback to each student. Good feedback must meet certain criteria including regular occurrence, promptness, and delivery in a calm, caring, and sensitive manner. Instructors can give thought to adopting an internal "checklist" for all feedback that they will provide to the students. This list, which should have criteria similar to the characteristics listed above, may become a powerful tool in difficult scenarios.

Student Presentations
- One way to assist the students in their educational and professional development is to assign a ten-minute oral presentation that can be part of the post-conference agenda.
- During the orientation day, assign each student a specific week of the clinical. Many instructors do not start the presentations until week three to allow each student ample time to select a topic.
- The topic should benefit the entire group and may include drug information, disease processes, new skills, etc. Encourage the students to use visuals, i.e., handouts, or PowerPoint slides.

Faculty Pearls
Faculty Locator Magnet
- Create a magnet that states, "The instructor is in this

room" to put on the patient's doorframe; it will assist the students in locating you in an efficient manner.

Mid-clinical conference

- Provide ten to fifteen minutes for students to ask any questions that may have developed or share an interesting event that happened with their patient.
- The instructor could also gather specific information from your students. One student may have a patient who has an arteriovenous fistula that is positive for bruit and thrill. Other students in the group may have never assessed an arteriovenous fistula before and would benefit from this opportunity.

Charge Nurse for a Day

- This assignment is best suited for advanced clinical students. Select a student to act as either the "float nurse" or "charge nurse" for the clinical day versus standard patient assignment. For example, the student who is the float nurse can assist other students with various interventions, i.e., dressing changes, ambulation, checking lab results, emptying Foley catheters, etc. Instruct other students to utilize the "float nurse" for at least one activity.
- The student designated as the charge nurse should report all new orders to other student nurses and ask specific questions about their patients' activity, elimination, and appetite, etc. The student charge nurse should delegate certain activities to the other students. These ideas provide the student with experience in organization and delegation; essential skills a nurse needs.

Help for the Instructor!

- If this is your first experience as a clinical instructor, find out what assistance is available to you. Is there a faculty member who you can call with questions as they arise? Is there any orientation provided for you? Does faculty meet regularly to discuss the progression of the students? Do you have any co-workers who also function as clinical instructors? Knowing in advance about available resources will help in planning.
- The hospital and specific unit or area may also be new to you. Contact the nurse manager and introduce yourself. Scheduling a tour of the floor or unit is ben-

eficial. Knowing the layout and how things are done are necessary. If you are not comfortable or appear nervous during clinical, this will only aggravate the students' fear and anxiety.

- Let the students know that they need to communicate any problems they have to you immediately.
- As the clinical progresses, you may develop different ideas for using the pre- and post-conference time. Invite a staff nurse, respiratory therapist, or another discipline to speak to the group. Continue to ask the students to reflect on each clinical and assess their strengths and weaknesses. What did they truly enjoy and what presented a challenge during this specific clinical? What one event had the most significance to them regarding patient care?
- Like the students, take some time to reflect on each clinical experience. What is working well with the students? What are the areas that need improvement? Can you verbalize each student's strengths or weaknesses for that day? Helping the students with their professional and educational goals while instilling the ideal of compassionate and competent care is an extremely rewarding benefit of teaching.

—Regina Rose Demasi, MSN, BSBA, RN
Instructor of Nursing
Wheeling Jesuit University
Wheeling, West Virginia

I keep note cards in my pocket with abnormal vital signs, lab values, abnormal assessment findings, and primary care provider orders that I hand to a student whose patient may have left the floor for a procedure, has been discharged, or any student who has down time for some other reason. I might ask them, "These are the most recent vital signs and labs on your patient, what would you do now?" or "These are the most recent primary care provider orders, prioritize how you would carry them out?"

—Becky Craig, RNC, MN, EdS, PhD
Nursing Instructor, Nursing Tutorial Lab
Perimeter College
Clarkston, Georgia

This is how I encourage my students to think about caring and apply this to our discussion and reflections on their own nursing practice to become more purposeful in demonstrating caring for the individual and families. Jason Kent, an incarcerated Christian, described some beautiful caring behaviors from an experienced nurse while he was in the hospital following emergency surgery. His letter to his mother shared in her book, *Between a Rock and a Grace Place,* is read to students in post-conference.

Using open-ended questions to elicit reflection and discussion, the students are encouraged to identify caring behaviors by the nurse. We spend some time considering if caring can be taught, developed, or is it innate. Usually our group of eight students evolve from several points insisting that "you either have it or you don't" to sharing how caring can be demonstrated, developed, and modeled for others. Many times, there are exciting moments for me as I watch the developing awareness of students who are able to offer specific examples of caring in their clinical day. We conclude by challenging each other to reflect on our own ways of showing caring to patients, families, and the other team members in clinical. I attempt to talk with each student individually in the clinical day to encourage specific caring behaviors and reflection on ways this can be developed in their nursing practice.

—Kathy Kilen, MA, RN, CNE
Nursing Faculty
St. Ambrose University,
Davenport, Iowa

Simulation Pearls

I used Keith's Clinical Reasoning 1-2-3 case studies with my second semester nursing students with simulation. The simulation scenario was of a patient with CHF. I utilized the following steps in this case based scenario:

- I had them complete step #1 of the case study and the "pre-clinical" portion of the clinical reasoning questions ("Clinical Reasoning Questions to Develop Nurse Thinking") after we went over their pre-clinical prep assignment (this was a case study I wrote to prepare them for the patient they would be taking care of in the simulation).
- The students went through skills stations where they did a respiratory and a cardiovascular focused assessment and an SBAR report.
- Students reviewed the lab values of the simulated patient and learned how to teach the patient about their disease process.
- We then went over step #1 of the case study, which

emphasizes recognizing relevant clinical data and nursing priorities. The first group then went into the simulation room to treat their patient. (We had three groups go through the simulation scenario.) They were to use all the tools that they had practiced in the skills labs as well as deliver 0800 medications and a nebulizer treatment.

- The "during clinical" portion of the clinical reasoning case study was worked through and students completed step #2 of the case study, which addressed recognizing clinical relationships of data.
- We reviewed step #2 together and debriefed together, using the scenario.
- At this point I discovered that students did not integrate or have a clear understanding of holistic care, so we went through step #3 that addressed psychosocial priorities so they could understand how to incorporate holistic care into the simulated experience.
- They then answered the "caring and the art of nursing" questions. This application worked well to get them to think out of the box of just doing tasks. I felt that they left with a better understanding of all aspects required to care for a patient, just like in the clinical setting.

—Gwen Reed MS, RN, Paramedic, CEN
Nursing Instructor
Gillette College
Gillette, Wyoming

I use case studies in classroom lecture and then as part of the lecture I integrate one of the patients in the case study in simulation using manikins weekly. I have a team of five students per one SIM person (primary nurse, medication nurse, and observer) who use an observation sheet to evaluate the team, a family member, and "The Voice" who initially gives an I-SBAR-R report and then becomes the voice of SIM man. The students have DocuCare available ahead of time with labs/diagnostics, orders, medications to help prepare themselves, but they do not always know the setting, such as their patient is in the ED (the beginning of the case study), or returning from PACU, or being discharged.

They must give medications (IV or oral), perform procedures such as starting IVs, draw blood work, administer oxygen (or correct the flow of a Venti mask), or contact the primary care provider with an allergy to an ordered medication or abnormal lab using I-SBAR-R. This helps bring the didactic material to the bedside. The most informative aspect is the debriefing afterward where everyone participates and learns by reflection. The students stay on the same teams every week so they can see an improvement in the performance by the end of the course.

—Mary Burns-Coral, MSN, RN, CNE
Nursing Faculty
Washtenaw Community College
Ann Arbor, Michigan

Students are assigned the reading before simulation. They enter the lab and are asked to go to their respective patient area. I demonstrate how to do a procedure to the class. I then ask for questions. After questions have been answered, the students go around the lab reciting how to do each step of the procedure.

For example:

- First student begins with checking order, patient identification, and explaining the procedure.
- Second student identifies the equipment involved, prepping of patient, and any special preparation required by the nurse such as hand washing.
- Third student begins with first step of procedure such as opening the sterile kit.
- Each student proceeds until the final step has been completed (while all students are responding to direction and doing the procedure themselves).
- Last student ends with cleanup and documentation details.

I begin with a different student each time so all will remember what is expected in addition to the procedure itself. Each student is expected to participate. This teaches about not only the procedure but teaches the patient and fellow students, too. If a student does not know the answer, they "pass" and the lesson continues with the next student. Obviously, they don't want to "pass" too often. It gets them prepped for clinical and helps me know who is not comprehending the information. A grade is not assigned to this particular activity to allow students to work under less pressure. Return demonstrations are performed at a later time.

—Pam Hays, RN, MSN, FCN
Nursing Faculty
John A. Logan College
Carterville, Illinois

I teach Health Assessment to first semester nursing students. I find my students' attention span waxing and waning during my lecture even though I make it interactive with skills. Our university has 50-minute length classes with 10 minute breaks; however, I decided to implement the "Pomodoro Technique" for class. I lecture for 25 minutes and we take a 5-minute "brain break" and then alternate class and break. For more info on the Pomodoro Technique, go to http://pomodorotechnique.com/.

- I also do clinical simulations with the first semester nursing students. We began using your Fundamental Reasoning for simulations, aka "campus clinicals." The students have an opportunity to review the patient's EMR chart (we use Simulation Learning System with Elsevier) ahead of time and they complete the Fundamental Reasoning paperwork as a "pass for clinical."
- I also integrated a virtual patient simulation, called Shadow Health, into my Health Assessment course. This semester, I began incorporating one of your questions into the debriefing portion. Each week, students need to identify what health assessment data from the virtual patient was relevant and explain its clinical relevance. I think this will be a big help in developing their critical thinking skills.

–Christy Dubert, PhD, RN,
Assistant Professor
Georgia Southern University
Statesboro, Georgia

Reflect

1. What "pearls" did you find helpful that you can incorporate into your program?

TRANSFORMING
NURSING EDUCATION

Though the classroom and clinical settings require radical transformation in nursing education, from my perspective, this is only the beginning. To see the entirety of nursing education transformed, we must acknowledge the "elephant in the room" regarding the ongoing persistence and prevalence of bullying and incivility in clinical practice as well as nursing education.

Men in nursing have been marginalized in the past and experienced institutional gender bias when the modern era was ushered in by Florence Nightingale. Nursing literature continues to document ongoing barriers that men continue to experience in nursing education.

25

Transforming Academia by Restoring Civility

Keith Rischer, RN, MA, CEN, CCRN

"I cannot put into words what it feels like to have nurses laugh in your face and belittle you when you ask a clinical question, roll their eyes and walk out on your report before it is finished...or to be scolded or yelled at in front of your other colleagues until you are apologizing profusely with tears streaming down your cheeks."
—Nurse in practice

"Being personally targeted and directly experiencing incivility has caused me to hate the job that I once loved. If it wasn't for the students, I would leave academia in a heartbeat."
—Nurse educator

Nursing has one of the highest rates of incivility of any profession (Johnson & Rea, 2009). Incivility is defined as a disregard for others that creates an atmosphere of disrespect and conflict that can progress to more threatening situations (Clark, 2013). How endemic is incivility in nursing? In clinical practice, 93 percent of nurses have witnessed bullying and 85 percent reported that they were victims of bullying (Coursey, Rodriguez, Dieckmann, & Austin, 2013). In a recent national study, 68 percent of nursing faculty reported moderate to severe levels of faculty to faculty incivility. But when mild levels of faculty to faculty incivility are included, the prevalence of incivility in nursing academia rose to 96 percent (Clark, Olender, Kenski, & Cardoni, 2013).

Is there a RELATIONSHIP between the high prevalence of incivility in the profession and nursing education? Is the uncivil culture of nursing education normalizing through role modeling this disrespectful and unprofessional behavior to students? Though curriculum is needed to structure what students are taught, Tanner (1990) recognized the power of the "hidden curriculum" that represents the values and example that are role-modeled by faculty to students. The "hidden curriculum" shapes and influences student formative development as much as what is taught and tested. What does the "hidden curriculum in your program teach students?

Incivility in nursing education is complex and has threads like a web that can adversely impact the relationship between faculty and students. To untangle this web and identify the unique dynamics present in nursing education, the following contexts of incivility will be explored:

- Student to faculty
- Faculty to student
- Faculty to faculty
- Incivility in clinical practice

Incivility in nursing education can be likened to a "dance." One leads and the other follows. It is not only a student or a faculty problem. Uncivil behavior does not exist in a vacuum, but both student and faculty are partners and interdependent in this "dance" (Clark, 2008). When both student and faculty engage, communicate, and seek resolution of conflict before it digresses to incivility, a culture of RESPECT and the "dance" of civility is present.

But if opportunities to promote engagement by both faculty and student are missed, the root of DISRESPECT is established and a "dance" of incivility is perpetuated. Once this dance has begun, regardless of who may be responsible for initiating it, incivility can escalate and become a blame game with no end in sight (Clark, 2008).

Student to Faculty Incivility

Entitlement and incivility have become increasingly pervasive in American society and contribute to incivility in nursing education (Clark & Springer, 2010). Unfortunately, students reflect these attitudes as they enter nursing education. Students may come to your program with a sense of entitlement; since they paid for an education, they believe the college "owes" them a degree. Student "entitlement" is exhibited by those who expect high grades for modest amounts of work, assume a "consumer" mentality toward education, refuse to accept responsibility, and make excuses for their failures.

The most common behaviors of student incivility include (Clark, 2008; Clark & Springer, 2010) :

- Rude comments, engaging in side conversations, dominating class
- Cell phone use, texting, inappropriate computer use in class
- Late to class and leaving early
- Sleeping in class
- Anger or excuses for poor performance
- Inadequate preparation
- Pressuring faculty until they get what they want
- Bad-mouthing other students, faculty, and the nursing program

Contributing Factors

Are there other factors that influence incivility in nursing students? Could the highly competitive and academically rigorous culture of nursing education itself be a contributing factor to student incivility? In one qualitative study, students felt that incivility was influenced by burnout from demanding workloads and competition in a high-stakes academic environment (Clark, 2008). By decreasing content overload and emphasizing what is most important, this will not only transform nursing education, but can also decrease student stress, which can help mitigate one of the influencing factors of student incivility.

Faculty to Student Incivility

Though the majority of nursing literature addressing incivility focuses on students, uncivil behavior by faculty to students is also a problem (Clark & Springer, 2007). In one study, uncivil behavior by faculty was most common in the classroom (60 percent), followed by the clinical setting (Marchiondo, Marchiondo, & Lasiter, 2010). When incivility is experienced and directed toward students in nursing education, it is "often very hostile and soul destroying" (Heinrich, 2010).

Preeminent nurse educator and researcher on incivility Dr. Cynthia "Cindy" Clark, has published over 40 articles in the nursing literature on incivility in nursing education. What influenced her to passionately pursue this topic? Incivility that she experienced as an 18-year-old nursing student.

Cindy explains her painful experience in her own words with Professor "Sour."

"For some reason, which still perplexes me today, Professor Sour took a particular dislike toward me. Being only 18 years old, I was ill-equipped and inexperienced with dealing with rude and demeaning teachers. She would find reasons to berate me and often in full view and in earshot of other students, nurses, physicians, and sometimes even patients. My classmates were supportive, but they experienced the wrath of Professor Sour as well and tried to avoid her as much as I did. Over time the incivility grew and deepened. Professor Sour found unique ways to demean and degrade me, until her bullying behaviors hit new heights when she attempted to publicly embarrass me in front of several physicians and nurses when I asked to leave the clinical unit to use the restroom. There I stood in front of everyone, filled with the deep humiliation that only a teenager can feel when being publicly chastised and demeaned especially about a private and personal matter. It was a defining moment in my professional life and one that I have never forgotten"
(Clark, 2013a, p.3-4).

Though there is no excuse for the types of behaviors Cindy experienced, what is it that influences nursing fac-ulty to demonstrate incivility toward their students? In the same qualitative study, faculty identified STRESS as the primary reason. Just like students, faculty are highly stressed from their demanding workloads. Other causes of faculty stress include high faculty turnover, lack of quali-fied educators, role stress, and incivility from all sides: students, other faculty, and administration (Clark, 2008).

Though faculty may not be aware of perceived uncivil behaviors toward students, any verbal/nonverbal communication that conveys a perception of the student of disrespect, abruptness, or rudeness must be guarded against by faculty because this is perceived as incivility by students.

Behaviors of incivility by faculty toward students include (Clark, 2008; Clark, 2011):

- Faculty superiority that is demonstrated by:
  - Exerting position and control over students
  - Setting unrealistic student expectations
  - Assuming a "know-it-all" attitude
  - Being rigid, unapproachable, or rejecting students' opinions
- Devaluing students' prior life experiences that can include work and academic experiences
- Ineffective educators who cannot manage the classroom
- Making condescending remarks or put-downs to students
- Showing favoritism to certain students
- Refusing or reluctance to answer questions

How to Change Academic Culture

Nurse educators must model the core values of the profession, which include caring, compassion, nurturing of the other, and respect. The ANA code of ethics states: *"The principle of RESPECT for persons extends to all individuals with whom the nurse interacts."* Educators can change the culture of academia and make it a place where support and nurturing in a high stress/stakes environment is possible. To create a healthy culture, there must first be a healthy relationship between faculty and students. This includes open/honest communication, working together, and establishing boundaries that are clearly defined and enforced.

Civility can become normative as a culture of respect is cultivated. The following are practical steps that educators can implement to make a goal of civility possible (Clark & Springer, 2010):

1. Model caring and respect in all that you do so students can see what true professionalism looks like in practice!
2. Provide opportunities to dialogue with students in open formats, such as a town hall meeting. This can provide needed dialogue and understanding.
3. Establish clearly written policies or place expectations in student codes of conduct that address incivility, and its consequences. Enforce them consistently.
4. Incorporate time management/stress reduction/self-care in the curriculum.
5. Listen carefully; give students positive feedback.
6. Encourage students to do their part to create a culture of civility. Encourage and EXPECT students to live out the highest standards of professionalism (Clark, 2011):
   - Be prepared, respectful, and engaged in your learning.
   - Do not speak in a negative, derogatory manner openly about other STUDENTS, FACULTY, or the nursing PROGRAM.
   - Abide consistently by the standards of student conduct of your institution.
   - Communicate your needs, and what you need/expect from faculty.
   - Work toward a common goal of civility and respect.

The Rest of Cindy's Story

Cindy goes on to explain how another educator whom she calls Professor "Sweet" lived out caring and respect and as a result made a lasting impact:

"One evening, after a particularly challenging day with Professor Sour, I was sitting alone studying in the cafeteria when I was approached by another member of the nursing faculty. After a bit of small talk she asked me how I was doing. She seemed genuinely interested but I learned long ago to keep my thoughts to myself and to avoid rocking the boat. So I made some lame comment like, 'I'm fine.' But that response did not satisfy Professor Sweet. She let me know that I could trust her and that it was safe for me to speak candidly and from the heart. Professor Sweet helped rebuild my fractured self-esteem and restored my confidence. She mentored me and cultivated a love for nursing that had been nearly destroyed by Professor Sour. As I grew stronger under the healing guidance of Professor Sweet, I began to trust again and to heal from the torment heaped upon me by Professor Sour" (Clark, 2013a, p.4-5).

Incivility in Clinical Practice

Incivility is an assault on human dignity and self-worth, and the effects can be devastating, debilitating, and enduring(Clark, 2013b). In the clinical setting, it is widely accepted that "nurses eat their young," which uninten-

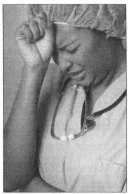

tionally normalizes incivility as something that should be tolerated. Incivility in the clinical setting is endemic. Sixty-four percent of nurses cited incivility as the primary reason for leaving their current job (Stagg, Sheridan, Jones, & Gabel Speroni, 2011). New nurses as well as men (Dellasega, 2009) are more likely to experience incivility most often from other more experienced or senior nurses (Griffin, 2004).

The most common overt bullying behaviors include patterns of fault-finding, intimidation, gossip, put-downs, and nonverbal innuendo such as raising eyebrows or sighing. More subtle bullying behaviors include isolation, exclusion, ignoring/refusing to help, and unfair assignments (Bartholomew, 2006). Other categories of bullying behavior include the resentful nurse who holds grudges and encourages others to join in as well as the cliquish nurse who intentionally excludes others from the "group" (Dellasega, 2009).

Other specific examples from the literature most commonly seen in the clinical setting include:

- Having information withheld so it affects your performance
- Having your views and opinions ignored
- Being personally ignored or excluded
- Micromanaging your work
- Persistent criticism of your work and effort
- Having insulting/offensive remarks made about you
- Repeated reminders of your errors and mistakes
- Having false allegations or accusations made against you (Johnson & Rea, 2009)

The most common examples of incivility I have experienced in clinical practice consisted of being marginalized and isolated by nurses who were unwilling to help. If I asked for help, they would sigh and make it clear that I was asking too much from them. During report, some nurses appeared disinterested, distracted, and asked numerous questions not even relevant to the patient's priority problem. When I didn't have this nonessential information, the nurse would look at me in a demeaning manner that clearly communicated disrespect.

I have witnessed new nurses break down and begin to cry when I asked before report how they were doing. On one unit, the nurse described how she felt that she had to prove herself, feeling belittled if she asked a question because the nurse would respond sarcastically, *"You don't know that?"* in a demeaning tone of voice. New nurses routinely overheard gossip about themselves or others and did not feel safe asking questions of certain nurses.

One New Nurse's Pain

One new nurse shared with me her experience with incivility and the emotional pain she experienced:

"I had heard of 'horizontal violence' in nursing school, but I never expected that it would happen to me, regularly in my own career and with my first position. I can honestly say that I cried every shift I worked for the first six months, and the only reason I stopped crying was not because it got any better, but because I had to change my expectations about the unit and accept my reality. I cannot put into words what it feels like to have nurses laugh in your face and belittle you when you ask a clinical question, roll their eyes and walk out on your report before it is finished, to literally have a back turned on you when trying to discuss a concern, or to be scolded or yelled at in front of your other colleagues until you are apologizing profusely with tears streaming down your cheeks.

"There have been countless times that I have overheard slanderous things said about me or some of my other colleagues, and the unit has accepted this kind of behavior as acceptable. Individuals, including management, have chosen to turn a blind eye to the dysfunction on the unit, which then gives individuals the false impression that this kind of behavior is acceptable. In order to survive on the unit I have had to learn which of my colleagues I can utilize as resources and positive resources and those that I cannot have contact with under any circumstances because they are toxic to me and toxic to the unit. I need to get off of the unit before I lose my passion for nursing altogether."

Consequences

This open letter validates the devastating consequences of a hostile work environment that creates feelings of inadequacy in a new nurse. Incivility is like putting gas on this fire, and feelings of failure, decreased self-esteem, self-doubt, anger, depression, burnout, and even post-traumatic stress disorder (PTSD) are common (Bartholomew, 2006). This can lead to decreased morale, low job satisfaction, increased absenteeism, and ulti-mately leaving the unit or even nursing entirely (Murray, 2008). Thirty percent of new nurses leave their first job after the first year when bullying is personally experi-enced (Johnson & Rea, 2009).

Incivility among nurses also adversely impacts pa-tient care. The Joint Commission has taken the position that incivility is a safety issue and has issued a standard to that effect. It has been shown that a unit that has a prevalence of incivility can lead to increased medical errors, adverse patient outcomes, and lower rates of nurse retention. By creating an environment that does not make it safe to ask questions, incivility poses a se-rious threat to patient safety and overall quality of care (Tillman Harris, 2011).

Root Causes

Why is incivility so endemic in nursing and nursing ed-ucation? One perspective in the literature is that incivility can be defined as RELATIONAL aggression, which is a feminine form of aggressive behavior. In comparison, men most often resort to PHYSICAL aggression with conflict. But because women comprise the majority of nurses, in-civility can manifest as relational aggression and is com-mon in the nursing profession (Dellasega, 2009).

Just as relational aggression among young women is normalized in adolescence through such vernacular as "mean girls," this accepted norm then becomes a self-fulfilling prophecy of what to expect in a profession where women are the majority. This may explain in part why there is an acceptance or tolerance of incivility in nursing. This pattern continues unchallenged because nurses do not challenge the status quo but are willing to put up with a hostile work environment to avoid conflict at all costs (Szutenbach, 2013).

Though bullying typically involves student peers or colleagues in the profession, it is also present when there is an unequal power relationship. In academia, this can be typified by the dean, department chair, or senior fac-ulty who bullies a new faculty member or when faculty members bully students.

Clinical Incivility

Nursing students are vulnerable to incivility because of inexperience and powerlessness as outsiders to the health care team. They are also under a tremendous amount of stress that can be exacerbated if incivility of any kind is experienced in the nursing program (Bowllan, 2015). Since the quality of student-staff nurse relationships is one of the most important factors that determine the qual-ity of the clinical learning experience (Levett-Jones, 2009), when incivility is directed towards students, it ad-versely impacts student learning. In one study, the ma-jority (88.7 percent) reported that they had experienced bullying in some context in the clinical setting. The most frequent bullying behaviors included (Clarke, Kane, Ra-jacich, & Lafreniere, 2012):

- Undervaluing student efforts (60.2%)
- Negative comments about becoming a nurse (45.3%)
- Unrealistic expectations (42.1%)
- Being treated with hostility (41.8%)
- Placed under pressure to produce work (41.5%)
- Being isolated or excluded (40.3%)

Clinical educators were identified as the greatest source of bullying behaviors (30.2 percent) followed by staff nurses (25.5 percent), classmates (15 percent), and patients and families (14 percent). Students were much more likely to consider leaving the nursing pro-gram (13 percent) as a result of having experienced bullying behaviors. In one study, 57.7 percent consid-ered leaving the program because of incivility (Celik & Bayrakatar, 2004).

Clinical Educators and Incivility

What is most concerning about the findings of Clarke's, et al., study is that nurse educators were responsible for role modeling incivility. Clinical faculty were responsi-ble for the following examples of incivility (Clarke, Kane, Rajacich, & Lafreniere, 2012):

- Undervaluing efforts
- Placing undue pressure to produce work
- Setting unrealistic expectations
- Intimidation with disciplinary measures
- Unjustly critical
- Changing clinical expectations without notice
- Threatening with a poor evaluation

If you are a clinical educator, reflect to determine if you may inadvertently be perceived by your students to be uncivil. For example, having high expectations for students is a good thing, but are they realistic, based on the professional development of the students you teach? If a student receives only persistent criticism and negative feedback, but nothing affirming, this could be perceived as uncivil by the student, though it may not be intentional. Effective communication skills can lessen the perception of uncivil behaviors. Be aware of any behaviors that could be perceived as uncivil so that you authentically role model caring and the professionals we want our students to become.

Staff nurses are also a primary source of incivility in the clinical setting. One study identified the following uncivil behaviors students experienced (Smith, Gillespie, Brown, & Grubb, 2016):

- Being ignored, intimidated, avoided, or isolated
- Nonverbal innuendo (sighs, eye rolling)
- Experiencing negative comments
- Being denied opportunities to learn
- Being hazed. Nurses who communicated that they liked to see students squirm.

If incivility by a staff nurse to a student occurs, it is the responsibility of the educator to advocate and address the concern directly with the nurse. This is never easy, but advocate for students by communicating what the student observed and perceived and allow the staff nurse to respond. Do not hesitate to use the chain of command and go to the charge nurse or nurse manager if you are unable to successfully resolve incivility directly.

Preparing Students to Change Culture

If your program uses the QSEN competencies, emphasize the competency of Teamwork and Collaboration. This competency situates the importance of CIVILITY by emphasizing the importance of respect and teamwork. Teamwork and collaboration is defined as the nurse who "functions effectively within nursing and inter-professional teams, fostering open communication, mutual respect, and shared decision making to achieve quality patient care" ("Pre-Licensure KSAS," 2014).

The attitudes needed to role-model teamwork include:

- VALUE the perspective and expertise of ALL health care team members.
- RESPECT the unique attributes that members bring to a team, including variations in professional orientations and accountabilities.
- APPRECIATE the importance of all professional collaboration.
- VALUE TEAMWORK and the relationships upon which it is based.
- VALUE different styles of communication used by patients, families, and health care providers.
- Contribute to resolution of conflict and disagreement ("Pre-Licensure KSAS," 2014).

Though these QSEN attitudes are important, what matters is what the nurse does. Be sure to emphasize the following ACTIONS and behaviors that must be lived out:

- Act with integrity, consistency, and respect for differing views.
- Demonstrate awareness of one's strengths and limitations as a team member.
- Initiate requests for help when needed.
- Function competently within one's scope of practice as a member of the health care team.
- Communicate with team members, adapting one's communication style to needs of the team and situation.
- Solicit input from other team members to improve individual, as well as team, performance.
- Initiate actions to resolve conflict.
- Assert one's position/perspective in discussions about patient care ("Pre-Licensure KSAS," 2014).

Power of Cognitive Rehearsal

The article "Teaching Cognitive Rehearsal as a Shield for Lateral Violence: An Intervention for Newly Licensed Nurses" is a must-read for every nurse educator. It defines professional behaviors as well as the most common uncivil behaviors. But more importantly, "cognitive rehearsal" teaches nurses to have a prepared plan to respond respectfully when specific uncivil behaviors are directed toward them. Because incivility thrives in an environment of passivity where it has become normalized, incivility can often be stopped in its tracks when it is addressed in an assertive, direct, and respectful way (Griffin, 2004).

In one study where nurses were empowered by this strategy, 100 percent of the nurses reported that when the perpetrator was confronted, the bullying behavior stopped (Coursey, Rodriguez, Dieckmann, & Austin, 2013). This strategy can be implemented when the nurse experiences incivility personally. For example, if a nurse has a pattern of raising eyebrows or sighs when asked for help, the empowered nurse has practiced and is prepared to respond in the following manner, "I sense (I see from your facial expression) that there may be something you wanted to say to me. Please speak directly to me" (Griffin, 2004).

Incivility Essentials

To strengthen the ability of students to respond appropriately when they experience incivility as a nurse in practice, this skill must also be practiced and contextualized to practice. I was asked by my hospital to do an incivility presentation for the new nurse residency program and created four practice-based scenarios that consist of uncivil encounters of nurses and physicians that demand an appropriate response. Here is a scenario with three questions the nurse must reflect upon, based on Griffin's article (2004):

You need to contact the physician for a clinical concern regarding a patient in your care. This physician is well known to other nurses to become angry and even verbally abusive towards nurses when he is called during the night. As you communicate your concern, the physician states in a harsh and angry tone of voice, "Why did you feel you had to address this in the middle of the night? This could have waited until morning!"

There are three questions that Griffin (2004) identified that need to be asked with any uncivil encounter to correctly process what just happened. These questions provide an opportunity for dialogue and practice of cognitive rehearsal that will directly translate to the practice setting:

1. Pause and process…what just happened?
2. What behaviors were uncivil in this encounter?
3. How should the nurse respond using cognitive rehearsal?

In addition to directly addressing incivility, encourage students to embrace the power of being a role model by living out respect, embracing diversity, and forming meaningful relationships with their fellow students and colleagues. Demonstrate professionalism in practice by never criticizing another student or colleague publicly, stand up for the absent colleague when they are not present, work as a team, and accept your share of the workload (Griffin, 2004).

I have observed from my own experience that patient care units are like families. Some are healthy and functional, while others are clearly dysfunctional and in need of intervention. Incivility is a toxic behavior that tends to be contagious and affects everyone on that unit. Remind your students that being a new nurse can feel like being in middle school again. You will want to do whatever it takes to fit in and be a part of the new group, even if it means being passive or indifferent to incivility around you. By being passive and doing nothing, you become part of the problem. Instead, encourage your students to hold themselves to the highest standards of professionalism in practice and be the change that is so desperately needed in nursing today!

The Elephant in the Room

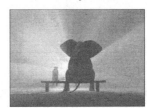

There is an elephant in the room of nursing education. What is this elephant that is not openly discussed yet present in most nursing education departments? The elephant is faculty-to-faculty incivility and how it steals the joy (Heinrich, 2006) of all too many nurse educators.

I recently received the following letter from a nurse educator that illustrates the problem.

One Educator's Story

"My transition from clinical practice into the academic setting has been one of the most rewarding, yet must frustrating and difficult experiences of my life. I entered academia and initially experienced a high level of professionalism and collegiality. Over time, things began to change and I began to feel targeted by uncivil behaviors after I received my doctorate two years ago.

"Being personally targeted and experiencing incivility has caused me to hate the job that I once

loved. If it wasn't for the students that I get to teach on a daily basis, I would leave academia in a heartbeat. It has now gotten to the point where I think of leaving my position all the time knowing that there has got to be a better educational environment out there than this.

"As a result of incivility, I have disengaged from my department. I currently keep my head down, stay under the radar, and keep quiet so I won't be noticed. Right now I continue to find myself bitter and extremely angry over how I have been unfairly treated and am completely ambivalent regarding my future in nursing education."

This nurse educator's experience is hardly unique. Varying levels of incivility are present in the majority of nursing education departments around the country (Clark, 2011). In one study, only 5 percent felt that faculty worked well together in their department (Heinrich, 2006).

Leading nurse educator and scholar Patricia Benner and the co-authors of *Educating Nurses* made it clear that nursing education is currently in need of RADICAL TRANSFORMATION. But to see this vision realized, our nursing departments must also be transformed by eliminating all vestiges of incivility because of its painful and destructive effects on colleagues. Incivility in academia has been shown to lower job satisfaction, decrease productivity, and increase turnover (Lester, 2009). The consequences of the anticipated nursing shortage will be exacerbated because of the inability to retain educators who may have a viable plan B of going back to clinical practice if academia remains an uncivil and hostile work environment.

CIVILITY must be the vision that educators strive to realize in their interactions with others. CIVILITY is RESPECT for others while honoring differences and seeking common ground with colleagues. It requires tolerating, listening, and being able to discuss differing viewpoints respectfully and treating one another with dignity and honor. (Clark & Carnosso, 2008).

Continuum of Incivility

Clark (2013) has identified that uncivil behaviors exist along a continuum that can range from subtle or more insidious behaviors to more active, aggressive behaviors that, if left unaddressed, can progress to threatening or violent

behaviors. According to Randle (2003), bullying is an ongoing, systematic pattern of behavior designed to intimidate, degrade, and humiliate another person through vicious words and cruel acts. Some examples of bullying behaviors include using threatening and abusive language and issuing constant and unreasonable criticism. Over time, an ongoing bullying culture can lead to acceptance of workplace mobbing, which is an even more aggressive type of bullying where more than one person collectively targets an individual with the intent to control, harm, and ultimately remove them from their current position.

In some cases, mobbing targets may be very good at what they do. Westhues (2004) identified that an "envy of excellence" and resultant jealousy of colleagues can occur when peers excel. Instead of celebrating the achievements and excellence of others, this jealousy can lead to creating an uncivil environment and workplace mobbing. In addition to the targeted colleague, students and their learning suffer when excellent faculty choose or are forced to leave academia because of endemic incivility.

Faculty to Faculty Incivility

In a recent study (Goldberg, Beitz, Wieland, & Levine, 2013), researchers identified the following unique aspects of incivility in academia:

Most likely targets

- **Promoters of change.** Faculty who do things differently or advocate for needed transformational change. If you plan to implement any of the recommendations from this book, consider yourself warned… You may have increased the likelihood that you may now have a target on your back!
- **Those who speak up/question status quo.**

Bullying tactics

- Withholding information
- Setting up to fail
- Gossip/personal slander
- Intentionally marginalizing or isolating targeted faculty

Bullying culture

- **Lack of teamwork and inability to work together.** This is a RED FLAG that a toxic, uncivil culture is present in clinical practice and academia.

- **Well-established cliques among faculty.** Most common clique is the old guard of senior faculty vs. new faculty who often see the need to change and do things differently.

Psychological responses by those targeted

- Humiliation
- Depression
- Feeling distracted, loss of concentration, diminished capacity for clinical judgment, anxiety, and physical sequelae such as G.I. disturbance, headaches, loss of appetite, and lack of sleep.
- Fearful/feelings of defenselessness because of isolation and lack of advocacy in the department
- **Self-blame.** What is wrong with me? This response is reinforced when a targeted colleague experiences similar patterns of incivility in other settings.

How targeted faculty fight back/cope

- Leave academia physically and never return to teaching, or mentally leave by disengaging from the department. Instead of packing their physical bags, they pack their mental bags and check out.
- Identify supportive colleagues who are safe.
- Stay invisible and fly beneath the radar.
- Use the pain of incivility as an opportunity for personal growth.

When incivility is experienced, though it may result in emotional scars, by choosing to leave a toxic environment, it provides an opportunity for healing to begin anew in a different department or setting.

Additional Themes of Academic Incivility

The literature has also identified the following additional themes of incivility that are unique to nursing education.

- Persistent gossip, criticism, and insulting, demeaning remarks (Clark & Springer, 2010)
- Nonverbal disapproval in staff meetings that include eye rolling, arm crossing, walking out of meetings, and the use of the "silent treatment" (Clark, 2013)
- Avoidant, isolative, and exclusionary behaviors that marginalize (Clark & Springer, 2010)
- Being blamed and falsely accused for something

they did not do (Clark, 2013)
- Setting others up to fail and intentional sabotage (Clark & Springer, 2010)
- Exerting superiority and rank over others/abuse of power (Clark & Springer, 2010)
- Not performing one's share of the workload (Clark & Springer, 2010)
- Power imbalance. Department chair or senior tenured faculty who use positional power to bully colleagues who are vulnerable because of their lower status in the department (Lester, 2009)
- Ingrained culture. Instead of seeing incivility as toxic and unhealthy, incivility is tolerated and even excused by leadership (Peters & King, 2017).

Are any of these additional examples of incivility in nursing education present in your department? Even if you are not experiencing incivility personally, but are passive or tolerant when gossip or other uncivil behaviors are expressed toward other colleagues, you, too, are part of the problem. I have also observed that when an uncivil culture is present, faculty who may not be currently bullied are fearful to speak up because they are afraid of becoming targeted as a result. Edmund Burke, an Irish political philosopher, once said, *"The only thing necessary for the triumph of evil is for good men to do nothing."* Incivility is a dark human behavior that I would consider evil. It must be confronted or it will continue to flourish unchallenged in your department. Culture can be changed when good men and women decide to take a stand and do something about it.

Do NOT minimize incivility because there are only one or two faculty who are a problem in your department. Incivility is like any cancer. Only a couple of cancerous cells can quickly replicate and destroy healthy cells and ultimately kill the host. In the same way, incivility has the power to replicate and be perpetrated by others, which can lead to the emotional destruction of previously healthy faculty (Clark, 2013). Therefore, ZERO tolerance for incivility and a cancer-free department is the goal for academia and ultimately the profession!

I have been amazed at the awareness and insightfulness nursing students have regarding detecting incivility and a lack of respect among faculty. Though it may be thought to be successfully "hidden" from students' awareness, it typically is not. It is "caught" and an object of discussion among students. What is the "hidden" curriculum in our programs and what are we really teaching our students? Tanner (1990) identified that it is NOT what is in the syllabus, but the verbal/nonverbal communication that is most important in what students really learn (Tanner, 1990).

Do You Still Have the Joy?

When incivility is experienced in the academic setting, one theme that Heinrich identified in her survey of nurse educators was that it causes "joy stealing." Her published article "Joy Stealing: 10 Mean Games Faculty Play and How to Stop the Gaming" must be read by every nurse educator. See if you can identify with the most common uncivil experiences and "games" in academia.

1. **The Set-Up Game.** Being set up to fail by lack of support or inequitable treatment by colleagues.
2. **The Devalue and Distort Game.** Your accomplishments are devalued or faculty turn your assets and strengths into liabilities.
3. **The Misrepresent and Lie Game.** Intentionally misrepresent/lie to prevent advancement or hire of targeted faculty.
4. **The Shame Game.** Private/public shaming with the intent to control.
5. **The Betrayal Game.** Being betrayed by colleague you thought was your friend.
6. **The Broken Boundaries Game.** When personal office space or professional boundaries are violated. For example, when your content is stolen by another or not given credit for your work that other faculty use.
7. **The Splitting Game.** When factions and division are present (new vs. senior faculty, adjunct vs. full-time, etc.).
8. **The Mandate Game.** Abusive use of power using win-lose tactics.
9. **The Blame Game.** When faculty make harsh or false accusations, ask questions later, and never apologize.
10. **The Exclusion Game.** Feeling isolated/marginalized for no obvious reason. (Heinrich, 2006)

Heinrich also identified that the emotional and psychological toll of incivility not only steals joy, but also impacts the zest, clarity, productivity, feelings of worth, and desire to be connected to a team or department (Heinrich, 2006). In addition to the personal impact of these games, a joy stealing environment can make it difficult to accomplish and bring needed change to your department because of the resistance and barriers that are encountered.

How to Change Academic Culture

To change department culture, the "elephant in the room" must be identified and called by its true name…incivility. Each faculty member must make a renewed commitment to treat one another with dignity and respect (Clark, 2011). More importantly, if you have been a sword that has wounded others with your sharp words, be humble and request forgiveness from those you have wounded.

To change the culture of a department where incivility is present takes time, patience, courage, and commitment to change by all in the department. The first, but also most difficult, step to bring healing is to respectfully address your concerns in private to an uncivil colleague. It can put an end to the problem by directly addressing the behavior (Clark, 2013). But to restore and maintain a culture of civility leadership needs to be directly involved and engaged to hold faculty accountable to be consistently civil and respectful.

In one report, the key to changing culture by cultivating civility in academia came down to three T's, truth telling, transparency, and tending to relationships (Heinrich, 2010).

1. **Truth telling.** Be direct and honest in all communication.
2. **Transparency.** Place in writing the standards you want to establish regarding how to support one another during the school year or scholarly pursuits.
3. **Tending to relationships.** Do not let the sun go down if you are still angry with a colleague. Deal with it that same day! Make the relationships in your department a priority, and nurture them so that the joy and passion that led you to become a nurse educator does not become derailed by incivility and hostile relationships.

WWFD?

What would Florence do (WWFD) to address incivility

in nursing? In her address to probationer nurses at St. Thomas Hospital in 1883, she said the following that provides insight:

"Let us run the race where all may win: rejoicing in their successes, as our own, and mourning their failures wherever they are, as our own. We are all one nurse." (Attewell, 2012, p. 76)

Nightingale's vision of professional nursing was to see that we are all ONE nurse as we care for patients in clinical practice or teach together in nursing departments. If this paradigm shift is lived out, the pain and struggles of others become our own. If a colleague is experiencing the pain of incivility, as ONE nurse I, too, share in her pain and will do whatever is needed to support or advocate if needed. This is also the essence of the timeless truth that was communicated in the parable of the Good Samaritan. When a fellow human being needs help, do something that demonstrates caring motivated by a heart of compassion.

Many are unaware of their own "blind spots" and cling to a view of reality that is not in accordance with the way things are. I have witnessed faculty, who were perpetrators of incivility, act as if they were the victim, expressing how mean and uncivil the other colleague was when in fact they were the uncivil perpetrators! Beware of triangulation and do not take sides with any conflict, but encourage direct communication between the parties responsible and avoid accelerating the drama in your department!

My Story

When I began my first position as a nurse educator several years ago, I was totally unprepared for the intensity and severity of incivility in the department. It was unlike anything I had experienced in the clinical setting. The uncivil behaviors that I observed included polarizing faculty attitudes toward the department chair, faculty denigrating one another openly in faculty staff meetings, and making it very clear they did not like or value one another. When these behaviors began to be directed toward me, it left a residual, painful "slime" that at times sticks to me even to this day.

When I applied for a tenure track position at the

end of the school year in a program where I had been hired as a temporary replacement, I was sure that I would be able to continue pursuing my love for teaching. I had positive student feedback and a lack of obvious problems. But to my shock and surprise I received the formal letter that told me I would not be coming back. Desperate to make sense of what just happened, I obtained a copy of the official notes of the faculty team who interviewed me.

What I read was shocking. My record was misrepresented and serious concerns about my performance were now in writing, but were NOT addressed to me personally during the school year. In the language of the nursing literature, I had "information withheld" that as a result "set me up to fail." I said to myself, "Never again! I can make more money with less stress in clinical practice."

I was distraught as I packed my bags and left my office at the end of the year, not sure if I would ever teach again. I knew that teaching was something I was very good at and enjoyed doing. But a shift had taken place that I was not consciously aware of. I had become unbalanced. Teaching was not only my passion, it had become my life! Doing what was needed to help my students learn gave me a sense of worth, value, and identity. As I painfully processed my future and next steps over the summer, Psalm 23:1–3 became very personal.

The Lord is my shepherd; I shall not want.
He makes me lie down in green pastures.
He leads me beside still waters.
He restores my soul.

Because I was not teaching, I was forced to take a much needed break and LIE DOWN. I did not realize it at the time, but I was emotionally and physically exhausted at the end of the school year. Our family could not afford me to rely on an educator salary so I continued to work 24 hours every weekend in clinical practice in addition to a full academic load. After I was forced to lie down, I was able to rest, which, over time, led to my RESToration.

Knowing that I am loved by God who is also a Good Shepherd restored my sense of true identity and worth. I realized that my true identity as a child of God can never be taken from me. I am secure. By the grace of God I am still standing but my path has changed. I am now engaged to serve the needs of educators to help bring needed transformation. But there is more to my story. It is how God used one person to encourage me and who was also instrumental to my healing when I needed it most.

If you have experienced the slime of incivility, you know that it has a way of "sticking" to you long after the event occurs. Though I always value the opportunity to share how educators can integrate clinical reasoning in the class and clinical settings at conferences, I was still struggling with the residue of incivility I had recently encountered when I presented at Elsevier's Faculty Development Institute in 2013. Dr. Patricia Benner was the keynote speaker, and I brought my well-marked copy of Educating Nurses to be signed by her, which she graciously did. I had a well-received breakout session that situated clinical reasoning and the recommendations from Patricia Benner and her co-authors from *Educating Nurses*. I finished my session and several educators made their way up front to talk with me afterward.

Another educator approached from a distance, making her way up front. Other educators who saw her coming moved out of the way to allow her to come to meet me. All she said was, "We need to talk, and I 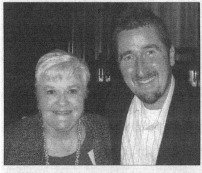 would like to know if we could meet for lunch." Since it was time for the lunch break, I quickly said yes because I recognized her from our prior meeting. It was Patricia Benner! Unknown to me, she had been in the audience for my session and wanted to let me know how much she appreciated my insights that made her work on clinical reasoning practical for nurse educaors to implement. Patricia Benner validated, encouraged, and affirmed me and recognized my contributions as an educator. She even left the door open to possible collaboration together in the future. The residue of incivility that had been sticking to me melted in a puddle at my feet, and I have since moved on, kept my head up, and have not looked back. Though the memory remains, its power was broken!

Takeaways

I share my story to illustrate a powerful life principle; the power of validation and encouragement to one another in stress-filled nursing departments. There are three takeaways I don't want you to miss.

1. **Be a Benner.** Patricia Benner took the time to recognize what I had done well and encouraged me in our time together. Do the same by communicating caring, support, and words of encouragement to those you work with regularly. It is needed and appreciated! Respect, appreciation, and validation can create a culture of civility and bring healing to hearts that have been wounded by incivility or provide needed support in a stressful work environment. "Be a Benner" and follow her powerful and professional example to go out of your way to encourage and affirm your colleagues whenever and as much as possible.

2. **Give no one the power to steal your joy, passion, and talent that you possess as a nurse educator.** Remain true to your ideal and give no one the power to steal your joy. Do NOT run away if incivility has wounded you, but take your stand and do NOT allow this villain to keep you from your calling. Persevere in the midst of any adversity incivility may bring. Stay faithful to the reasons that influenced your decision to become an educator and do not look back!

3. **Those who are uncivil do not define you or have the last word on your worth.** My passion is teaching others. I thought it would be in the context of teaching nursing students, but since I was not asked to return to teach in academia, doors have since opened to continue to teach, by instructing educators through my work and case studies on clinical reasoning and through my website, blog, YouTube channel, and presentations across the country. If your journey has taken an unexpected turn because of the incivility of others, be confident that God is in control of your life and story. Just keep

moving forward! As I share my story and the incivility I experienced, I often see educators wiping away tears. I know that they can all too easily identify with the pain of my experience because they have lived and experienced it as well. If you have been wounded by incivility, do not take the assessment of others personally! Step back to see the bigger picture of your life and story and do NOT let the villain of incivility derail your calling and purpose as an educator. Find supportive colleagues and persevere to make a difference in the students you teach!

Overcoming the Villain

What do *Cinderella*, the *Wizard of Oz*, and the *Lion King* all have in common? These popular fairy tales and stories all have a villain (Evil Stepmother, Wicked Witch of the West, and Scar) that almost succeeded in derailing the purpose and destiny of Cinderella, Dorothy, and Simba. These stories are mythic and communicate timeless truths. Your life is also an unfolding story. You, too, have a unique purpose and destiny to fulfill as a nurse or nurse educator. It is not a coincidence that you are in your current role. But your story also has a villain.

In nursing or nursing education, incivility and bullying behaviors have the power to be the villain of your story. It can be so painful, joy stealing, and relentless that some will throw in the towel and allow incivility and bullying behaviors to keep them from pursuing their passion and calling. Despite adversity, these characters overcame and did NOT allow the villain to win. The purposes of their lives were realized and fulfilled. The same can and needs to be true for you as well.

The Power of Words

Words that are spoken are a two-edged sword. They can bring healing, as Patricia Benner demonstrated, or they can deeply wound. In childhood, there was a common saying, "Sticks and stones may break my bones but words can never hurt me!" Unfortunately, this statement is a lie, because words do hurt, and disrespectful words or words spoken in anger can have a power to become our identity and the way we view ourselves. Because so much hinges on our words and how we communicate with one another, we must strive to be QUICK to listen and SLOW to speak!

Solomon, the wisest man of ancient history, wrote the following words of wisdom in Proverbs that, if put into practice, will recapture civility in nursing and nursing education. I have found the following principles of communication life-giving and restorative if they are put into practice with all that we say and do.

Our words have power. *"There is one whose rash words are like sword thrusts, but the tongue of the wise brings healing."* Proverbs 12:18

We must learn to listen. *"The ear that listens to life-giving reproof will dwell among the wise."* Proverbs 15:31

Be SLOW to anger. *"Whoever is slow to anger is better than the mighty, and he who rules his spirit than he who takes a city."* Proverbs 16:32

Speak less. *"The more talk, the less truth; the wise measure their words."* Proverbs 10:19

Our tone matters. *"A soft answer turns away wrath, but a harsh word stirs up anger."* Proverbs 15:1

Reflect

1. What "dance" between students and faculty currently exists in your program…respect or disrespect?

2. What are the most common examples of STUDENT to FACULTY incivility that are prevalent in your program? How have you addressed them?

3. What are the most common examples of FACULTY to STUDENT incivility that you or your colleagues may have demonstrated? How have you addressed them?

4. What are the most common examples of FACULTY to FACULTY incivility present in your department? How have you addressed them?

5. Who do you need to forgive or offer forgiveness to in your department in order to bring needed healing?

6. If you have experienced incivility, what are you doing, or need to do to overcome this villain?

References

Attewell, A. (2012). *Illuminating florence: Finding nightingale's legacy in your practice.* Indianapolis, IN: Sigma Theta Tau International.

Bartholomew, K., (2006), *Ending nurse to nurse hostility: Why nurses eat their young and each other.* Marblehead, MA: HCPro Incorporated.

Bowllan, N.M. (2015). Nursing students' experience of bullying: Prevalence, impact, and interventions. *Nurse Educator, 40*(4), 194-198.

Celik, S.S., & Bayraktar, N. (2004). A study of nursing student abuse in turkey. *Journal of Nursing Education, 43,* 330-336.

Clark, C. M. (2008). The dance of incivility in nursing education as described by nursing faculty and students. *Advances in Nursing Science, 31,* E37–E54.

Clark, C. M. (2011). Pursuing a culture of civility: An intervention study of one program of nursing, *Nurse Educator, 36*(3), 98–102.

Clark, C. (2013a). *Creating & sustaining civility in nursing education.* Indianapolis, IN: Sigma Theta Tau.

Clark, C. M. (2013b). National study on faculty-to-faculty incivility: Strategies to foster collegiality and civility. *Nurse Educator, 38*(3), 98–102.

Clark, C. M., & Carnosso, J. (2008). Civility: A concept analysis. *Journal of Theory Construction & Testing, 12,* 11–15.

Clark, C., & Springer, P. (2007a). Incivility in nursing education: A descriptive study of definitions and prevalence. *Journal of Nursing Education, 46,* 7-14.

Clark, C. M., & Springer, P.J. (2010). Academic nurse leaders' role in fostering a culture of civility in nursing education, *Journal of Nursing Education, 49*(6), 319–325.

Clark, C. M., Olender, L., Kenski, D., & Cardoni, C. (2013). Exploring and addressing faculty-to-faculty incivility: A national perspective and literature review. *Journal of Nursing Education, 52*(4), 211–218.

Clarke, C.M., Kane, D.J., Rajacich, D.L., & Lafreniere, K.D. (2012). Bullying in undergraduate clinical nursing education. *Journal of Nursing Education, 51*(5), 269-276.

Coursey, J. H., Rodriguez, R.E., Dieckmann, L.S., & Austin, P.N. (2013). Successful implementation of policies addressing lateral violence. *AORN Journal, 97*(3), 101–109.

Dellasega, C. A. (2009). Bullying among nurses. *American Journal of Nursing, 109,* 52–58.

Griffin, M. (2004). Teaching cognitive rehearsal as a shield for lateral violence: An intervention for newly licensed nurses. *The Journal of Continuing Education in Nursing, 35,* 257–263.

Goldberg, E., Beitz, J., Wieland, D., & Levine, C. (2013). Social bullying in nursing academia. *Nurse Educator, 38*(5), 191–197.

Heinrich, K. T. (2006). Joy-stealing games. Retrieved from the Reflections on Nursing Leadership Web site: http://www.reflectionsonnursingleadership.org/pages/ vol32_2_heinrich.aspx

Heinrich, K.T. (2010). An optimist's guide for cultivating civility among academic nurses. *Journal of Professional Nursing, 26*(6), 325–331.

Johnson, S. J., & Rea, R. E. (2009). Workplace bullying: Concerns for nurse leaders. *The Journal of Nursing Administration, 39*(2), 84–90.

Lester, J. (2009). Not your child's playground: Workplace bullying among community college faculty. *Community College Journal of Research and Practice, 33,* 444–462.

Levett-Jones, T., Lathlean, J., Higgins, I., & McMillan, M. (2009). Staff-student relationships and their impact on nursing student's, belongingness and learning. *Journal of Advanced Nursing, 65,* 316-324.

Marchiondo, K., Marchiondo, L.A., & Lasiter, S. (2010). Faculty incivility: Effects on program satisfaction of BSN students. *Journal of Nursing Education, 49*(11), 608-614.

Murray, J. S. (2008). No more nurse abuse. *American Nurse Today,* 17–19.

Peters, A.B, & King, L. (2017). Barriers to civil academic work environments: Experiences of academic faculty leaders. *Nurse Educator, 42*(1), 38-41.

Pre-Licensure KSAS. (2014). QSEN.com. Retrieved from http://qsen.org/competencies/pre-li censure-ksas/#patient-centered_care

Randle, J. (2003). Bullying in the nursing profession. *Journal of Advanced Nursing, 43*, 395–401.

Smith, C.R., Gillesoie, G.L., Brown, K.C., & Grubb, P.L. (2016). Seeing students squirm: Nursing students' experiences of bullying behaviors during clinical rotations. *Journal of Nursing Education, 55*(9), 505-513.

Stagg, S. J., Sheridan, D., Jones, R., & Gabel Speroni, K. (2011). Evaluation of a workplace bullying cognitive rehearsal program in a hospital setting. *The Journal of Continuing Education, 12*(9), 395–401.

Szutenbach, M. (2013). Bullying in nursing: Roots, rationales, and remedies. *Journal of Christian Nursing, 30*(1), 16–23.

Tanner, C. A. (1990). Clinical education, circa 2010. *Journal of Nursing Education, 41*(2), 51–52

Tanner, C. A. (1990). Caring as a value in nursing education. *Nursing Outlook, 38*(2), 70–72.

Tillman Harris, C. (2011). Incivility in nursing. Retrieved from Tips to improve patient education skills (2015). *Bold Voices, 7*(8), 14.

Westhues, K. (2004). *The envy of excellence: Administrative mobbing of high-achieving professors.* Lewis ton, NY: Edwin Mellen Press.

Transforming Academia by Improving Male Student Success

Keith Rischer, RN, MA, CEN, CCRN

"Men have no place in nursing "except where physical strength was needed."
—Florence Nightingale

Quantitative research has shown that the barriers men face in nursing education are "pervasive, consistent, and have changed little over time."
—Chad O'Lynn, PhD, RN

Author's note: Gender as well as ethnic diversity is needed in nursing education. International students also have unique struggles that need to be addressed to remedy their high failure-to-complete rates in academia as well. I have included recommended resources in the appendix. As a graduate nursing student I did my thesis on the topic of men in nursing and performed an exhaustive review of the nursing literature. This chapter is a reflection of what I discovered. I have found that most nurse educators are unaware of the history, legacy, and current struggles of men in nursing and nursing education. It is my hope that this chapter will shine light to bring needed change.

Male nursing students have one of the highest failure-to-complete nursing education rates of any demographic in nursing education today. In one study, the failure to complete rate for men was almost 30 percent; in comparison, women had a 10 percent failure to complete rate. The statistical relationship of gender and course completion in this same study was p=0.009 (McLaughlin, Muldoon, & Moutray, 2010). These findings have been replicated where male failure to complete rates remain as high as 40-50 percent in some programs. What are the contributing factors to this finding? What can be done in nursing education to promote the success of men in nursing education? In order to understand this current dynamic, it needs to be put in his-

torical perspective to understand how the recent past may continue to influence the present.

Historical Legacy of Men as Caregivers

Nursing has not always been primarily a woman's profession. From the beginning of recorded history, caring for the sick was primarily the responsibility of male caregivers. In the BC era, the following are historical examples:

- 400 BC: In Hippocratic writings in ancient Greece, public nursing care was provided by men (Brown, 2000).
- 400 BC: In ancient Rome, the best possible care was provided to soldiers in military hospitals by male caregivers called "nosocomi" (O'Lynn & Tranbarger, 2007). Unfortunately, this legacy has been tarnished because it is also the root word for "hospital" or "nosocomial" acquired infection!
- 250 BC: In India, the first public hospitals were developed where only men were taught and trained as primary caregivers (O'Lynn & Tranbarger, 2007).
- In the AD era, this historical trend continued as caring for the sick became a ministry of the early Christian church. Both men and women served as caregivers in this era. Examples of the ongoing legacy of male caregivers include the following:
- AD 100: Male deacons as well as female dea-

conesses were responsible for ministering and caring for those who were ill (Anthony, 2004).

- AD 100–476: Roman Empire–Men continued to serve as nosocomi in military hospitals until the fall of the Roman Empire in AD 476.

- AD 300: In early Christian Greece and Rome, orders of monks known as Parabolani sacrificially cared for victims of the plagues. As a result, many monks lost their lives (Anthony, 2004).

- AD 324–1453: Byzantine period in Eastern Europe– Both men and women were caregivers in the hospitals that provided care (O'Lynn & Tranbarger, 2007).

- AD 400–1600: Historical accounts of the monastic movement show that men were responsible for the nursing care of the sick, wounded, and dying (O'Lynn & Tranbarger, 2007).

- AD 1100: Brothers of St. Anthony developed hospitals in France, Spain, and Italy (O'Lynn & Tranbarger, 2007).

- AD 1400: Alexian Brothers cared for victims of the plague and buried the dead. They became a religious community that continues to serve the needs of the sick today (O'Lynn & Tranbarger, 2007).

- AD 1500: St. Camillus de Lellis, a Franciscan monk who founded the male caregiving order of the Camellians, created the symbol of the red cross that remains the universal symbol of health care today. His order serves in 35 countries today (O'Lynn & Tranbarger, 2007).

- AD 1600: Men also participated in nonmilitary orders during this time up until the sixteenth century when monastery orders were dissolved (Evans, 2004).

Nightingale and the Modern Era

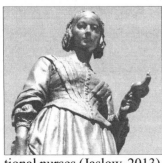

Despite the rich historical legacy that men have experienced as caregivers, why are there so few men in nursing today? Men currently comprise 9.6 percent of registered nurses and 8.1 percent of licensed vocational nurses (Jaslow, 2013). In order to put the currently low participation rates of men in nursing in perspective, we have to go back 150 years. Though I admire Nightin-

gale for her passion and vision to pioneer the modern era of nursing, she had a philosophical worldview regarding men in nursing that continues to influence the present.

"No one individual was more responsible for ushering in a period of female domination of nursing than Nightingale" (O'Lynn & Tranbarger, 2007, p. 323). When Nightingale instituted the modern era of nursing, she chose to firmly establish nursing as a woman's occupation. To her, *"every woman was a nurse,"* and a woman who entered nurse training was doing only what came naturally (Evans, 2004). European religious sisterhoods also embraced Nightingale's reforms, which by their very nature were exclusive to women (Anthony, 2004).

Nightingale believed that men have no place in nursing "except where physical strength was needed" (Villeneuve, 1994) and that men's "hard and horny" hands were not fit to touch, bathe, and dress wounded limbs, however gentle their hearts may be (Brown, 2000).

In England during the late 1800s, men who remained in nursing were excluded from general nursing practice as well as Nightingale's schools of nursing. The only practice environment available to men at this time was in the insane asylums where men were needed because of their physical strength to restrain violent patients. The psychiatric education of men was considered inferior in length and quality in comparison to the women who attended Nightingale's schools of nursing. If a man wanted to expand his learning to include obstetrics and maternal-child nursing, he was perceived as a pervert and threatened with expulsion (Evans, 2004).

There were also other social and cultural forces in the mid-1800s that contributed to the lack of men who chose to enter the nursing profession. These social forces included the decline of male monastic orders that began in the 1500s with the Protestant Reformation, the increase in the number of convents and female nursing orders, and the Industrial Revolution of the 1800s that attracted men for its higher pay and no demand for formal education (O'Lynn & Tranbarger, 2007).

Institutional/Educational Bias

Because men were not allowed to be trained as general nurses, by 1900 in England, general hospitals were dominated by female nurses. By 1919, the General Nursing Council (the equivalent of our current state boards of nursing) offered full membership only to women who were "general trained." Since most men were not able to be admitted to these schools, nursing consolidated its position as the first self-determining female profession (Mackintosh, 1997). Men comprised only 0.004 percent of nurses in England from 1921–1938; the laws were changed to allow general nursing schools to accept men in 1947 (Mackintosh, 1997).

In the United States, men in nursing were excluded from membership in professional organizations such as the American Nurses Association (ANA) that was founded in 1897. African-American nurses faced no similar bias. Men continued to be barred from the ANA until 1930 when the official position of the ANA was changed to strongly support men in nursing (O'Lynn & Tranbarger, 2007). National laws that were in place between 1901 and 1955 prevented men from serving as nurses in the United States Army Nurse Corps. It was only after the Korean War that this policy was changed. This continued to lower male participation in nursing in the United States so that by 1930, less than 1 percent of nurses were men (Anthony, 2004).

Men in Nursing: By the Decades

In order to put this past gender bias and discrimination that men have experienced in historical context, the small but incremental increases over the decades validates the early struggles that men experienced in the modern era and suggest the power of ongoing social, cultural, and educational barriers that persist today. These were the participation percentages of men in nursing 100 years later after the modern era was instituted by the reforms of Nightingale:

- 1950: 1%
- 1960: 1%
- 1970: 2.7%
- 1980: 4.1%
- 1990: 5.7%
- 2000: 7.6%
- 2011: 9.6%

In comparison, female participation in the once male- dominated profession of medicine demonstrated dramatic movement to participation parity. But it wasn't always that way. Women had comparably low percentages of participation in the 1950s but achieved gender parity with dramatic increases in the last 20 years.

- 1950: 5.7%
- 1970: 9.4%
- 1980: 28.2%
- 1990: 39.2%
- 2000: 45.6%
- 2014: 47.0

Lingering Bias

Though gender bias and discrimination toward men in nursing was evident in the past, is this bias still evident today? Would it surprise you to know that up until the 1960s only 15 percent of public nursing schools were willing to admit men into their program? As recent as 1981, a public school of nursing continued to exclude men because of their gender (Jaslow, 2013). As recently as 2004, a hospital in West Virginia had a policy that prevented qualified male nurses from working in obstetrics due to concerns of patient privacy. This case was appealed all the way to the Supreme Court (Kouta & Kaite, 2011). It is ironic that male obstetricians are widely accepted in this clinical area, but male nurses typically are not.

Social/Cultural Barriers

Though the discriminatory policies of the past have been a contributing factor to the low participation rates of men in nursing, why don't more men seriously consider entering the nursing profession today? Numerous studies have addressed this topic and some of the barriers that men most commonly identified include the following (Roth & Coleman, 2008).

Traditional Feminine Image of Nursing

- Because nursing remains a female-dominated profession, the perception that nursing is "women's work" is not inherently attractive to most men. Combine this perception with an adolescent male who may be struggling to establish a sense of gender identity and what it means to be a man, and nursing will not be seriously considered as an option by most.

Gender Role Strain

- Masculine role strain can be defined as the tension that is experienced when a man chooses to pursue a gender role that is perceived as being incompatible with being a man. This ties in closely with the first social barrier of nursing being a woman's profession.

- Depending on the degree of social support that a male student receives, if strong social support is not present, this will influence whether he will complete the program.

Lack of Male Role Models/Mentors

- Because the current participation of men in nursing remains less than 10 percent, men who decide to become a nurse have few if any male role models in the nursing profession. This influence is taken for granted by women who have mothers or other family members who are nurses and can look to them for guidance and affirmation in pursuing nursing as a career option.
- Consider the influence of media. What examples of men in nursing are positive role models that men can aspire to be like? One that comes to mind is Gaylord Focker from *Meet the Parents*. Though this movie was at times very funny, it reinforced the majority of negative stereotypes about men who choose to enter the nursing profession.

The Name of the Profession…NURSE!

- Words do have power and carry strong associations. In one study of 100 male high school students, the number of male students who would consider nursing increased from six to twenty-one when nursing was renamed by the gender neutral title "registered clinician" (Gorman, 2003).
- Recognizing the implications of this finding, as well as the feminine overtones of the word "nurse," will nursing be willing to consider a gender-neutral title to remove this barrier for male participation? This is not unthinkable and has been done in other contexts. The airline industry changed the name of the overtly feminine title "stewardess" to the inclusive and gender-neutral title of "flight attendant" when men began to enter this female-dominated profession.
- Professions that were once male dominated have changed their names to be gender-inclusive. For example, when women began to enter male-dominated occupations such as police and fire protection, the prior title of policeMAN and fireMAN were replaced with the gender-neutral titles of police OFFICER and fireFIGHTER.

Stereotypes

Stereotypes in nursing have the power to distort reality about what is true about those who are members of the profession. The power of distorted assumptions cuts both ways for men and women in nursing. For women, the most common stereotype is the "naughty nurse" who uses her position to seduce and meet the sexual needs of her male patients. This stereotype demeans and degrades women as well as the nursing profession.

Unfortunately, the stereotypes that men experience are just as prevalent and just as powerful to distort reality (McLaughlin, Muldoon, & Moutray, 2010). Listed below are the most common assumptions and stereotypes that men encounter if they choose to enter the nursing profession. Was it just a coincidence that the lead character from *Meet the Parents* was named GAYlord (emphasis mine) Focker and played off the top three stereotypes that men in nursing are homosexual, effeminate, and not smart enough for medical school?

The following are the most common stereotypes that men encounter:

- Homosexual
- Effeminate
- Underachievers–not smart enough for medical school
- Sexual predators
- Not as caring/compassionate

Educational Barriers

Though nursing education has little control over the broader social/cultural barriers of men who enter the nursing profession, it does have control over its academic culture. Unfortunately, nursing educational barriers continue to exist that directly impact the success of men in academia. Quantitative research has shown that the barriers men face in nursing education are "pervasive, consistent, and have changed little over time" (O'Lynn, 2004). Though overt bias is rare, COVERT discrimination is much more common.

One way this more subtle form of discrimination manifests itself is the feminine emphasis on how to provide care. The underlying message to male students is that in order to be a nurse, you have to behave like a woman (Carol, 2006). In addition, fundamental nursing textbooks have limited or excluded historical male contributions to nursing while emphasizing those of women. This revision of nursing history perpetuates the myth that nursing has always been a female-dominated profession (Anthony, 2004).

Nursing faculty may also be inadvertently part of the problem. Men perceive an inherent bias in nursing education with feelings of isolation and loneliness exacerbated by the lack of male faculty who serve as role models, as well as the use of the pronoun "she" and assumption that nursing is a feminine profession. In addition, the pedagogies used in education emphasize feminine learning styles, communication strategies, personal reflection, and methods of caring (Dyck, Oliffe, Phinney, & Garrett, 2009).

Male students quickly realize that if they are assertive or question faculty (traditional masculine traits) they are stigmatized and targeted as a potential problem. As a result, they temper their masculine behavior and act more feminine to "fit in." Though there is an assumption by some faculty that men who enter nursing are doing so primarily for financial gain, the motivation for men to enter nursing is similar to women: the desire to help others, a sense of calling, and job security (Harding, 2009).

A National League for Nursing (NLN) core competency for nurse educators is creating an environment that facilitates student learning. This is done by recognizing the influence of gender, experience, and other factors to learning ("Core Competencies of Nurse Educators with Task Statements," 2005). In essence, the NLN holds every nurse educator to a standard that breaks down perceived or actual barriers to learning. Therefore, every nurse educator has a responsibility to directly address and confront the educational barriers toward men that continue to be documented in the literature and persist in nursing education today.

The following themes from the literature identify barriers that persist in nursing education that may influence the ability of men to successfully complete nursing education.

1. No history of men in nursing (McLaughlin, Muldoon, & Moutray, 2010)
2. Lack of guidance on masculine styles of caring (O'-Lynn, 2003)
3. No guidance on "intimate touch" (Harding, North, & Perkins, 2008)
4. Lack of guidance on how men and women communicate differently (O'Lynn, 2004)

5. "Chilly" classroom climate (Bell-Scriber, 2008)
6. Exclusive use of lecture in classroom (O'Lynn, 2004)
7. Feelings of isolation/loneliness (Stott, 2007)
8. Lack of male mentoring/role modeling (O'Lynn, 2004)

No History of Men in Nursing

If men have no knowledge of their historical legacy and identity as caregivers and have an inaccurate perception that nursing has always been "women's work," this may prevent some men from considering the nursing profession and completing nursing education. Most fundamental nursing textbooks continue to limit or exclude the male contributions to nursing while emphasizing those of women (McLaughlin, Muldoon, & Moutray, 2010). This revision of nursing history perpetuates the myth that nursing has always been a female-dominated profession (O'Lynn & Tranbarger, 2007). If the historical legacy of men as caregivers was clearly presented in textbooks and widely known by nurse educators, this barrier could be eliminated immediately!

This obstacle is one of the most important barriers to bring down and also one of the easiest. Faculty who recognize the need to make this legacy known can present this content in their classroom or create a handout for their students to address the current gap in nursing education regardless of what textbook publishers choose to publish.

I have been impressed with the accuracy and extensive inclusion of men in nursing history found in Kozier & Erb's *Fundamentals of Nursing*. Unfortunately, this textbook is the exception. The following are examples of bias and even revision of nursing history in others:

In a former but recent edition of a top-selling fundamental textbook, the "Milestones in Nursing History" table begins with this entry: "AD 400, entry of women into nursing." They were off by almost 1,000 years and cited the wrong gender (Potter & Perry, 2004)!

The current edition of this fundamental textbook begins nursing history with Florence Nightingale, ignoring more than 2,000 years of caregiving that included male participation and male nursing leaders (Potter & Perry, 2012).

ACTION Points for Educators
- Present and address both the BC and AD eras in

your nursing history lecture as well as examples of men as caregivers. I highly recommend Chad O'Lynn's recent book, *A Man's Guide to a Nursing Career,* because of its thorough documentation of the history of men in nursing. It includes relevant role models of male caregivers who served sacrificially as they cared for others.

- Closely examine the fundamentals of nursing textbook that your program uses. If the history of men in nursing is inaccurate, minimal, or nonexistent, contact your book representative and express your concern! If an error is found in a textbook, it is typically addressed and corrected for the next edition. In the same way, any inaccurate or lack of information about men as caregivers should also be addressed and will hopefully be included in the next edition.

Lack of Guidance on Masculine Styles of Caring
Men Care Differently
Certain masculine traits have been perceived as being incompatible with caring. Florence Nightingale believed that men were incapable of caring and advocated for the removal of men from traditional patient care settings (Dossey, 1999). This inaccurate assumption has been reinforced by feminists including Gilligan and Chodorow, who have tied caring behaviors as belonging exclusively to woman (Thompson, 2002).

As a male member of the nursing profession, I can personally attest to the truth that men do care and are fully capable of caring behaviors. But just as there are distinct gender styles related to communication, there are also masculine styles of caring. In one qualitative study of male nursing students (Patterson, et al., 1996) men communicated caring by establishing a rapport with patients that was not dependent on the use of touch. In another study, men used humor in their interactions with patients to develop a caring rapport.

Women are much more likely to use physical touch as they provide care. Since most nurse educators are women, they emphasize a feminine style of caring (O'-Lynn, 2003) when evaluating caring for both men and women. In one quantitative study (O'Lynn, 2003), 30.9 percent of men reported that nursing faculty emphasized feminine styles of caring, while 53.6 percent reported that they received no guidance or instruction of the masculine styles of caring that are documented in the literature.

ACTION Point for Educators
- Provide content and instruction in your curriculum on masculine styles of caring and how it differs from women.

No Guidance on "Intimate Touch"
When men use touch with a woman, it can be interpreted as potentially sexual regardless of the context. When women use touch, it is typically interpreted as an act of caring. The use of physical touch for men in nursing becomes a cause of potential concern when men perform intimate cares or procedures on women. Men also experience stress and vulnerability when providing intimate care because of the potential need to explain and defend themselves in the no-win situation of "my word against hers" should an allegation of inappropriate touch be made, even if the patient is confused.

Because most nurse educators are women, this aspect of male vulnerability is not recognized or considered, but it is documented in the literature (Evans, 2002). Addressing the vulnerability that some men may experience is also not addressed in most fundamental textbooks. Provide your male students with practical strategies to DECREASE stress and vulnerability and provide a sense of safety when providing intimate care in the clinical setting.

The following strategies will help provide needed support and decrease your male students' stress while providing intimate care or procedure such as catheterization (Harding, North, & Perkins, 2008).

- **Establish and build trust by being professional in all aspects of patient care.** This will decrease the likelihood for intimate touch to be misinterpreted.
- **Obtain permission to do intimate care/procedure.** This communicates professionalism and respect for women who may not say no unless given an opportunity to do so.
- **Use a female chaperone if there is a potential for being vulnerable.** The most common example of this intervention is when a female patient is confused. Also utilize if the patient expresses this preference.
- **Communicate and explain everything that you will do ahead of time and while you are doing it.** This will decrease the likelihood of any touch being misinterpreted, especially when the labia are being cleansed and separated to prepare for insertion of the

catheter. Communicate in a calm and confident manner that is free of anxiety while engaging the patient in conversation (Evans, 2013).

- **Modify techniques to limit personal exposure and ensure privacy.** Limiting exposure will allow the woman to feel safe and respected and ensure her dignity, and she will likely not misinterpret intimate touch.
- **Delegate intimate care to women.** If a female patient prefers a woman to provide intimate care, then have a female colleague do so.

ACTION Point for Educators

- Provide content and instruction in your curriculum HOW to practically provide intimate touch while providing care especially from the male perspective.
- Provide opportunities for male students to practice these best-practice principles in the skills lab when performing perineal care. This strategy was found to improve the comfort that men experienced when providing intimate touch (O'Lynn & Krautscheid, 2014).

Lack of Guidance on How Men and Women Communicate Differently

Men and women are different and unique in many ways. This includes differences in the communication styles of men and women. To strengthen communication in the clinical setting, men and women need to be aware of these differences so there is greater understanding and more effective communication between men and women. One barrier that men in nursing education experience is a lack of instruction on communicating more effectively with women (O'Lynn, 2004).

Women tend to emphasize the relational nature of communication, using verbal and nonverbal cues to establish "rapport talk" to connect with others. This may include sharing information about their family, children, significant others, or more intimate details of their life. In comparison, men tend to emphasize the content aspects of communication that focus on "just the facts" to accomplish needed tasks. Men tend to wonder when female nurses will get to the point, and women may make the inaccurate assumption that men are unfriendly or withdrawn because they do not reciprocate with "rapport talk" (O'Lynn & Tranbarger, 2007).

Another area that men and women communicate dif-

ferently is how they give and receive praise. Women tend to liberally give and receive praise regularly to others. Praise communicates that their efforts are appreciated and noticed. The norms of masculine communication emphasize goals and getting things done. Men tend to give praise when something significant was accomplished or done very well, not routinely. This can lead to misunderstandings in the workplace when the male nurse receives praise from women and may think that he is above average. Conversely, because men do not tend to offer praise for ordinary efforts, women may feel that he does not value or appreciate her efforts and make the assumption that he is cold or arrogant as a result (O'Lynn & Tranbarger, 2007).

Men and women tend to make judgments differently. While women tend to be nonjudgmental, men are more likely to rush to judgment and reach a decision more quickly. This has important implications in clinical practice, where men may be more likely to make premature clinical judgments. Clinical educators need to be aware of this tendency and model critical thinking that ensures that male students have addressed and examined all alternatives before making a decision (Brady & Sherrod, 2003).

ACTION Point for Educators

- Provide content and instruction in your curriculum regarding differences in communication styles to promote understanding and develop greater teamwork and understanding between men and women in your program and ultimately in practice (O'Lynn & Tranbarger, 2007).

"Chilly "Classroom Climate

"Chilly" can be defined by the degree of support that students experience in nursing education. Though this is needed for all students, men in nursing often do not feel supported, but singled out and held to a different standard because of their gender (Bell-Scriber, 2008). In one study, researchers observed faculty interactions with students over an entire semester and then interviewed both male and female students.

Male students reported the following perceptions and behaviors of nurse educators:

- Faculty were harsh. *"It's not the words they say; it is how they say it."*

- Men observed that faculty spent more time with female students in the clinical setting.
- Men experienced prejudicial comments from faculty such as, *"Men are going into nursing for the wrong reason. They only want to be a CRNA."*

When researchers asked, "Describe an experience that was personally meaningful to you as a student," ALL of the men reported an experience that they had with a PATIENT in the clinical setting. In comparison, 75 percent of female students described an experience with nursing FACULTY (Bell-Scriber, 2008).

ACTION Point for Educators

- Reflect to see if you have any stereotypes or inaccurate assumptions toward male students that may influence the way you respond to them in your program.

Exclusive Use of Lecture in Classroom

Just as there are individual differences in learning styles, there are differences between men and women and how they most effectively learn and process new information. Women tend to have a preference for auditory learning and prefer a more traditional learning environment such as a formal classroom. This could be a reason why female students may resist efforts to change the classroom when educators introduce active learning or "flip" the classroom.

In contrast, men tend to be visual as well as kinesthetic learners who prefer a more informal classroom that emphasizes active and applied learning strategies. Male nursing students prefer to be independent and self-directed in their learning (Brady & Sherrod, 2003). Men also prefer to have reading assignments as well as lecture content kept to a minimum with examples and application to real-world practice (Keri, 2002). O'Lynn (2004) identified that one of the most frequent barriers that male students identified was a lecture-only format in the classroom. Men also have a preference and gain mastery of content when the technical aspects of nursing are emphasized (Stott, 2007).

ACTION Points for Educators

- Mix it up! Combine lectures with active learning strategies.
- Emphasize teamwork and collaborative learning.

- Use real-life scenarios such as case studies to situate learning.
- Limit required reading assignments by emphasizing NEED to know content.
- Integrate the applied sciences of pathophysiology and pharmacology into content lectures.
- Emphasize the technical knowledge and skills of nursing. Pursue clinical internships in ED and ICU. Make these available to male students who tend to have a preference for these settings.

Feelings of Isolation/Loneliness

Because men are currently a minority in nursing education, the lack of male camaraderie and support is limited. As a result, men experience isolation and feelings of loneliness in nursing education. This can lead to men becoming ambivalent about becoming a nurse and cause them to question their desire and motivation to complete nursing education (Stott, 2007). The isolation that men experience can be a contributing factor to the high failure to complete rates in nursing education. This finding reinforces the importance of placing male students together in the same clinical group to decrease feelings of isolation and provide needed support (Meadus & Twomey, 2011).

ACTION Points for Educators

- Make it a priority to check in regularly with male students in your program and ask them how they are doing. Allow them to express their feelings and provide needed support. Knowing that an educator cares goes a long way toward alleviating isolation and loneliness that some men may experience.
- Provide opportunities for male students to discuss problems or struggles. Consider organizing a local student chapter of the American Assembly for Men in Nursing (AAMN). It is a national professional organization whose purpose is to provide a framework for nurses (both men and women) to meet and discuss the factors which affect men as nurses, support men within nursing, and encourage them to grow professionally by recognizing the contributions men make within the nursing profession ("About Us," 2014).
- Place male students in the same clinical group.
- Encourage group learning and activities in your classrooms. But be sure to mix it up by having students who may not normally interact together do so.

- To increase the recruitment of men and other minorities in your program, examine your school's recruitment material to make sure it contains men, women, and ethnic minorities. Collaborate with the guidance counselors at the high school in your community to ensure that they are providing accurate information to male students regarding nursing as an appropriate career choice so that men are not discouraged from considering nursing (Meadus & Twomey, 2011).

Lack of Male Mentoring/Role Modeling

Male nursing students need role models they can identify with and who validate their decision to enter the nursing profession. Because male faculty are a minority in nursing education, this role modeling and support is lacking. Clinical nurse educators must make it a priority to identify male nurses in the practice setting who can be assigned to a male student in clinical (Meadus & Twomey, 2011). This is a simple but effective strategy that will provide male students with a role model and needed support whenever possible.

ACTION Point for Educators

- Place male students with a male instructor or a male nurse on the floor if possible to promote needed role modeling and additional support (Brady & Sherrod, 2003).

How's the Climate Today?

Though the barriers that men have experienced in nursing education have been documented in the literature for years, is the current climate warmer toward male students in nursing education? It depends on your program. Incivility thrives where it is tolerated and becomes an accepted unit or academic norm. Gender bias can also become an accepted norm that adversely impacts the success and retention of male students in that setting. When a culture of bias is present, the "hidden curriculum" (Tanner, 1990) of nursing education communicates to students that faculty bias against men is acceptable and female students can be influenced as a result.

Pursuing "Gender Competence"

Cultural competence is taught to nurture and cultivate an attitude of respect and appreciation for those from other cultures. Since students from other countries are entering nursing education, to best serve their unique needs, cultural competence is not optional. In the same way, this chapter provides a crash course from the literature on "gender competence" in nursing education. This becomes a higher priority as more men enter the profession. Just as cultural ethnocentricity and the tendency to see your cultural lens as best must be recognized and resisted, many of the barriers that men experience in nursing education are a result of gender ethnocentricity by female nursing faculty.

Women in nursing education need to step back and recognize that the construct of their feminine lens of caring, communication, and learning styles will be different— complementary— but not superior to men. When these differences are not only recognized, but respected and valued, many of the current barriers that men experience can be eliminated. As a result, men will feel valued and supported, which will influence their success in nursing education.

Men Have a Place

There are a wide variety of practice settings that are an excellent fit for men. Though men practice in almost every clinical setting, the highest concentration of male participation is found in the ED, critical care, and nurse anesthetists. Though men make up only 9.6 percent of registered nurses in the United States, they comprise 41 percent of nurse anesthetists (Jaslow, 2013).

What do these three clinical areas have in common? They are HIGH tech, LOW touch specialties. They have high degrees of technology, adversity, autonomy, and acuity where the nurse can make a difference and literally save a life. Deep in the male psyche is the need to have a battle to fight and an adventure to live by (Eldredge, 2001), which each of these clinical areas represent.

Following are general principles that I have found effective as a male member of the profession to help men successfully transition to a work culture that is predominantly female.

- **Find common ground with the women you work with.** Though you may not be able to identify with some of the intimate, personal details that women often share with one another, be intentional to find common ground. You may be tempted at times to disengage because female colleagues do not show an interest in sports, hunting, or fishing. But if you have children or pets, these topics are areas of common interest.

- **Be a team player.** Make yourself available by offering help whenever possible. Though men sometimes get asked to literally do the literal "heavy lifting" on the unit, this assistance is always appreciated and is a practical way to build a bridge with female co-workers.
- **Celebrate diversity!** Incivility in nursing is a result of not valuing and respecting the unique gender differences of men and women. The direct communication styles of men may create an offense to some women. Accept the gender distinctives of the opposite sex. Do not be critical of men because they are not more like women, and vice versa!

Looming Nursing Shortage

Because of the current nursing faculty shortage, in 2014-15, more than 68,000 qualified nursing students were turned away in part because of lack of qualified faculty. Almost two-thirds of nursing programs surveyed indicated this was the primary contributing factor to not admitting all qualified students ("Nursing Faculty Shortage Fact Sheet," 2015). There is a "perfect storm" brewing. The average age of professors is 57 and the mean age of practicing registered nurses is 46 ("Nursing Faculty Shortage Fact Sheet," 2015). It is imperative that these findings instill a sense of urgency to proactively address the barriers that prevent faculty recruitment in academia to ensure that students who enroll and then graduate are well prepared for professional practice.

More than one million nurses will be needed in the next several years to address a looming nursing shortage ("Nursing Shortage," 2014). There is only one way that this potential crisis can be averted: INCREASE the participation of current underrepresented demographic groups in nursing. Though men make up the largest underrepresented demographic (49.2% of population, 9.6% in nursing), Hispanics (16.9% of population, 3.6% nursing) and African-Americans (13.1% of population, 5.4% nursing) are also underrepresented ("The U.S. Nursing Workforce: Trends in Supply and Education," 2013).

Reflect

1. What is the current percentage of men in your program? (Compare to current percentage in the RN workforce is about 10 percent)

2. What is the failure to complete rates of men and other high-risk groups such as ESL students in your program?

3. What was previously unknown to you regarding the historical aspect of men in nursing?

4. What will you do to communicate this history to your students?

5. What educational barriers currently exist in your program that may impede the success of men in your program?

6. What can you do to address these barriers to support male students in your program?

References

American Assembly for Men in Nursing (2014). About us. Retrieved from http://aamn.org/aamn.shtml

Anthony, A. S. (2004). Gender bias and discrimination in nursing education: Can we change it? *Nurse Educator, 29,* 121–125.

Bell-Scriber, M. J. (2008). Warming the nursing education climate for traditional-age learners who are male. *Nursing Education Research, (29)*3, 143–150.

Brady, M. S., & Sherrod, D. R. (2003). Retaining men in nursing programs designed for women. *Journal of Nursing Education, 42*(4), 159–162.

Brown, B. (2000). Men in nursing: Ambivalence in care, gender and masculinity. *International History of Nursing Journal, 5,* 4–13.

Carol, R. (2006). Discrimination in nursing school: Thing of the past or alive and well? *Minority Nurse,* 56–62.

Core Competencies of Nurse Educators with Task State ments (2005). Retrieved from http://www.nln.org/docs/default-source/default-document-library/core-competencies-of-nurse-educators-with-task-statements.pdf?sfvrsn=

Dyck, J. M., Oliffe, J., Phinney, A., & Garrett, B. (2009). Nursing instructors' and male students' perceptions of undergraduate, classroom nursing education. *Nurse Education Today, 29,* 649–653.

Dossey, B. M. (1999). *Florence Nightingale: Mystic, visionary, healer.* Springhouse, PA: Springhouse Corporation.

Eldredge, J. (2001). *Wild at heart: Discovering the secret of a man's soul.* Nashville, TN: Thomas Nelson.

Evans, J. (2004). Men nurses: A historical and feminist perspective. *Journal of Advanced Nursing, 47,* 321–328.

Evans, J. A. (2002). Cautious caregivers: Gender stereotypes and the sexualization of men nurses' touch. *Journal of Advanced Nursing, (40)*4, 441–448.

Gorman, D. (2003). A nurse by any other name…*Nursing Spectrum, 7*(10), 10 [northeast edition.]

Harding, T. (2009). Swimming against the malestream: Men choosing nursing as a career. *Nursing Praxis in New Zealand, 25*(3), 4–16.

Harding, T., North, N., & Perkins, R. (2008). Sexualizing men's touch: Male nurses and the use of intimate touch in clinical practice. *Research and Theory for Nursing Practice: An International Journal, 22*(2), 88–101.

Jaslow, R. (2013). Number of male U.S. nurses triple since 1970. Retrieved from http://www.cbsnews.com/news/number-of-male-us-nurses-triple-since-1970/

Keri, G. (2002). Male and female college students' learning styles differ: An opportunity for instructional diversification. *College Student Journal, 36*(3), 433.

Kouta, C., & Kaite, C. P. (2011). Gender discrimination and nursing: A review of the literature. *Journal of Professional Nursing, (27)*1, 59–63.

McLaughlin, K., Muldoon, O.T., & Moutray, M. (2010). Gender, gender roles and completion of nursing education: A longitudinal study. *Nurse Education Today, 30,* 303–307.

Mackintosh, C. (1997). A historical study of men in nursing. *Journal of Advanced Nursing, 26,* 232–236.

Meadus, R. J., & Twomey, J. C. (2011). Men student nurses: The nursing education experience. *Nursing Forum, 46,* 269–279.

Nursing Faculty Shortage Fact Sheet (2015). Retrieved from http://www.aacn.nche.edu/media-relations/FacultyShortageFS.pdf

Nursing Shortage (2014). Retrieved from http://www.aacn.nche.edu/media-relations/fact-sheets/nursing-shortage

O'Lynn, C. (2003). *Defining male friendliness in nursing education programs: Tool development.* Unpublished dissertation, Kennedy-Western University, Cheyenne, WY.

O'Lynn, C. E. (2004). Gender based barriers for male students in nursing education programs: Prevalence and perceived importance. *Journal of Nursing Education, 43*(5), 229–236.

O'Lynn, C. E., & Tranbarger, R. E. (2007). *Men in nursing: History, challenges, and opportunities.* New York, NY: Springer Publishing Company.

O'Lynn, C., & Krautscheid, L. (2014). Evaluating the effects of intimate touch instruction: Facilitating professional and respectful touch by male nursing students. *Journal of Nursing Education, 53*(3), 126-135.

Paterson, B. L., Tschikota, S., Crawford, M., Saydak, M., Venkatesh, P., & Aronowitz, T. (1996). Learning to care: Gender issues for male nursing students. *Canadian Journal of Nursing Research, 28*(1), 25–39.

Potter, P. A., & Perry, A. G. (2004). *Fundamentals of nursing.* (6th ed.). St. Louis, MO: Mosby.

Potter, P. A., & Perry, A. G. (2012). *Fundamentals of nursing.* (8th ed.). St. Louis, MO: Mosby–Elsevier.

Roth, J. E., & Coleman, C. L. (2008). Perceived and real barriers for men entering nursing: Implications for gender diversity. *Journal of Cultural Diversity, 15*(3), 148–152.

Stott, A. (2007). Exploring factors affecting attrition of male students from an undergraduate nursing course: A qualitative study. *Nurse Education Today, 27(*4), 325–332.

Tanner, C. A. (1990). Caring as a value in nursing education. *Nursing Outlook, 38*(2), 70–72.

The U.S. nursing workforce: Trends in supply and education (2013). Retrieved from http://www.ananursespace.org/blogs/peter-mcme-namin/2013/05/06/the-us-nursing-workforce-trends-in-supply-and-education?ssopc=1

Thompson, E. H. (2002). What's unique about men's caregiving? In B. J. Kramer & E. H. Thompson (Eds.), *Men as caregivers: Theory, research, and service implications* (20–50). New York: Springer.

Villeneuve, M. J. (1994). Recruiting and retaining men in nursing: A review of the literature. *Journal of Professional Nursing, 10,* 217

A New Paradigm for Nursing Education

Keith Rischer, RN, MA, CEN, CCRN

"One whose life makes a great difference for all: All are better off than if he had not lived."

—Florence Nightingale

When I created my clinical reasoning case studies in 2011, my only goal was to promote my students' learning by incorporating the educational best practice recommendations from *Educating Nurses*. As I shared my work around the country and saw that other educators could successfully transform their classrooms and clinical settings as well, I began to realize that these tools could communicate a new vision and paradigm shift that could transform nursing education and even the nursing profession.

What is this transformational vision that I am calling forth? It is nothing new, but an emphasis that needs to be recovered from our past as technology, ever increasing amounts of information, and emphasis on NCLEX pass rates have distracted nurse educators from recognizing what is unique and MOST important about the nursing profession and preparing students for clinical practice. The seeds of this vision were planted by Cindy Clark, Chris Tanner, Patricia Benner, and the co-authors of *Educating Nurses*.

As you read this book, were you able to get a glimpse of what this new vision and direction needs to be for nursing education? I am championing a vision that all educators can embrace to realize the reformation and radical transformation that is currently needed in nursing and nursing education:

Restore the centrality and value of caring, civility, and clinical reasoning that leads to correct clinical judgments so nurses are better prepared for practice and patient outcomes are improved.

But a vision and mission to restore the values of the past and embrace today's practice challenges are powerless. They are simply words on a page regardless of how powerful or inspirational they may be. One thing is needed…you! This book was written to provide a spark, to reignite your passion, and to encourage you to make a difference right where you are. You are the hero of this story. You are on the frontlines and can bring this needed change. What legacy are you currently creating? Begin today to leave a legacy that makes a difference for others to follow long after you leave academia!

Next Steps

Though you have come to the end of this book, your journey and decision to embrace this vision and become a transformational nurse educator and reformer of the nursing profession has just begun. An ancient Chinese proverb captured this dynamic perfectly. A journey of a thousand miles begins with a FIRST STEP. It is now time to take that first step to do something differently to bring needed change to your program. The following steps will provide a framework to help you initiate and successfully implement transformational change.

Step 1:
Have a Sense of Urgency.

The time is NOW, not next semester. What will be the consequences if you delay? How will student learning be impacted and how will this affect the patients your students will eventually care for?

Step 2:
Have a Vision for Transformational Change.

Change is possible. Dare to dream and think big. It is my hope that the vision presented in this book will inspire you to do the same in your program.

Step 3:
Don't Be a Lone Ranger.

Share your vision with your teaching team and then the entire department. Be prepared to persuade reluctant colleagues. Use the essential shifts of integration from *Educating Nurses* as a starting point and what you found helpful from this book to guide you.

Step 4:
Do Something!

Just as a nursing care plan will not advance the plan of care unless it is implemented, the same is true regarding transformational change. The numerous practical strategies are meant to be a "buffet" that any transformational nurse educator can pick and choose from and implement or adapt to their program.

Step 5: Evaluate the Impact of Any Changes.

Be willing to "tweak" and refine as needed along the way. Expect some student resistance, but do NOT let this be the determining factor to change course and go back to the old ways of doing things. Do not forget the vision and WHY you are doing things differently. It all comes back to developing nurses who care, critically think, and clinically reason by recognizing the need to rescue when a change of status becomes apparent.

Transforming the Profession

Transforming nursing education is only the beginning. The profession and health care systems that deliver care are also in need of transformation. Nurse educators who serve students can role model the values nursing embodies. Serving others is not valued in our culture. The unique intangibles that nurses provide are not always recognized by the health care systems that employ nurses. Nurses are all too often viewed as a bottom line expense and though respected by the public, this respect and value is not always reciprocated by health care corporations. As a result some have lost sight of the dignity, value. and pride that should be inherent as a member of the nursing profession.

Nurses do not consistently value and respect one another. The devaluing and disrespectful behaviors of incivility and bullying are all too common, and a cancer and blight on a profession that is known for its virtues of caring and compassion. Before caring can be given to patients, it must first be given to one another.

Nursing education must lead the way and positively role model to the next generation of nurses what caring, compassion, and civility look like, instead of perpetuating the ongoing cycle of incivility in the profession, our graduates must be empowered and equipped to be the needed change. The power to transform academia and even health care itself is possible. This transformation begins with each nurse educator restoring the identity, values, and legacy the profession was founded upon, and instilling this in every nursing student we touch in our program.

To empower nurses with a transformational vision of the profession that can be clearly communicated and championed by nurse educators to the next generation of nurses, this is where I would start…

Nurses care, but they first care for one another.
Nurses bring healing as they demonstrate caring in all they do.
Nurses are powerful. They can save a life.
Nurses serve, and as a result become greatest of all.

Following Florence

Florence Nightingale was not only a transformational nurse educator, she chose to become a reformer and transformer of the nursing profession. The following quote captures her spirit that needs to be distilled to nursing students today:

"Are we proud to be Nurses? To be called Nurse? Let us run the race where all may win: rejoicing in their successes, as our own, and mourning their fail-ures, wherever they are, as our own. We are all one Nurse." (Attewell, 2012, p. 74, 76)

Though she has been dead for over 100 years, Nightingale continues to speak. She wrote the following that remains relevant to nurse educators today. Let these words inspire you to follow in her steps and embrace the responsibility of becoming a transformational nurse and nurse educator in this generation:

"I think one's feelings waste themselves in words; they ought all to be distilled into actions which bring results...data is passive; only people can act" (Attewell, 2012, p. 8, 22).

Reflect

1. What first step(s) will you take after reading this book to ACT and bring transformational change?

2. How will you communicate a transformational vision of nursing to your students?

References

Attewell, A. (2012). *Illuminating florence: Finding nightingale's legacy in your practice*. Indianapolis, IN: Sigma Theta Tau International.

Acknowledgements

I (Keith) am indebted to nurse educators across the country who have embraced a transformational vision for nursing education and be a part of the needed change by helping to make this resource a reality.

To Patricia Benner—Thank you for your lifelong contributions to the profession of nursing that you so clearly love. May your past, present, and future work continue to transform nursing. Your assistance in helping me rescue my static "house" metaphor of nursing education with a "vibrant, living house" was needed and appreciated. Words cannot express my appreciation for encouraging me when I needed it most.

To Pat Pence—I am indebted to have your collaboration and contributions to my original manuscript. You have demonstrated the highest level of professionalism through your willingness to share your knowledge and experience in this book despite your current full-time load in academia.

To Carol Huston—Thank you for your willingness to give the gift of your time to help and guide a fellow colleague and author despite a very busy schedule. Your perspective and experience as a nurse educator and author made this book the best it could possibly be. I am thankful and appreciative for your advocacy and willingness to open doors for me to present my work on clinical reasoning to others.

To Cindy Clark—Thank you for using your lens as an expert on incivility in nursing and reviewing the chapter on incivility to ensure it clearly and concisely communicates the problem, but more importantly, the solution. You truly practice caring and respect! I so appreciate your input.

To those nurse educators who reviewed my manuscript despite their own busy schedule in academia: Cindy Clark, Carol Huston, Patricia Pence, Julie Hogue, Lin Rauch, Barb Hill, Janice Eilerman, Becky Craig, Judith Rudokas, and Jill Lawson. Thank you for your contributions to refine and polish what I have written.

A very special thank you to those educators who contributed their educational "pearls" and words of encouragement. There are far too many to list here, but listed by name in the book! Your contributions have strengthened and supported what has been written.

To the staff nurse and nurse educator who shared their personal stories of incivility and wished to remain anonymous. You know who you are. Thank you for your willingness to be transparent and share your story, so others may see the impact of incivility on others.

To my wife Rhonda–Thank you for your ongoing love and support over our 35 years of marriage. You encouraged me to pursue my passion as a nurse educator, and provided the stability in our home to see my dream become a reality. I could not have done it without you! I am forever grateful

Appendix A

Recommended Resources

New Nurse Educator
- **Journal**: *American Journal of Nursing*
- **Journal:** *Journal of Nursing Education*
- **Journal:** *Nurse Educator*
- **Journal:** *Teaching and Learning in Nursing*
- **Website:** American Association of Colleges of Nursing (AACN). The essentials of baccalaureate education: Faculty tool kit.
  http://www.aacn.nche.edu/faculty/faculty-development/faculty-toolkits/BacEssToolkit.pdf
- **Website:** National League for Nursing. Professional Development resources available at
  http://www.nln.org/professional-development-programs
- **Website:** Organization for Associate Degree Nursing. Resources for nurse educators available at
  https://www.oadn.org
- **Website:** Nurse.com (http://www.nurse.com/) is an excellent web-based resource to keep abreast of regional and national news relevant to nursing and much more.
- **Website:** Center for Courage Renewal: http://www.couragerenewal.org by Parker Palmer, a world-renowned writer, speaker, and activist on issues in education. His website has an abundance of resources for educators that will help you reflect on your teaching practice and bring about change to transform your nursing classroom.
- **Website:** National League for Nursing (http://nln.org) is national organization website that provides resources and tools to advance excellence, innovation, and integrity in nursing education. Within the Professional Development section are innovative teaching and simulation resources, hallmarks of excellence, competencies for nurse educators, and a CNE certification section that including a link to order the Official NLN CNE Review Book.

General
- **Book:** *Illuminating Florence: Finding Nightingale's Legacy in Your Practice* (2012) by Alex Attewell
- **Book:** *The Nurse's Reality Gap: Overcoming Barriers Between Academic Achievement and Clinical Success* (2013) by Leslie Neal-Boylan
- **Book:** *The Courage to Teach: Exploring the Inner Landscape of a Teacher's Life* (2007) by Parker Palmer
- **Book:** *Let Your Life Speak: Listening for the Voice of Vocation* (2000) by Parker Palmer

Art of Nursing
- **Case Studies:** Clinical Dilemmas: Case Studies that Cultivate Caring, Civility and Clinical Reasoning: http://www.keithrn.com/home/store/
- **Book:** *Nursing the Spirit: The Art and Science of Applying Spiritual Care* (2001) by Dorothy Wilt and Carol Smucker
- **Book:** *Spiritual Care: A Guide for Caregivers* (2000) by Judith Allen Shelly
- **Book:** *The Nurse with an Alabaster Jar* (2006) by Mary Elizabeth O'Brien
- **Book**: *Spirituality In Nursing: Standing on Holy Ground* (2013) by Mary Elizabeth O'Brien
- **Book:** Primacy of Caring (1989) by Patricia Benner
- **Book:** *Margin: Restoring Emotional, Physical, Financial, and Time Reserves to Overloaded Lives* (2004) by Richard Swenson
- **Website:** Caring for the Human Spirit emagazine
  http://bit.ly/2rIXViL

Applied Sciences of Nursing
- **Book:** *Memory Notebook of Nursing Vol. 1* 6th ed. JoAnn Zerwekh
- **Book:** *Memory Notebook of Nursing: A Collection of Visual Images and Mnemonics to Increase Memory and Learning, Vol. 2* (2010) by JoAnn Zerwekh, Jo Carol Claborn, and C.J. Miller
- **Flashcards:** *Mosby's Pathophysiology Memory NoteCards: Visual, Mnemonic, and Memory Aids for*

Nurses, 2nd ed. (2010) by JoAnn Zerwekh, Jo Carol Claborn, and Tom Gaglione

- **Flashcards:** *Mosby's Pharmacology Memory Note Cards: Visual, Mnemonic, and Memory Aids for Nurses* (2014) by JoAnn Zerwekh and Jo Carol Claborn
- **Website:** Pathophysiology and treatment of any medical problem. "Medscape:"
  http://emedicine.medscape.com/
- **Website:** Khan Academy/NCLEX-RN:
  https://www.khanacademy.org/test-prep/nclex-rn#table-of-contents
  - Excellent pathophysiology review of all body systems as well as NCLEX practice questions
- **YouTube channel:** Think Like a Nurse:
  https://www.youtube.com/user/ThinkLikeANurse
- **YouTube channel:** Simple Nursing:
  https://www.youtube.com/user/SimpleNursing
- **Internet PDF:** "Lab Values: Interpreting Chemistry and Hematology for Adult Patients"
  http://www.rn.com/getpdf.php/1754.pdf

Nurse Thinking

- **Book:** *Educating Nurses: A Call for Radical Transformation* (2009) by Patricia Benner, Molly Sutphen, Victoria Leonard, & Lisa Day
- **Book:** *Expertise in Nursing Practice: Caring, Clinical Judgment, and Ethics* (2009) by Patricia Benner, Christine Tanner, & Catherine Chesla
- Book: *Clinical Wisdom and Interventions in Acute and Critical Care, Second Edition: A Thinking-in-Action Approach* (2011) by Patricia Benner, Patricia Hooper Kyriakidis, & Daphne Stannard
- **Book:** *Clinical Reasoning: The Art & Science of Critical & Creative Thinking* (1999) by Daniel Pesut and JoAnne Herman
- **Book:** *Critical Thinking, Clinical Reasoning, and Clinical Judgment a Practical Approach*, 5th ed. (2013) by Rosalinda Alfaro-LeFevre
- **Book:** *Teaching for Critical Thinking: Tools and Techniques to Help Students Question Their Assumptions* (2012) by Stephen Brookfield

Clinical Teaching

- **Book:** *Teaching in Nursing: A Guide for Faculty* by Diane Billings and Judith Halstead

- **Website:** QSEN Institute-Reformulating SBAR to "I-SBAR-R" http://qsen.org/reformulating-sbar-to-i-sbar-r/
- **Book:** *The Eight-Step Approach to Teaching Clinical Nursing* (2011) by Joanne Herman, Loretta Manning, Lydia Zager
- **Book:** *Clinical Teaching Strategies in Nursing* (2015) by Kathleen Gaberson, Marilyn Oermann, Teresa Shellenbarger
- **Book:** *Creative Teaching Strategies for the Nurse Educator* 2nd ed. (2016) by Judith Herrman

Classroom Teaching

- **Book:** *Creative Teaching Strategies for the Nurse Educator* (2016) 2nd ed. by Judith Herrmann
- **Book:** *Classroom Assessment Techniques: A Handbook for College Teachers* (1993) 2nd ed. by Thomas Angelo and K. Patricia Cross
- **Book:** *What the Best College Teachers Do* (2004) by Ken Bain
- **Book:** *Make it Stick: The Science of Successful Learning* (2014) by Peter Brown, Henry Roediger, and Mark McDaniel
- **Book:** T*eaching in Nursing: A Guide for Faculty* by Diane Billings and Judith Halstead

Simulation

- **Website**: The International Nursing Association for Clinical Simulation and Learning: http://www.in-acsl.org/
- **Article:** Dreifuerst, K. (2010). Using debriefing for meaningful learning to foster development of clinical reasoning in simulation, *Journal of Nursing Education, 51*(6), 326-333.

Testing

- **Website**: Evolve website on educational trends and testing policy development:
  https://evolve.elsevier.com/education/educational-trends/
- **Website:** National Council of State Boards of Nursing (2016). NCLEX-RN® detailed test plan: Item writer/item reviewer/nurse educator version. Retrieved from
  https://www.ncsbn.org/RN_Test_Plan_2016_Final.pdf

- **Website:** National League for Nursing Center for Assessment and Evaluation: http://www.nln.org/centers-for-nursing-education/nln-center-for-assessment-and-evaluation
- **Website:** Blooms Taxonomy-University of Waterloo/Centre for Teaching Excellence http://bit.ly/2qIjFqu

Incivility
- **Book:** *Pickle Pledge: Creating a More Positive Healthcare Culture—One Attitude at a Time* (2010) by Joe Tye and Bob Dent
- **Book:** *Creating & Sustaining Civility in Nursing Education* (2013) by Cynthia Clark
- **Book:** *Ending Nurse-to-Nurse Hostility: Why Nurses Eat Their Young and Each Other,* 2nd ed. (2014) by Kathleen Bartholomew
- **Website:** "Civility Matters: Creating and sustaining communities of civility": http://hs.boisestate.edu/civilitymatters/
- **PDF:** Incivility Essentials: http://www.keithrn.com/product/incivility/

Men in Nursing
- **Book for students:** *A Man's Guide to a Nursing Career* (2012) by Chad O'Lynn
- **Book for educators:** *Men in Nursing: History, Challenges, and Opportunities* (2007) by Chad O'Lynn and Russell Tranbarger
- **Website:** American Assembly for Men in Nursing: www.AAMN.org

Diversity/International Students
- **Book:** *The Light in Their Eyes: Creating Multicultural Learning Communities* (2009) by Sonia Nieto
- **Book:** *Multicultural Course Transformation in Higher Education: A Broader Truth* (1996) by Ann Morey and Margie Kitano
- **Book:** *The Spirit Catches You and You Fall Down: A Hmong Child, Her American Doctors, and the Collision of Two Cultures* (2012) by Anne Fadiman

Appendix B

Serving the Poor through Medical Missions

To put the needs of the developing world in context, if 100 jetliners crashed today killing 26,500 people, it would get the world's attention. If this happened day after day, you would demand that something be done to stop this ongoing loss of human life! But a tragedy of this scope occurs every day in the developing world. Every day, 26,500 children die of preventable causes related to their poverty. Over one year, this equates to 10,000,000 lives lost (Shah, 2013).

After the massive earthquake struck Haiti in January 2010, I felt powerless and helpless yet wanted to do something to help with my ED clinical background. The news reports dramatically witnessed the urgency of medical needs of thousands who were dead and wounded with minimal resources to care for the suffering. I was eventually able to serve as part of a medical mission team through our church in May 2010. Though the critically wounded were by then cared for, our team was able to provide much-needed clinic care for those living in tent cities in Port-au-Prince. Though our team accomplishments may seem small and a proverbial "drop in the bucket," the "drop" matters, because every person matters to God and each of us have equal worth as we are created in His image.

Haiti has the highest rates of infant, under-age-five, and maternal mortality in the Western Hemisphere. The infant mortality rate is 57 per 1,000 in 2007; in the US, it is 6.7 deaths per 1,000. Maternal mortality is 523 deaths per 100,000 births in Haiti, compared with 13 per 100,000 in the US. Diarrhea, respiratory infections, malaria, tuberculosis, and HIV/AIDS are the leading causes of death. Not coincidentally, Haiti has the lowest number of nurses/1000 population in the world: 0.11 nurses/1000.

Though we lament the nursing shortage here in the US (16th in the world at 9.37/1000), nothing compares to the tragic shortages of nurses in Haiti and the developing world. As a nurse or nurse educator, you have a skill that can serve others wherever you choose to practice.

Don't Waste Your Life

One book that continually challenges me is *Don't Waste Your Life* by John Piper. Each one of us has a finite amount of time to live our life for what really matters. The greatest tragedy is to come to the end of your days realizing that you wasted the one life you have been given on this earth. In addition to not wasting my life, I also do not want to waste this opportunity to encourage anyone who is reading this book to help those in the developing world in a variety of ways.

I have listed organizations that specialize in short-term medical mission outreach in the developing world. I also have a medical missions tab on my website that has numerous resources for those who may be interested in serving in this context as well.

Though the needs of the poor in the developing world are profound, there are people in your community that you can also serve through medical mission. Though it takes time, energy, and financial resources to go to another country, you can make a difference right in your own community. Partner with ministries that serve the homeless, or the poor in free medical clinics. There is no shortage of work to be done. Just open your eyes to see how you can be used to make a difference wherever you decide to serve.

Don't Throw Away Your Textbooks!

Liberia, an English-speaking West African country is in desperate need of nursing textbooks because of a prolonged civil war that has devastated the country. It is not uncommon to have an entire nursing class of 80 students

To put the needs of the developing world in context, if 100 jetliners crashed today killing 26,500 people, it would get the world's attention. If this happened day after day, you would demand that something be done to stop this ongoing loss of human life! But a tragedy of this scope occurs every day in the developing world. Every day, 26,500 children die of preventable causes related to their poverty. Over one year, this equates to 10,000,000 lives lost (Shah, 2013).

After the massive earthquake struck Haiti in January 2010, I felt powerless and helpless yet wanted to do something to help with my ED clinical background. The news reports dramatically witnessed the urgency of medical needs of thousands who were dead and wounded with minimal resources to care for the suffering. I was eventually able to serve as part of a medical mission team through our church in May 2010. Though the critically wounded were by then cared for, our team was able to provide much-needed clinic care for those living in tent cities in Port-au-Prince. Though our team accomplishments may seem small and a proverbial "drop in the bucket," the "drop" matters, because every person matters to God and each of us have equal worth as we are created in His image.

Haiti has the highest rates of infant, under-age-five, and maternal mortality in the Western Hemisphere. The infant mortality rate is 57 per 1,000 in 2007; in the US, it is 6.7 deaths per 1,000. Maternal mortality is 523 deaths per 100,000 births in Haiti, compared with 13 per 100,000 in the US. Diarrhea, respiratory infections, malaria, tuberculosis, and HIV/AIDS are the leading causes of death. Not coincidentally, Haiti has the lowest number of nurses/1000 population in the world: 0.11 nurses/1000.

Though we lament the nursing shortage here in the US (16th in the world at 9.37/1000), nothing compares to the tragic shortages of nurses in Haiti and the developing world. As a nurse or nurse educator, you have a skill that can serve others wherever you choose to practice.

Don't Waste Your Life

One book that continually challenges me is *Don't Waste Your Life* by John Piper. Each one of us has a finite amount of time to live our life for what really matters. The greatest tragedy is to come to the end of your days realizing that you wasted the one life you have been given on this earth. In addition to not wasting my life, I also do not want to waste this opportunity to encourage anyone who is reading this book to help those in the developing world in a variety of ways.

I have listed organizations that specialize in short-term medical mission outreach in the developing world. I also have a medical missions tab on my website that has numerous resources for those who may be interested in serving in this context as well.

Though the needs of the poor in the developing world are profound, there are people in your community that you can also serve through medical mission. Though it takes time, energy, and financial resources to go to another country, you can make a difference right in your own community. Partner with ministries that serve the homeless, or the poor in free medical clinics. There is no shortage of work to be done. Just open your eyes to see how you can be used to make a difference wherever you decide to serve.

Don't Throw Away Your Textbooks!

Liberia, an English-speaking West African country is in desperate need of nursing textbooks because of a prolonged civil war that has devastated the country. It is not uncommon to have an entire nursing class of 80 students have just a few textbooks that are shared by all. A nurse colleague who is native to Liberia has an organization, Liberian Health Initiative, that coordinates shipments of nursing textbooks and other needed supplies for nursing education in Liberia. If you have older edition textbooks (<10 years old), please send them by USPS media mail to:

> **Liberian Health Initiative**
> **P.O. Box 29628**
> **Minneapolis, MN 55429**

Additional Resources
Medical Missions

- Bulk Medications for Medical Ministry: Blessings International: http://www.blessing.org/
- Medical Mission Outreach: Medical Teams International: http://www.medicalteams.org/
- Medical Mission Outreach: Global Health Outreach: http://cmda.org/missions/detail/global-health-outreach
- Mercy Ships/Youth With a Mission:

http://www.mercyships.org/
- Nursing Education: Haiti Nursing Foundation: http://haitinursing.org/
- Medical Missions: Liberian Health Initiative: http://www.liberianhealthinitiative.org/
- Book: *When Helping Hurts: Alleviating Poverty Without Hurting the Poor...and Yourself* (2012) by Steve Corbett & Brian Fikkert
- Book: *Let the Nations Be Glad* 3rd ed. by John Piper

Faith Based
- Nurses Christian Fellowship: http://ncf-jcn.org/
- Book: Called to Care: *A Christian Worldview for Nursing* by Judith Allen Shelly & Arlene B. Miller
- *Book: The Nurse with an Alabaster Jar: A Biblical Approach to Nursing by Mary Elizabeth O'Brien & Judith Allen Shelly*
- Journal: *Journal of Christian Nursing (JCN)*
- Book (free PDF download!): *Don't Waste Your Life* by John Piper:
  http://www.desiringgod.org/books/dont-waste-your-life
- Booklet: "For Your Joy" by John Piper:
  http://www.desiringgod.org/books/for-your-joy

Reflections
1. Do you have a desire to serve others through medical missions? If so, what country are you drawn to?

2. What ministries serve the poor in your community where you and/or students could serve others?

3. What can you do today to educate yourself on what is required to serve effectively in the country you are interested in?

Appendix C

Transformation Toolbox
Clinical Reasoning Tools and Resources to
TEACH Students to THINK Like a Nurse!

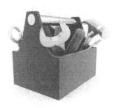

Teaching the Art of Nursing

1. **Clinical Dilemma Case Study:** Anxiety or Spiritual Distress? Practice the "art" of nursing with this dilemma that emphasizes the importance of holistic and spiritual care.

Teaching the Applied Sciences

1. **Worksheet: Medications to Master.** Blank worksheet that uses the "Pharm. 5" questions to guide student learning of what is most important.
2. **Worksheet: "Lab Planning."** Blank worksheet that guides student learning of most important lab data and develops a "lab plan of care" by identifying essential nursing assessments for relevant abnormal labs.

Teaching Clinical Reasoning

1. **Template: Clinical Reasoning Questions to Develop Nurse Thinking.** The foundational tool to develop clinical reasoning in students. This template can be the primary care planning tool for advanced clinical instead of a traditional care plan.

Teaching in Clinical

1. **Template: DEEP Learning of MOST Important in Clinical.** Prepares students for your clinical rotation by identifying what meds, labs, problems, complications, and nursing skills need to be known.
2. **Worksheet: Patient Preparation.** Simplified clinical prep tool for advanced students. Like the worksheet I use in my clinical practice.

Pearls from Clinical Educators

1. **Quick Medication Guide:** Nancy Delmont, MSN, RN
2. **Patient Assessment Form.** Patricia Pence, EdD, MSN, RN
3. **Care Web:** Claudette Abounder, MS, ANP

Teaching in the Classroom

1. **Template: Transform My Lecture.** Quickly identify eight essential components of a concise NEED to know presentation.
2. **Heart Failure Clinical Reasoning 1-2-3 Case Studies.** Three clinical reasoning case studies on heart failure.

   The first case study emphasizes identifying RELEVANT clinical data and nursing PRIORITIES.

   The second uses the same scenario but emphasizes identifying PATTERNS or relationships of clinical data to make connections to recognize how clinical data is related.

   The final case study uses the same scenario but adds the psychosocial history so psychosocial nursing priorities are identified and the "art" of nursing is emphasized to provide holistic nursing care.

Clinical Dilemma
Anxiety or Spiritual Distress

STUDENT Worksheet

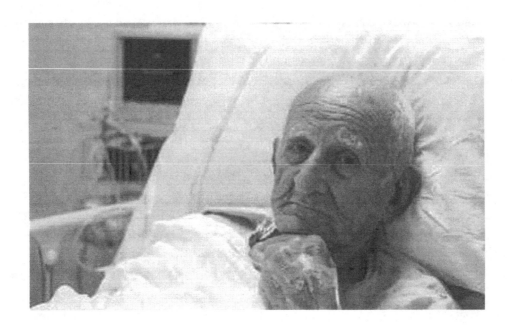

John James, 77 years old

Overview

When a patient is anxious, could this represent something more than a primary problem of anxiety? In this dilemma, a patient who almost died after surgery is making excellent progress, but something may be wrong. Does his sudden onset of shortness of breath and feelings of anxiety represent a physical, emotional, or a spiritual problem? The nurse needs to think in action and determine the current nursing priority to provide needed care and support.

Clinical Dilemma Activity: STUDENT

Anxiety or Spiritual Distress

I. Scenario

History of Present Problem:

John James is a 77-year-old man who had coronary artery bypass graft (CABG) x 4 vessels three days ago for multi-vessel coronary artery disease. He lost over 1000 mL of blood shortly after surgery due to a bleeding graft site and almost died as a result. He is currently off all vaso-active drips, his arterial line has been discontinued and he is clinically stable. John is scheduled to transfer to the cardiac step-down unit later today.

Personal/Social History:

John's wife died six months ago after fifty years of marriage. He lives alone in his own apartment. He has one son who lives in the area and checks in at least once a week to see how he is doing. He is a Vietnam War veteran who has not been active in his church since he returned from the war over forty years ago.

What data from the histories is important & RELEVANT; therefore it has clinical significance to the nurse?

.RELEVANT Data from Present Problem:	Clinical Significance:
RELEVANT Data from Social History:	Clinical Significance:

II. The Dilemma Begins…

Current Concern:

John puts on his call light and as you enter the room he states that he feels short of breath and is visibly anxious. His breath sounds are clear and his O2 saturation is 98% on 2 liters n/c. His respiratory rate is 20/minute and his heart rate is 78/minute-sinus rhythm. He acknowledges that he is anxious and feels like he is having a panic attack and has never felt like this before. When you ask him if there is anything that he may be anxious about, he shares the following, "I used to go to church when I was little, but when I saw so many of my friends die in Vietnam and was helpless to save them, how could I believe in a God who allowed such horrible things to happen. Before the war I could not even kill a cat or dog. In Vietnam I killed so many people. How can I be forgiven for what I have done?"

What data from the current concern is important & RELEVANT; therefore it has clinical significance to the nurse?

RELEVANT Data from Current Concern:	Clinical Significance:

© 2015 Keith Rischer/www.KeithRN.com

III. Resolving the Dilemma

1. Identifying data that is RELEVANT, what is the essence of this current dilemma?

2. What additional information is needed by the nurse that would help clarify the current dilemma?

3. What additional members of the healthcare team could be used in this situation? Why?

4. What is the nursing priority?

5. What nursing interventions and/or principles can the nurse use to successfully resolve this clinical dilemma?

6. What is the expected response of the patient that indicate the nursing interventions were effective?

7. What response by the patient would indicate that a change in the plan of care and nursing interventions are needed?

8. What is the patient likely experiencing/feeling right now in this situation?

9. What can I do to engage myself with this patient's experience, and show that he matters to me as a person?

10. What was learned from this case study that you will incorporate into your practice?

Medications That Must Be Mastered Worksheet

Name	Dose: High-low-avg.?	Pharm. Class	Therapeutic Use/Mechanism of Action	Adverse Actions (most common SE)	Nsg Considerations (what must be known before)

Lab Planning Worksheet

Lab:	Normal Value:	Clinical Significance:	Nursing Assessments/Interventions Required:
Value:	Critical Value:		

Lab:	Normal Value:	Clinical Significance:	Nursing Assessments/Interventions Required:
Value:	Critical Value:		

Lab:	Normal Value:	Clinical Significance:	Nursing Assessments/Interventions Required:
Value:	Critical Value:		

Lab:	Normal Value:	Clinical Significance:	Nursing Assessments/Interventions Required:
Value:	Critical Value:		

Lab:	Normal Value:	Clinical Significance:	Nursing Assessments/Interventions Required:
Value:	Critical Value:		

Clinical Reasoning Questions to Develop Nurse Thinking

(Formulate and reflect before and after report, but **BEFORE** seeing patient the first time)

1. *What is the primary problem and what is its underlying cause or pathophysiology?*

2. *What clinical data from the chart is RELEVANT and needs to be trended because it is clinically significant?*

3. *List all relevant nursing priorities. What nursing priority captures the "essence" of your patient's status and will guide your plan of care?*

4. *What nursing interventions will you initiate based on this priority and what are the desired outcomes?*

5. *What body system(s), key assessments and psychosocial needs will you focus on based on your patient's primary problem or nursing care priority?*

6. *What is the worst possible/most likely complication(s) to anticipate based on the primary problem?*

7. *What nursing assessments will identify this complication EARLY if it develops?*

8. *What nursing interventions will you initiate if this complication develops?*

While Providing Care (Review and note after initial patient assessment)

1. What clinical assessment data did you just collect that is RELEVANT and needs to be TRENDED because it is clinically significant to detect a change in status?

2. Does your nursing priority or plan of care need to be modified in any way after assessing your patient?

3. After reviewing the primary care provider's note, what is the rationale for any new orders or changes made?

4. What educational priorities have you identified and how will you address them?

DEEP Learning of MOST Important in This Clinical Setting

Medications:
1.
2.
3.
4.
5.
6.
7.
8.
9.
10.

Labs:
1.
2.
3.
4.
5.

Most Common Illnesses/Surgeries:
1.
2.
3..

Nursing Skills:
1.
2.
3.

Patient Preparation Worksheet

Time	Meds/Care Priorities	Misc.

Adm. Date _____ Days since adm. _____ POD# _____

<u>Chief Complaint/Primary Problem:</u>

<u>Past Medical History</u>

	CV	Resp	Neuro	GI	GU	Skin/Pain	Misc.	VS
Prior Nursing Assessment >>>								
Current Nursing Assessment >>>								

Lab Test	Current	Most Recent
Na+		
K+		
Mg+		
Creat.		
WBC		
Neut. %		
Hgb.		

Allergies _____
Code Status _____
IV site _____
IV Maintenance _____
IV Drips _____
Activity _____
Fall Risk/Safety _____
Diet _____
Bladder/Bowel _____

End of Shift SBAR to Oncoming Nurse

Situation:
Background:
Assessment:
Recommendation:

Quick Medication Guide

Prefix/Suffix	Class	Use	Ex: Generic	Trade
pril	ACE inhibitor	HF, HTN	lisinopril	Zestril
sartan	ARB	HF, HTN	valsartan	Diovan
triptan	Antimigraine	acute migraine h/a	sumatriptan	Imitrex
ergot	Ergotamine Deriviative			
statin	Antihyperlipidemic Agent	Lower cholesterol	atorvastatin	Lipitor
dipine	Calcium Channel Blocker	Manage arrhythmias Treat angina	amlodipine	Norvasc
tidine	Histamine 2 Blocker	Acid Reflux GERD	ranitidine	Zantac
prazole	Proton Pump Inhibitor		omeprazole	Prilosec
conazole	Antifungal Agent	Fungal Infections	Fluconazole	Diflucan
afil	Erectile Dysfunction Agent	ED	Sildenafil	Viagra
osin	Alpha Adrenergic Blocker	HTN, BPH	terazosin	Hytrin
olol	Beta Adregenic Blocker	HTN, Angina, Arrythmias	metoprolol	Lopressor
mab	Monoclonal antibody	Autoimmune Diseases/Immune Suppression	adalimumab	Humira
setron	5HT Blocker Antiemetic	Nausea	ondansetron	Zofran
tide	Incretin Mimetic	Type II Diabetes	exenatide	Byetta
gliptin	Antidiabetic Agent	Type II Diabetes	sitagliptin	Januvia
Zepam or zolam	Antianxiety Agent	Anxiety, Sedation	lorazepam	Ativan
barbital	Sedative	Sedation/seizures	phenobarbital	Luminal
vir	Antiviral agents	Viral Infections	acyclovir	Zovirax
cycline	Tetracycline Antibiotic	Bacterial Infection	doxycycline	Doryx
cillin	Penicillin Antibiotic		amoxicillin	Amoxil
floxacin	Fluoroquinolone Antibiotic		ciprofloxacin	Cipro
Ceph or cef	Cephalosporin Antibiotic		cephalexin	Keflex
sulfa	Sulfonamide Antibiotic or derivative		sulfasalazine	Azulfidine
nitro	Vasodilator	Treat/prevent angina	nitroglycerin	Nitrobid
dronate	Bone reabsorption	Osteoporosis	risedronate	Actonel

Patient Assessment Form

Student: Resident/Patient initials:

BP: T: P: R:

Mental status:

Any type of discomfort at present time:

Level of orientation: (Person, place, time, and situation)

Skin color and temperature:

Breathing effort:
Lungs sounds:
Cough/sputum:

Apical pulse:
Radial pulses bilaterally:

Pulse ox:

Capillary refill:
Any clubbing:

Abdominal:

Lower extremities:
    Skin condition:
    Pulses:
    Edema:

Any other observations or subjective data:

Top 3 priorities for this resident/patient based on your assessment:
1.

2.

3.

Assessment comparison:

1. Assess two residents/patients with a partner.
2. Remember to use handwashing before and after care and to provide privacy.
3. After assessments are completed, compare your assessments and make a problem list for each resident/patient based on relevant data.
4. Write an appropriate nursing diagnosis, including RT and AMB sections.
5. List what nursing interventions are *done currently by staff* to address this nursing diagnosis. You may need to check the medical record for plan of care and current orders. The nursing interventions should be realistic for your *residents/patients*. Include a *time factor* in each nursing intervention.

Resident/Patient initials:	**Resident/Patient initials:**
Problem list	**Problem list**

	Resident/Patient initials:	Resident/Patient initials:
Top Nursing diagnosis		
Priority nursing interventions		

CARE WEB

1. Assessment(s)/ Intervention(s)

Anticipated Outcome:
The patient will...

Patient Response (at time of care)

1.

2.

Patient Issues/Concerns

1.

2.

3.

4.

2. Assessment(s)/Intervention(s)

Anticipated Outcome:
The patient will…

3. Assessment(s)/Intervention(s)

Anticipated Outcome:
The patient will…

Patient Response (at time of care)

3.

4.

4. Assessment(s)/Intervention(s)

Anticipated Outcome:
The patient will…

Transforming My Lecture Template

Pathophysiology Review:

Most Important Medications:

Most Important Lab Values:

Nursing Priorities/Plan of Care:

Worst Possible/Most Likely Complications:

Assessments to Identify Complication:

Interventions to Rescue:

Patient Education Priorities:

Active Learning Strategy to Contextualize Content:

Step #1: THINK Like a Nurse by Recognizing RELEVANCE and PRIORITIES

Four Principles of Clinical Reasoning:

1. Identify and interpret RELEVANT clinical data.
2. TREND relevant clinical data to determine current status (stable vs. unstable).
3. Grasp the "essence" of the current clinical situation.
4. Determine nursing PRIORITY and plan of care.

History of Present Problem:

JoAnn Smith is a 72-year-old woman who has a history of myocardial infarction (MI) four years ago and systolic heart failure secondary to ischemic cardiomyopathy with a current ejection fraction (EF) of only 15%. She presents to the emergency department (ED) for shortness of breath (SOB) the past three days. Her shortness of breath has progressed from SOB with activity to becoming SOB at rest. The last two nights she had to sleep in her recliner chair to rest comfortably upright. She is able to speak only in partial sentences and then has to take a breath when talking to the nurse. She has noted increased swelling in her lower legs and has gained six pounds in the last three days. She is being transferred from the ED to the cardiac step-down where you are the nurse assigned to care for her.

What data from the PRESENT PROBLEM are RELEVANT and must be interpreted as clinically significant by the nurse?

RELEVANT Data from Present Problem:	Clinical Significance:

Patient Care Begins:

Current VS:	P-Q-R-S-T Pain Assessment (5th VS):	
T: 98.6 F/37.0 C (oral)	Provoking/Palliative:	
P: 92 (irregular)	Quality:	Denies Pain
R: 26 (regular)	Region/Radiation:	
BP: 162/54 MAP: 90	Severity:	
O2 sat: 90% (6 liters n/c)	Timing:	

What VS data is RELEVANT and must be recognized as clinically significant by the nurse?

RELEVANT vs. Data:	Clinical Significance:

Current Assessment:	
GENERAL APPEARANCE:	Appears anxious, restless
RESP:	Breath sounds have coarse crackles scattered throughout both lung fields ant/post, labored respiratory effort, patient sitting upright
CARDIAC:	Rhythm: atrial fibrillation, pale, cool to the touch, pulses palpable throughout, 3+ pitting edema lower extremities from knees down bilaterally, S3 gallop, irregular, no jugular venous distention (JVD) noted
NEURO:	Alert and oriented to person, place, time, and situation (x4)
GI:	Abdomen soft/nontender, bowel sounds audible per auscultation in all four quadrants
GU:	Voiding without difficulty, urine clear/yellow
SKIN:	Skin integrity intact, skin turgor elastic, no tenting present

What assessment data is RELEVANT and must be recognized as clinically significant by the nurse?

RELEVANT Assessment Data:	Clinical Significance:

RELEVANT Assessment Data:	Clinical Significance:
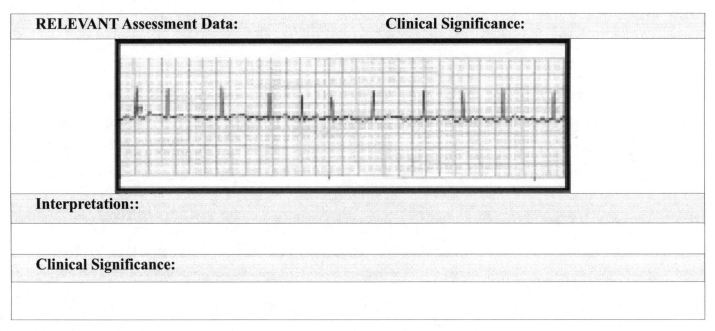	
Interpretation::	
Clinical Significance:	

Radiology Reports: Chest x-ray
What diagnostic results are RELEVANT and must be recognized as clinically significant by the nurse?

RELEVANT Results:	Clinical Significance:
Bilateral diffuse pulmonary infiltrates consistent with pulmonary edema	

Lab Results:

Complete Blood Count (CBC):	Current:	High/Low/WNL?	Previous:
WBC (4.5-11.0 mm 3)	4.8		5.8
Hgb (12-16 g/dL)	12.9		13.2
Platelets (150-450x 103/μl)	228		202
Neutrophil % (42-72)	68		65

What lab results are RELEVANT and must be recognized as clinically significant by the nurse?

RELEVANT Lab(s):	Clinical Significance:	TREND: Improve/Worsening/Stable:

Basic Metabolic Panel (BMP):	Current:	High/Low/WNL?	Previous:
Sodium (135-145 mEq/L)	133		138
Potassium (3.5-5.0 mEq/L)	4.9		4.2
Glucose (70-110 mg/dL)	105		118
Calcium (8.4-10.2 mg/dL)	8.8		9.5
Creatinine (0.6-1.2 mg/dL)	2.9		2.2

What lab results are RELEVANT and must be recognized as clinically significant by the nurse?

RELEVANT Lab(s):	Clinical Significance:	TREND: Improve/Worsening/Stable:

Misc. Chemistries:	Current:	High/Low/WNL?	Previous:
Magnesium (1.6-2.0 mEq/L)	1.9		1.8
PT/INR (0.9-1.1 nmol/L)	2.5		2.4

What lab results are RELEVANT and must be recognized as clinically significant by the nurse?

RELEVANT Lab(s):	Clinical Significance:	TREND: Improve/Worsening/Stable:

Cardiac Labs:	Current:	High/Low/WNL?	Previous:
Troponin (<0.05 ng/mL)	0.10		0.12
BNP (B-natriuretic Peptide) (<100 ng/L)	1855		155

RELEVANT Lab(s):	Clinical Significance:	TREND: Improve/Worsening/Stable:

Put it All Together to THINK Like a Nurse!

1. What is the primary problem that your patient is most likely presenting?

2. What nursing PRIORITY (ies) will guide your plan of care? (if more than one-list in order of PRIORITY)

3. What interventions will you initiate based on this PRIORITY?

Nursing Interventions:	Rationale:	Expected Outcome:

4. What educational/discharge PRIORITIES will be needed to develop a teaching plan for this patient and/or family?

STEP #2: How to THINK Like a Nurse by Recognizing Clinical RELATIONSHIPS

Six Essential Clinical Relationships:
1. RELATIONSHIP of the past medical history and current medications
2. RELATIONSHIP between RELEVANT present problem data and the primary medical problem
3. RELATIONSHIP between RELEVANT clinical data and the primary problem
4. RELATIONSHIP between the primary medical problem and nursing priority
5. RELATIONSHIP between the primary care provider's orders and primary problem
6. RELATIONSHIP between diseases in PMH that may have contributed to the development of the current problem

History of Current Problem:

JoAnn Smith is a 72-year-old woman who has a history of myocardial infarction (MI) four years ago and systolic heart failure secondary to ischemic cardiomyopathy with a current ejection fraction (EF) of only 15%. She presents to the emergency department (ED) for shortness of breath (SOB) the past three days. Her shortness of breath has progressed from SOB with activity to becoming SOB at rest. The last two nights she had to sleep in her recliner chair to rest comfortably upright. She is able to speak only in partial sentences and then has to take a breath when talking to the nurse. She has noted increased swelling in her lower legs and has gained six pounds in the last three days. She is being transferred from the ED to the cardiac step-down where you are the nurse assigned to care for her.

1. What is the RELATIONSHIP of the past medical history and current medications?
(Which medication treats which condition? Draw lines to connect)

Past Medical History	Home Meds:
Diabetes mellitus type II	1. ASA 81 mg PO daily
Hypertension	2. Carvedilol 3.25 mg PO daily
Atrial fibrillation	3. Lisinopril 5 mg PO daily
Hyperlipidemia	4. Ezetimide 10 mg PO daily
Chronic renal insufficiency (baseline creatinine 2.0)	5. Hydralazine 25 mg PO 4x daily
Cerebral vascular accident (CVA) with no residual deficits	6. Torsemide 20 mg PO bid
Heart failure (systolic) secondary to ischemic cardiomyopathy	7. KCL 20 meq PO daily
MI with stent x2 to LAD 4 years ago	8. Warfarin 5 mg PO daily
	9. Glyburide 5 mg PO daily

Patient Care Begins

Current VS:	P-Q-R-S-T Pain Assessment (5th VS):	
T: 98.6 F/37.0 C (oral)	Provoking/Palliative:	
P: 92 (irregular)	Quality:	Denies Pain
R: 26 (regular)	Region/Radiation:	
BP: 162/54 MAP: 90	Severity:	
O2 sat: 90% (6 liters n/c)	Timing:	

Current VS:	
GENERAL APPEARANCE:	Appears anxious, restless
RESP	Breath sounds have coarse crackles scattered throughout both lung fields ant/post, labored respiratory effort, patient sitting upright
CARDIAC:	Rhythm: atrial fibrillation, pale, cool to the touch, pulses palpable throughout, 3+ pitting edema lower extremities from knees down bilaterally, S3 gallop, ir regular, no jugular venous distention (JVD) noted
NEURO:	Alert and oriented to person, place, time, and situation (x4)
GI:	Abdomen soft/nontender, bowel sounds audible per auscultation in all four quadrants
GU:	Voiding without difficulty, urine clear/yellow
SKIN:	Skin integrity intact, skin turgor elastic, no tenting present

Radiology Reports: Chest x-ray
What diagnostic results are RELEVANT and must be recognized as clinically significant by the nurse?

RELEVANT Results:	Clinical Significance:
Bilateral diffuse pulmonary infiltrates consistent with pulmonary edema	

Lab Results:

Complete Blood Count (CBC):	Current:	High/Low/WNL?	Most Recent:
WBC (4.5-11.0 mm 3)	4.8		5.8
Hgb (12-16 g/dL)	12.9		13.2
Platelets (150-450x 103/µl)	228		202
Neutrophil % (42-72)	68		65

What lab results are RELEVANT and must be recognized as clinically significant by the nurse?

RELEVANT Lab(s):	Clinical Significance:	TREND: Improve/Worsening/Stable:

Basic Metabolic Panel (BMP):	Current:	High/Low/WNL?	Previous:
Sodium (135-145 mEq/L)	133		138
Potassium (3.5-5.0 mEq/L)	4.9		4.2
Glucose (70-110 mg/dL)	105		118
Calcium (8.4-10.2 mg/dL)	8.8		9.5
Creatinine (0.6-1.2 mg/dL)	2.9		2.2

What lab results are RELEVANT and must be recognized as clinically significant by the nurse?

RELEVANT Lab(s):	Clinical Significance:	TREND: Improve/Worsening/Stable:

Misc. Chemistries:	Current:	High/Low/WNL?	Previous:
Magnesium (1.6-2.0 mEq/L)	1.9		1.8
PT/INR (0.9-1.1 nmol/L)	2.5		2.4

What lab results are RELEVANT and must be recognized as clinically significant by the nurse?

RELEVANT Lab(s):	Clinical Significance:	TREND: Improve/Worsening/Stable:

What lab results are RELEVANT and must be recognized as clinically significant by the nurse?

Cardiac Labs:	Current:	High/Low/WNL?	Previous:
Troponin (<0.05 ng/mL)	0.10		0.12
BNP (B-natriuretic Peptide) (<100 ng/L))	1855		155

RELEVANT Lab(s):	Clinical Significance:	TREND: Improve/Worsening/Stable:

Make a clinical JUDGMENT. Is a PROBLEM present?

Based on your identification and TRENDING of RELEVANT clinical data, is a problem present?

If a problem is present, what is it?

What is the underlying cause/pathophysiology of this primary problem?

THINK Like a Nurse by Recognizing Clinical RELATIONSHIPS

2. What is the RELATIONSHIP between RELEVANT current problem data and the primary medical problem?

RELEVANT Current Problem Data:	How Does it Relate to Primary Medical Problem?

3. What is the RELATIONSHIP between RELEVANT clinical data and the primary problem?

RELEVANT VS Data:	How Does it Relate to Primary Problem?
RELEVANT Assessment Data:	How Does it Relate to Primary Problem?

4. What is the RELATIONSHIP between the primary medical problem and nursing priority(ies)?

Nursing Priority(ies):	How Nursing Priority will help Resolve Primary Medical Problem:

5. What is the RELATIONSHIP between the primary care provider's orders and primary problem?

Care Provider Orders:	How it Will Resolve Primary Problem:
Titrate oxygen to keep O2 sat >92%	
Furosemide 40 mg IV push	
Nitroglycerin IV drip: titrate to keep SBP <130	
Strict I&O	
Fluid restriction of 2000 mL PO daily	
Low sodium diet	

6. Is there a RELATIONSHIP between diseases in the patient's past medical history that may have contributed to the development of the current problem?
(Which disease likely developed FIRST, then started a "domino effect"?)

Past Medical History	What Came FIRST:
• Diabetes mellitus type II • Hypertension • Atrial fibrillation • Hyperlipidemia • Chronic renal insufficiency (baseline creatinine 2.0) • Cerebral vascular accident (CVA) with no residual deficits • Heart failure (systolic) secondary to ischemic cardiomyopathy • MI with stent x2 to LAD 4 years ago	**What Then Followed:**

STEP #3: Recognizing HOLISTIC Care

Holistic Care:

1. Integrate caring, empathy, engagement, and presence while providing care.
2. Care for the entire person (physical-emotional-spiritual).
3. Identify educational and psychosocial needs.
4. Determine psychosocial PRIORITY and plan of care.

History of Present Problem:

JoAnn Smith is a 72-year-old woman who has a history of myocardial infarction (MI) four years ago and systolic heart failure secondary to ischemic cardiomyopathy with a current ejection fraction (EF) of only 15%. She presents to the emergency department (ED) for shortness of breath (SOB) the past three days. Her shortness of breath has progressed from SOB with activity to becoming SOB at rest. The last two nights she had to sleep in her recliner chair to rest comfortably upright. She is able to speak only in partial sentences and then has to take a breath when talking to the nurse. She has noted increased swelling in her lower legs and has gained six pounds in the last three days. She is being transferred from the ED to the cardiac step-down where you are the nurse assigned to care for her.

Personal/Social History:

JoAnn is a retired math teacher who is unable to maintain the level of activity she has been accustomed to because of the progression of her heart failure the past two years. She has struggled with depression the past two years and has been more withdrawn since her husband of 52 years died unexpectedly three months ago from a myocardial infarction.

What data from the PERSONAL/SOCIAL history are RELEVANT and must be interpreted as clinically significant by the nurse?

RELEVANT Data from Social History:	Clinical Significance:

Put it All Together and CARE Like a Nurse!

1. Based on your identification of RELEVANT clinical data, is a psychosocial concern present?

2. If a psychosocial concern is present, what is it?

3. How does the psychosocial concern contribute to the primary medical problem or disease progression for this patient?

4. What are your PSYCHOSOCIAL nursing PRIORITY (ies)?

5. *What interventions can you initiate with each holistic category as well as address these psychosocial priorities?*

Nursing Interventions:	Rationale:	Expected Outcome:
CARE/COMFORT:		
EMOTIONAL:		
SPIRITUAL:		
CULTURAL (IF APPLICABLE):		

6. *What principles of therapeutic communication will be needed to encourage dialogue between the nurse, patient, and/or family?*

7. *What educational priorities will be needed to develop a teaching plan to limit disease progression for this patient and/or family?*

8. *What additional members of the health care team can be utilized to address psychosocial priorities with this patient and/or family?*

9. *What is the patient likely experiencing/feeling right now in this situation?*

10. *What can you do to engage yourself with this patient's experience, and show that he/she matters to you as a person*

Appendix D

A Nurse Educator's Prayer

Lord, let me bring Your presence into my classroom and clinical settings today.

I acknowledge my need for Your strength, patience, and perseverance.

Help me to see students I teach through Your heart and eyes.

Help me to be moved with Your heart of love and compassion for every student I come in contact with.

Help me to see Your presence in every student and educator I work with.

Help me remember that when I serve others in Your name, I am caring and touching you.

Thank you for this day and the opportunities I will have to share a vision of nursing that includes the importance of serving and caring for others.

Help me to live out and role model caring, compassion, and excellence in all that I do.

Help my students to handle the stress of nursing education and embrace the highest levels of professionalism and respect for others.

Help my students to see that greatness is not defined by the title that you hold, but serving those in need.

Help my students to give themselves grace to be a student learner and to desire to be the best possible nurse they can be.

Help me to remember that as I teach and serve others in Your name, I am making a difference and leaving a lasting legacy of Your love.

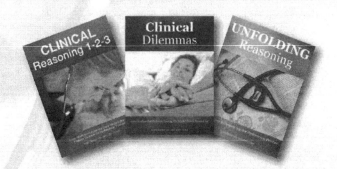

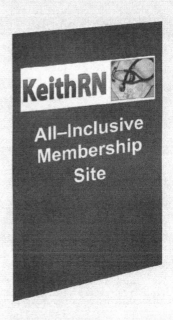
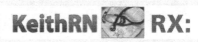
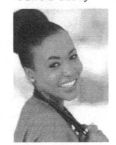

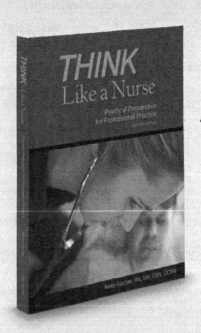
 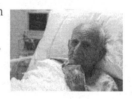